Handbook of Liver Diseases and Nutrition

Handbook of Liver Diseases and Nutrition

Editor: Lucinda Clopton

AMERICAN
MEDICAL PUBLISHERS
www.americanmedicalpublishers.com

AMERICAN
MEDICAL PUBLISHERS
www.americanmedicalpublishers.com

Cataloging-in-Publication Data

Handbook of liver diseases and nutrition / edited by Lucinda Clopton.
p. cm.
Includes bibliographical references and index.
ISBN 978-1-63927-682-0
1. Liver--Diseases. 2. Liver--Diseases--Nutritional aspects. 3. Diet in disease.
4. Liver--Diseases--Diet therapy. 5. Nutrition. I. Clopton, Lucinda.
RC846 .H36 2023
616.362--dc23

American Medical Publishers,
41 Flatbush Avenue,
1st Floor, New York,
NY 11217, USA

ISBN 978-1-63927-682-0 (Hardback)

Contents

Preface

Kidneys are two reddish-brown organs that are shaped like beans and are found in vertebrates. They are positioned on the right and left side of the retroperitoneal space. Kidney disease is a condition in which the kidneys get damaged. It often leads to kidney dysfunction to some extent and might become the reason for kidney failure, which results in complete damage of kidneys and their function. Kidney failure is called the final stage of kidney disease in which kidney transplant or dialysis is the only way to treat the damage. The patients of kidney disease which are in the initial stages must consume less amount of sodium. Some patients might be recommended to minimize the consumption of protein. Patients having kidney disease must take a diet containing vegetables, fruits, whole grains, nuts, poultry, fish, beans, and dairy products low in fat. This book contains some path-breaking studies on the role of nutrition in liver diseases. It is a valuable compilation of topics, ranging from the basic to the most complex advancements. Those in search of information to further their knowledge will be greatly assisted by this book.

This book has been the outcome of endless efforts put in by authors and researchers on various issues and topics within the field. The book is a comprehensive collection of significant researches that are addressed in a variety of chapters. It will surely enhance the knowledge of the field among readers across the globe.

It gives us an immense pleasure to thank our researchers and authors for their efforts to submit their piece of writing before the deadlines. Finally in the end, I would like to thank my family and colleagues who have been a great source of inspiration and support.

Editor

1

Muscle Loss in Chronic Liver Diseases: The Example of Nonalcoholic Liver Disease

Jean-Pascal De Bandt *, **Prasanthi Jegatheesan** and **Naouel Tennoune-El-Hafaia**

EA4466 PRETRAM, Faculté de Pharmacie de Paris, USPC, 75006 Paris, France; pira_jegatheesan@hotmail.com (P.J.); naouel.el-hafaia@parisdescartes.fr (N.T.-E.-H.)

* Correspondence: jean-pascal.de-bandt@parisdescartes.fr

Abstract: Recent publications highlight a frequent loss of muscle mass in chronic liver diseases, including nonalcoholic fatty liver disease (NAFLD), and its association with a poorer prognosis. In NAFLD, given the role of muscle in energy metabolism, muscle loss promotes disease progression. However, liver damage may be directly responsible of this muscle loss. Indeed, muscle homeostasis depends on the balance between peripheral availability and action of anabolic effectors and catabolic signals. Moreover, insulin resistance of protein metabolism only partially explains muscle loss during NAFLD. Interestingly, some data indicate specific alterations in the liver–muscle axis, particularly in situations such as excess fructose/sucrose consumption, associated with increased hepatic de novo lipogenesis (DNL) and endoplasmic reticulum stress. In this context, the liver will be responsible for a decrease in the peripheral availability of anabolic factors such as hormones and amino acids, and for the production of catabolic effectors such as various hepatokines, methylglyoxal, and uric acid. A better understanding of these liver–muscle interactions could open new therapeutic opportunities for the management of NAFLD patients.

Keywords: sarcopenia; protein metabolism; insulin resistance; endoplasmic reticulum stress; hepatokine; amino acid; uric acid; methylglyoxal

---

1. Introduction

The loss in muscle mass, often wrongly referred to as sarcopenia, has long been largely neglected in liver diseases. This is probably partly because of possible difficulties in its assessment due, for example, to fluid retention. However, several recent studies have shown frequent loss of muscle mass associated with poor prognosis in various chronic liver diseases. The progressive deterioration of muscle trophicity in these diseases is therefore receiving increasing attention. Overall, studies demonstrate muscle loss in nearly 60% of patients with end-stage liver diseases and this is associated with a worse prognosis [1]. However, muscle loss is already present in the early stages of liver disease and worsens with its severity [2]. This is particularly the case of nonalcoholic fatty liver disease (NAFLD), which encompasses a broad spectrum of disorders ranging from simple steatosis to nonalcoholic steatohepatitis (NASH), cirrhosis, and hepatocellular carcinoma, and where loss of muscle mass can occur very early during the disease. Indeed, in addition to the disturbances in muscle homeostasis related to metabolic disorders, several pieces of evidence indicate a specific role of the alterations in liver function in muscle loss. This is particularly important as the progressive deterioration of muscle trophicity promotes NAFLD progression, given the role of the muscle in energy metabolism. The alterations in the liver–muscle axis, due to hepatic steatosis, initiate a vicious circle in which liver disease favors defective muscle protein accretion and in which muscle loss favors metabolic alterations as well as hepatic steatosis and inflammation.

After examining some epidemiological data on muscle loss in chronic liver diseases and NAFLD, the authors of this review focus on muscle homeostasis and the different mechanisms by which NAFLD can act on muscle protein metabolism, including the decreased peripheral availability and action of anabolic factors such as hormones and amino acids, and the production of catabolic effectors such as various hepatokines, methylglyoxal, and uric acid.

It should be noted that many authors speak of sarcopenia while patients present only this loss of muscle mass. Indeed, the European society for clinical nutrition and metabolism defines sarcopenia, a term first coined for geriatric patients, as "a syndrome of its own characterized by the progressive and generalized loss of skeletal muscle mass, strength and function (performance) with a consequent risk of adverse outcomes" [3].

2. Muscle Loss in Chronic Liver Diseases

The interest in muscle mass loss in liver diseases is the result of recent evidence of its frequency and its consequences in terms of morbidity and mortality. A meta-analysis of 7 Asian studies and 13 Western studies in patients with liver cirrhosis of various etiologies concluded that muscle loss was present in 48.1% of patients, more prevalent in men (61.6%) than in women (36%) [4]. Several studies have shown that muscle loss in liver transplant candidates is associated with increased mortality [2] and increased risk of complications [4] In a recent systematic review and meta-analysis, the pooled hazard ratios of muscle loss was 1.84 (95% CI: 1.11–3.05, $p = 0.02$) for post-transplantation mortality [5]. Moreover, muscle loss appeared to be associated with increased complications, such as infections [6], ascites, encephalopathy, and variceal hemorrhage [7].

More specifically for NAFLD, most data come from studies in the Korean population. Using data from the Korean National Health and Nutrition Examination Surveys (KNHANES), Lee et al. [8] showed that NAFLD was present in 2761 (28.5%) out of 9676 subjects, and that 337 NAFLD patients (12.2%) had low muscle mass. Hong et al. [9] studied the relationship between muscle mass and liver disease evaluated by serum gamma-glutamyl transferase (GGT) in 3193 adults aged over 50 years from the fifth KNHANES. They observed that patients in the highest GGT quintile were 2.3 times more likely to have low muscle mass than those in the lowest quintile. In a seven-year Korean longitudinal study [10] on 12,624 subjects without initial NAFLD, followed for occupational medicine purpose, 14.8% of the subjects developed NAFLD and the highest tertile of muscle mass was inversely associated with the incidence of NAFLD compared to the lowest tertile. Finally, in the study by Koo et al. [11] of 309 subjects with signs of hepatic steatosis, the prevalence of low muscle mass was 8.7% in patients without NAFLD and 17.9% and 35%, respectively, in biopsy-proven nonalcoholic fatty liver and NASH patients. In this study, as in Lee's study [8], low muscle mass was associated with fibrosis (OR: 2.05, 95% CI: 1.01–4.16, $p = 0.034$), independently of body mass index and insulin resistance. This relationship between low muscle mass and fibrosis has also been confirmed in a European cohort of biopsy-proven NAFLD patients [12].

Given the importance of muscle in energy and nitrogen homeostasis, this muscle loss negatively affects whole-body metabolism [13]. The consequences on hepatic metabolism are clearly shown, for example, in the study by Flannery et al. [14] of healthy sedentary elderly subjects. These authors observed, after a test meal, a twofold higher hepatic de novo lipogenesis (DNL), a threefold higher postprandial hepatic triglyceride (TG) content, and significantly increased plasma TG compared to healthy, young subjects. Note that, in a study of 452 apparently healthy adults from the Korean Sarcopenic Obesity Study [15], patients in the lowest quartile of muscle mass had a 5.2-fold increased risk of NAFLD compared to the highest quartile (95% CI: 1.63–16.33, $p = 0.041$). In this study, hepatic steatosis and skeletal muscle mass index were negatively correlated with insulin resistance, low grade inflammation, and arterial stiffness, and positively correlated with plasma TG and alanine aminotransferase.

3. Muscle Protein Homeostasis

To understand the mechanisms by which hepatic disorders may affect muscle protein homeostasis, the authors will first briefly review some main aspects of the control of protein metabolism in muscle.

Muscle homeostasis in healthy individuals depends on the fasting–feeding alternation and, at the cell level, on the balance between protein synthesis and catabolism. Protein synthesis is activated by anabolic factors such as hormones (insulin and insulin-like growth factor 1 [IGF-1]), and amino acid (AAs) availability (with AAs such as leucine and arginine playing specific regulatory roles), and it is inhibited by nutrient deficiency and inflammatory processes. Conversely, protein catabolism is activated by energy and AA deficiency and inflammatory processes, and it is inhibited by anabolic hormones [16].

During the postprandial period, anabolic effects of feeding result from increased protein synthesis and decreased catabolism due to increased availability and action of anabolic effectors. AAs stimulate protein synthesis; insulin has a permissive effect and increases the supply of nutrients to muscles through its vasodilatory properties. Insulin-induced inhibition of proteolysis is enhanced by AA availability [17]. In addition, the activation of protein synthesis depends on specific AAs such as leucine and arginine; thus, the anabolic effects of feeding also depend on specific qualitative variations in AA availability [18]. Finally, the vasodilatory effects of insulin play an important role in the physiological coupling between hemodynamic and metabolic homeostasis [19]. The increase in the metabolic activity of skeletal muscle requires adequate availability of the substrate for nitric oxide (°NO) synthesis (i.e., arginine) to increase blood flow for substrate supply.

On the long term, maintaining skeletal muscle mass also depends on the growth hormone (GH)/IGF-1 axis. Blood IGF-I is 80% dependent on its GH-induced liver production. Plasma IGF-I is associated positively with lean body mass and muscle function, and negatively with body fat mass. IGF-I action is also regulated by its binding to circulating IGF-1 binding proteins (IGFBP) produced by the liver [20].

Overall, the maintenance of muscle mass requires that the muscles be responsive to these anabolic effectors and that the anabolic effectors actually and quantitatively reach the muscles. As indicated below, NAFLD may be associated with a decrease in muscle mass as a consequence of (i) insulin-resistance; (ii) decreased IGF-1 production by the liver; (iii) decreased AA flows to the muscles due to increased splanchnic utilization; (iv) a defective postprandial peripheral vasodilatory response; or (v) the catabolic effect of various mediators, including hepatokines, produced by the liver in steatosis-induced situations of endoplasmic reticulum (ER) stress.

4. Insulin Resistance and Muscle Homeostasis

A first process that can promote muscle loss is insulin resistance. Depending on the pathophysiological situation, insulin resistance may either precede NAFLD, due to increased adiposity, or result from NAFLD as the steatotic liver is the site of increased glucose and TG production; in all cases, the two processes reinforce each other. Decreased sensitivity of protein turnover to insulin action has been described in both type 1 and type 2 diabetes [21]. This decrease in insulin sensitivity may result from several mechanisms such as lipotoxicity, glucotoxicity, and inflammation.

Increased circulating free fatty acid (FFA) concentration favors ectopic lipid deposition and altered insulin signaling due to the accumulation of TG deposition, for example, in muscle [22]. Moreover, specific FFAs (e.g., palmitate) and lipid metabolites (e.g., ceramide and diacylglycerol) may induce insulin resistance. It should be noted that palmitate also activates toll-like receptor 4 (TLR4) and triggers inflammatory processes [23].

Excess glucose induces oxidative stress in muscles and the production of advanced glycation end products (AGEs) that interact with the receptors of AGEs on muscle cells. These receptors induce the production of reactive oxygen species and cause inflammation via mitogen-activated protein kinases and nuclear factor κB pathways [24]. For example, Howard et al. [25] showed that high glucose and AGEs induce a defect in myocyte membrane repair.

Excess adipose tissue, particularly visceral adipose tissue, is associated with the increased secretion of pro-inflammatory cytokines, such as tumor necrosis factor α and interleukin-6, and adipokines (leptin and resistin, whereas insulin-sensitizing adiponectin production decreases) which promote insulin resistance [26]. Interestingly, in the authors' model of fructose-induced NAFLD in rats, muscle loss was associated with increased visceral adiposity and an inflammatory state [27].

A last mechanism by which insulin resistance may contribute to muscle loss is the above-mentioned defect in the postprandial peripheral vasodilatory response as it reduces the flow of anabolic factors to the muscle. Indeed, in addition to its essential metabolic actions, insulin stimulates the production of nitric oxide (°NO) by endothelial °NO synthase (eNOS). Therefore, in the post-prandial period, insulin induces vasodilation, increased blood flow and increased availability of substrates and hormones for target tissues. Insulin resistance is associated with impaired endothelium-dependent vasodilation and vascular function [19]. There is thus a reciprocal interaction between insulin resistance and the defect in endothelial °NO production. The pathophysiological mechanisms linking these two processes contribute to metabolic disorders and the cardiovascular features of the metabolic syndrome. Moreover, insulin resistance states are associated with decreased availability of an important AA, arginine, the substrate of eNOS for °NO synthesis.

5. Metabolic Disorders, Liver Steatosis, and Endoplasmic Reticulum Stress

Although insulin resistance may affect muscle function, it cannot by itself explain the defect in muscle protein accretion associated with NAFLD and, more specifically, with the excessive consumption of fructose. Therefore, another process must contribute to muscle protein loss. One explanation could be excess DNL, the cause of steatosis, leading to hepatic oxidative stress, inflammation, and ER stress.

Under normal conditions, at the hepatic level, FFAs come from white adipose tissue (WAT) lipolysis during the fasting period, from diet, and from DNL. FFAs will either be esterified into TG and then exported to the blood as very-low-density lipoproteins (VLDL) or degraded by β-oxidation. Pathological accumulation of lipids in the liver may result from the excessive entry of FFAs released by insulin-resistant WAT, particularly visceral adipose tissue, excessive activation of DNL, and alterations in β-oxidation and lipid excretion as VLDL. In NAFLD patients, approximately 60% of FFAs come from lipolysis in WAT, nearly 25% result from DNL, and the remainder come from diet [28]. Nutritional factors, such as a diet rich in sucrose/fructose and lipids, and the disequilibrium of the energy balance thus play a major role in the occurrence of this pathology.

Excessive sucrose or fructose consumption can significantly contribute to liver steatosis and disease progression. Experimental studies repeatedly demonstrated that a high-sucrose or high-fructose diet promotes subcutaneous and visceral obesity, insulin resistance, dyslipidemia, increased blood uric acid, and hypertension [29]. Even moderate doses of fructose can induce metabolic syndrome, fatty liver, and type 2 diabetes even in the absence of excess energy intake [30]. In humans, a high-fructose intake (>1.5 g/kg/day) can double the intrahepatic fat content within six days [31]. Conversely, in a pilot study of 15 NAFLD patients, Volynets et al. [32] showed that a dietary intervention focusing on a 50% reduction in fructose intake was associated with decreased hepatic steatosis and improved liver function and glucose tolerance. This can be at least in part explained by the specificities of fructose metabolism in the liver and the excessive activation of DNL. Indeed, fructose is both a substrate and an activator of DNL through the activation of carbohydrate-responsive element-binding protein (ChREBP) and sterol regulatory element-binding protein 1c, two transcription factors controlling the main enzymes involved in DNL [33]. Excess DNL causes oxidative stress in liver cells and is associated with the development of hepatic inflammation and insulin resistance [34,35]. It also induces ER stress, which contributes to the aggravation of NAFLD [34]. The superposition of ER stress and inflammation may lead to the production of various mediators, such as cytokines, hepatokines, and carbohydrate and lipid derivatives, which can act at the whole-body level and contribute to alterations in whole-body metabolism [36,37].

With respect to muscle mass loss, studies [27,38,39] have shown that excessive consumption of fructose or sucrose leads to changes in body composition with fat accumulation and alterations of muscle protein pool. Interestingly, in a study of community-dwelling elderly subjects, Laclaustra et al. [40] showed an association between added sugar consumption and the appearance of frailty. Several lines of evidence indicate that sucrose-related alterations in liver metabolism, at least in part due to the conversion of sucrose into lipids in the process of DNL, lead to changes in peripheral organ metabolism and muscle protein accretion. This is illustrated by the comparison of mouse models of primary steatosis, resulting from an increase in hepatic DNL, and secondary steatosis resulting from ectopic lipid deposition, primary steatosis being associated with significantly lower lean body mass [41].

6. Hepatic Endoplasmic Reticulum Stress and Muscle Homeostasis

The question therefore arises about the mechanisms by which these alterations in liver homeostasis may affect muscle protein metabolism.

6.1. Alterations of the GH/IGF-1 Axis

The bidirectional relationship between steatosis and insulin resistance has already been mentioned. Steatosis is also associated with alterations of the GH/IGF-1 axis. While data on plasma GH are inconsistent [42,43], studies agree on a decrease in plasma IGF-1 in NAFLD [42–44]. The liver being the main organ contributing to plasma IGF-1 concentration, this suggests that NAFLD alters IGF-1 production. Runchey et al. [45] showed in 4172 adults who participated in the NHANES III that the highest quartiles of IGF-1 and IGF-1/IGFBP-3 were associated with a lower likelihood and grade of NAFLD. Note that in an exploratory study of healthy volunteers on a high-sucrose diet, the authors observed an association between increased liver lipid content and decreased plasma IGF-1 [46]. In a model of Western diet-induced NAFLD in mice, steatosis was associated with a 40% decrease in IGF-1 hepatic expression [47]. This seems to be specific for liver steatosis, as suggested by Chishima et al. [43] in a study of Japanese patients with NAFLD or Hepatitis C virus (HCV) chronic liver disease where IGF-1 levels were decreased in patients with NAFLD but not with HCV. Moreover, serum IGFBP-3 levels were also decreased, indicating a reduction in blood half-life of IGF-1. Conversely, hepatic ER stress is associated with the stimulation of IGFBP1 secretion [48]. IGFBP1 is a modulator of IGF-1 action and its overexpression is associated with hyperinsulinemia and glucose intolerance [49]. Experimentally, hepatic steatosis-related alterations in GH/IGF-1 axis are associated with a decrease in muscle myofibrillar protein content and a reduction in muscle strength in the absence of significant inflammation [47].

6.2. Alterations of Amino Acid Interorgan Fluxes

Disorders of nitrogen homeostasis in situations of stimulated DNL may be an early event during the development of steatosis [33]. In an experimental model of fructose-induced NAFLD in rats, the prolonged administration of a fructose-rich diet was associated with a decrease in lean body mass, an increase in visceral fat mass, and changes in AA plasma levels, notably in arginine bioavailability. Conversely, an increase in AA availability enable to decrease DNL and associated alterations in body composition [27]. In healthy volunteers, an essential AA supplement reduced fructose-induced intrahepatic lipid accumulation [50]. Interestingly, based on their results showing alterations in blood AA profile in non-diabetic NAFLD patients with or without obesity, Gaggini et al. [51] concluded that the observed increase in AAs such as branched-chain and aromatic AAs resulted from an increase in muscle proteolysis. Finally, in overweight hypertriglyceridemic patients, fructose infusion was associated with altered AA plasma levels and increased splanchnic extraction [33]. Similarly, postprandial AA availability was impaired in healthy volunteers receiving a high-sucrose diet [46]. Taken together, these data suggest that excess hepatic DNL is associated with a reorientation of AA fluxes towards the liver at the expense of muscle protein homeostasis.

6.3. Hepatokines and Muscle Homeostasis

In situations of hepatic ER stress, induced for example by steatosis, an increased production of some hepatokines and inflammatory cytokines has been demonstrated [52]. In cultured hepatocytes, steatosis has been associated with changes in the secretion of approximately 30 hepatokines [53].

Some of these mediators may be involved in muscle loss through a direct effect or through the deterioration of insulin sensitivity. For example:

(1) Fetuin A is a glycoprotein associated with alterations in glucose and lipid metabolism. Both experimental and clinical studies showed increased hepatic expression and plasma levels of Fetuin A during NAFLD. Studies in humans showed a close relationship between plasma Fetuin A and the metabolic syndrome [54]. Its production by hepatocytes is strongly stimulated by ER stress [55]. This protein produced primarily by the liver is an endogenous inhibitor of the insulin receptor tyrosine kinase in skeletal muscle [56]. Fetuin A may also bind TLR4, stimulating inflammatory pathways [52].
(2) Fibroblast growth factor 21 (FGF21) is a mediator produced primarily by the liver that contributes to the regulation of energy metabolism and insulin sensitivity [57]. FGF21 is now recognized as a key player in the adaptive response to starvation and feeding [58]. Fructose induces FGF21 production by the activation of the transcription factor ChREBP [59]. ER stress modulates FGF21 expression in the liver [60]. FGF21 is an intriguing hepatokine as it is generally considered as beneficial [59]; however, some data indicate either states of FGF21 resistance or deleterious effects, as suggested by the very high FGF21 plasma levels observed in patients with insulin resistance [52]. In male and female rats fed a high-fat high-fructose diet, FGF21 was increased only in males and this was associated with marked liver damage, inflammation, and oxidative stress [61]. AA deprivation is also a potent inducer of hepatic FGF21 production via ER stress response [62]; very high levels of FGF21 could potentially alter nitrogen homeostasis in the context of NAFLD-associated muscle mass loss. It should be noted that transgenic mice overexpressing FGF21 exhibit increased gluconeogenesis in the fed state, and that acute treatment with FGF21 induces key enzymes in the gluconeogenic pathway [62], suggesting an increased hepatic utilization of AAs.
(3) Hepassocin (HPS, hepatocyte-derived fibrinogen-related protein 1 [HFREP1], fibrinogen-like protein 1 [FGL1]) is increased in NAFLD and induces insulin resistance in muscle [52]. Wu et al. have shown in humans that increased plasma HPS is independently associated with insulin resistance [63]. In primary hepatocytes or in vivo in mice, HPS expression is induced by ER stress. In differentiated myotubes, depending on the dose, HPS activated the c-Jun N-terminal kinase inflammatory pathway and altered insulin sensitivity [64]. In mice, hepatic HPS overexpression induced insulin resistance, while its knockdown was associated with improved insulin sensitivity in high-fat fed mice [63].

6.4. Hepatic Production of Catabolic Factors

Finally, carbohydrate metabolism may lead to the release by the liver of metabolites with significant peripheral effects.

During normal glycolysis, small amounts of methylglyoxal (MG) may be released. MG is produced by the fragmentation of the two products of aldolase B, namely glyceraldehyde-3-phosphate and dihydroxyacetone phosphate. MG is a powerful glycating agent leading to the generation of AGEs. Under normal conditions, its formation rate represents 0.1–0.4% of glycolytic flux [65], but the acceleration of glycolytic flux by fructose greatly increases MG formation. MG induces endothelial dysfunction [66]. Dhar et al. [67] showed an increase in MG formation associated with hypertension in fructose-fed rats. By acting on vascular function, MG may therefore contribute to a decrease in the peripheral availability of anabolic hormones and AAs.

A high-fructose intake results in an increased plasma uric acid level [39,68]. First, uric acid can contribute to fructose-induced metabolic disorders by impairing endothelial function, thereby decreasing insulin sensitivity by preventing insulin-induced muscle vasodilation. In addition, Zhu et al. [69] recently showed in mice that uric acid inhibits insulin signaling in muscle and induces insulin resistance. This effect may be related to uric acid-induced oxidative stress. In a study of severely obese subjects, Fabbrini et al. [70] observed a 40% decrease in insulin sensitivity in those with increased plasma uric acid. In an analysis of data from 7544 subjects who participated in the NHANES III, Beavers et al. [71] showed an association between increased blood uric acid levels and low muscle mass.

7. Conclusions

Chronic liver diseases contribute to alterations in muscle protein homeostasis, already at the stage of hepatic steatosis. While this review is limited to alterations in the liver–muscle axis, the situation is probably even more complex because NAFLD can be considered as a systemic disease affecting not only the liver and muscles, but also the gut and adipose tissue. High-fat and high-fructose diets, which promote the development of NAFLD, are associated with alterations in gut microbiota, increased gut permeability, and bacterial toxin translocation that can affect muscle homeostasis through systemic inflammation and insulin resistance [72]. Similarly, excessive sucrose consumption is associated with an increase in visceral adipose tissue in which has a higher production of pro-inflammatory factors and metabolic alterations than subcutaneous adipose tissue [26]. Muscle mass and function can be influenced by this adipose tissue dysfunction. The difficulty now becomes to establish the respective contribution of these different mechanisms in order to better define therapeutic targets.

Author Contributions: The three authors wrote the manuscript and approved the final content.

Acknowledgments: None.

Abbreviations

AA	amino acid
AGE	advanced glycation end products
ChREBP	carbohydrate-responsive element-binding protein
DNL	de novo lipogenesis
eNOS	endothelial °NO synthase
ER	endoplasmic reticulum
FFA	free fatty acid
FGF21	fibroblast growth factor 21
GGT	gamma-glutamyl transferase
GH	growth hormone
HCV	Hepatitis C virus
HPS	hepassocin
IGF	insulin-like growth factor
IGFBP	IGF binding protein
KNHANES	Korean National Health and Nutrition Examination Surveys
MG	methylglyoxal
NAFLD	nonalcoholic fatty liver disease
NASH	nonalcoholic steatohepatitis
NHANES	national health and nutrition examination survey
°NO	nitric oxide
TG	triglycerides
TLR4	toll-like receptor 4
VLDL	very-low-density lipoprotein
WAT	white adipose tissue

References

1. Bhanji, R.A.; Narayanan, P.; Allen, A.M.; Malhi, H.; Watt, K.D. Sarcopenia in hiding: The risk and consequence of underestimating muscle dysfunction in nonalcoholic steatohepatitis. *Hepatol. Baltim. Md.* **2017**, *66*, 2055–2065. [CrossRef] [PubMed]

2. Anand, A.C. Nutrition and muscle in cirrhosis. *J. Clin. Exp. Hepatol.* **2017**, *7*, 340–357. [CrossRef] [PubMed]
3. Cederholm, T.; Barazzoni, R.; Austin, P.; Ballmer, P.; Biolo, G.; Bischoff, S.C.; Compher, C.; Correia, I.; Higashiguchi, T.; Holst, M.; et al. ESPEN guidelines on definitions and terminology of clinical nutrition. *Clin. Nutr.* **2017**, *36*, 49–64. [CrossRef] [PubMed]
4. Kim, G.; Kang, S.H.; Kim, M.Y.; Baik, S.K. Prognostic value of sarcopenia in patients with liver cirrhosis: A systematic review and meta-analysis. *PLoS ONE* **2017**, *12*, e0186990. [CrossRef] [PubMed]
5. Van Vugt, J.L.A.; Levolger, S.; de Bruin, R.W.F.; van Rosmalen, J.; Metselaar, H.J.; IJzermans, J.N.M. Systematic review and meta-analysis of the impact of computed tomography-assessed skeletal muscle mass on outcome in patients awaiting or undergoing liver transplantation. *Am. J. Transplant.* **2016**, *16*, 2277–2292. [CrossRef] [PubMed]
6. Lucidi, C.; Lattanzi, B.; Di Gregorio, V.; Incicco, S.; D'Ambrosio, D.; Venditti, M.; Riggio, O.; Merli, M. A low muscle mass increases mortality in compensated cirrhotic patients with sepsis. *Liver Int.* **2018**, *38*, 851–857. [CrossRef] [PubMed]
7. Montano-Loza, A.J.; Duarte-Rojo, A.; Meza-Junco, J.; Baracos, V.E.; Sawyer, M.B.; Pang, J.X.Q.; Beaumont, C.; Esfandiari, N.; Myers, R.P. Inclusion of sarcopenia within MELD (MELD-Sarcopenia) and the prediction of mortality in patients with cirrhosis. *Clin. Transl. Gastroenterol.* **2015**, *6*, e102. [CrossRef] [PubMed]
8. Lee, Y.; Kim, S.U.; Song, K.; Park, J.Y.; Kim, D.Y.; Ahn, S.H.; Lee, B.W.; Kang, E.S.; Cha, B.S.; Han, K.H. Sarcopenia is associated with significant liver fibrosis independently of obesity and insulin resistance in nonalcoholic fatty liver disease: Nationwide surveys (KNHANES 2008–2011). *Hepatology* **2016**, *63*, 776–786. [CrossRef] [PubMed]
9. Hong, N.; Lee, E.Y.; Kim, C.O. Gamma-glutamyl transferase is associated with sarcopenia and sarcopenic obesity in community-dwelling older adults: Results from the Fifth Korea National Health and Nutrition Examination Survey, 2010-2011. *Endocr. J.* **2015**, *62*, 585–592. [CrossRef] [PubMed]
10. Kim, G.; Lee, S.E.; Lee, Y.B.; Jun, J.E.; Ahn, J.; Bae, J.C.; Jin, S.M.; Hur, K.Y.; Jee, J.H.; Lee, M.K.; et al. Relationship between relative skeletal muscle mass and non-alcoholic fatty liver disease: A 7-year longitudinal study. *Hepatology* **2018**. [CrossRef] [PubMed]
11. Koo, B.K.; Kim, D.; Joo, S.K.; Kim, J.H.; Chang, M.S.; Kim, B.G.; Lee, K.L.; Kim, W. Sarcopenia is an independent risk factor for non-alcoholic steatohepatitis and significant fibrosis. *J. Hepatol.* **2017**, *66*, 123–131. [CrossRef] [PubMed]
12. Petta, S.; Ciminnisi, S.; Di Marco, V.; Cabibi, D.; Cammà, C.; Licata, A.; Marchesini, G.; Craxi, A. Sarcopenia is associated with severe liver fibrosis in patients with non-alcoholic fatty liver disease. *Aliment. Pharmacol. Ther.* **2017**, *45*, 510–518. [CrossRef] [PubMed]
13. Rossi, P.; Marzani, B.; Giardina, S.; Negro, M.; Marzatico, F. Human skeletal muscle aging and the oxidative system: Cellular events. *Curr. Aging Sci.* **2008**, *1*, 182–191. [CrossRef] [PubMed]
14. Flannery, C.; Dufour, S.; Rabøl, R.; Shulman, G.I.; Petersen, K.F. Skeletal muscle insulin resistance promotes increased hepatic de novo lipogenesis, hyperlipidemia, and hepatic steatosis in the elderly. *Diabetes* **2012**, *61*, 2711–2717. [CrossRef] [PubMed]
15. Hong, H.C.; Hwang, S.Y.; Choi, H.Y.; Yoo, H.J.; Seo, J.A.; Kim, S.G.; Kim, N.H.; Baik, S.H.; Choi, D.S.; Choi, K.M. Relationship between sarcopenia and nonalcoholic fatty liver disease: The Korean Sarcopenic Obesity Study. *Hepatology* **2014**, *59*, 1772–1778. [CrossRef] [PubMed]
16. De Bandt, J.P. Leucine and mammalian target of rapamycin-dependent activation of muscle protein synthesis in aging. *J. Nutr.* **2016**, *146*, 2616S–2624S. [CrossRef] [PubMed]
17. Boucher, J.; Kleinridders, A.; Kahn, C.R. Insulin receptor signaling in normal and insulin-resistant states. *Cold Spring Harb. Perspect. Biol.* **2014**, *6*, a009191. [CrossRef] [PubMed]
18. Gryson, C.; Walrand, S.; Giraudet, C.; Rousset, P.; Migné, C.; Bonhomme, C.; Ruyet, P.L.; Boirie, Y. "Fast proteins" with a unique essential amino acid content as an optimal nutrition in the elderly: Growing evidence. *Clin. Nutr.* **2014**, *33*, 642–648. [CrossRef] [PubMed]
19. Muniyappa, R.; Quon, M.J. Insulin action and insulin resistance in vascular endothelium. *Curr. Opin. Clin. Nutr. Metab. Care* **2007**, *10*, 523–530. [CrossRef] [PubMed]
20. Song, Y.H.; Song, J.L.; Delafontaine, P.; Godard, M.P. The therapeutic potential of IGF-I in skeletal muscle repair. *Trends Endocrinol. Metab.* **2013**, *24*, 310–319. [CrossRef] [PubMed]

21. Short, K.R.; Irving, B.A.; Basu, A.; Johnson, C.M.; Nair, K.S.; Basu, R. Effects of type 2 diabetes and insulin on whole-body, splanchnic, and leg protein metabolism. *J. Clin. Endocrinol. Metab.* **2012**, *97*, 4733–4741. [CrossRef] [PubMed]
22. Masgrau, A.; Mishellany-Dutour, A.; Murakami, H.; Beaufrère, A.M.; Walrand, S.; Giraudet, C.; Migne, C.; Gerbaix, M.; Metz, L.; Courteix, D.; et al. Time-course changes of muscle protein synthesis associated with obesity-induced lipotoxicity. *J. Physiol.* **2012**, *590*, 5199–5210. [CrossRef] [PubMed]
23. Shen, H.; Eguchi, K.; Kono, N.; Fujiu, K.; Matsumoto, S.; Shibata, M.; Oishi-Tanaka, Y.; Komuro, I.; Arai, H.; Nagai, R.; et al. Saturated fatty acid palmitate aggravates neointima formation by promoting smooth muscle phenotypic modulation. *Arterioscler. Thromb. Vasc. Biol.* **2013**, *33*, 2596–2607. [CrossRef] [PubMed]
24. Ibrahim, Z.A.; Armour, C.L.; Phipps, S.; Sukkar, M.B. RAGE and TLRs: Relatives, friends or neighbours? *Mol. Immunol.* **2013**, *56*, 739–744. [CrossRef] [PubMed]
25. Howard, A.C.; McNeil, A.K.; Xiong, F.; Xiong, W.C.; McNeil, P.L. A novel cellular defect in diabetes: Membrane repair failure. *Diabetes* **2011**, *60*, 3034–3043. [CrossRef] [PubMed]
26. Trayhurn, P. Hypoxia and adipocyte physiology: Implications for adipose tissue dysfunction in obesity. *Annu. Rev. Nutr.* **2014**, *34*, 207–236. [CrossRef] [PubMed]
27. Jegatheesan, P.; Beutheu, S.; Ventura, G.; Nubret, E.; Sarfati, G.; Bergheim, I.; De Bandt, J.P. Citrulline and nonessential amino acids prevent fructose-induced nonalcoholic fatty liver disease in rats. *J. Nutr.* **2015**, *145*, 2273–2279. [CrossRef] [PubMed]
28. Fuchs, C.D.; Claudel, T.; Trauner, M. Role of metabolic lipases and lipolytic metabolites in the pathogenesis of NAFLD. *Trends Endocrinol. Metab.* **2014**, *25*, 576–585. [CrossRef] [PubMed]
29. Bizeau, M.E.; Pagliassotti, M.J. Hepatic adaptations to sucrose and fructose. *Metabolism* **2005**, *54*, 1189–1201. [CrossRef] [PubMed]
30. Roncal-Jimenez, C.A.; Lanaspa, M.A.; Rivard, C.J.; Nakagawa, T.; Sanchez-Lozada, L.G.; Jalal, D.; Andres-Hernando, A.; Tanabe, K.; Madero, M.; Li, N.; et al. Sucrose induces fatty liver and pancreatic inflammation in male breeder rats independent of excess energy intake. *Metabolism* **2011**, *60*, 1259–1270. [CrossRef] [PubMed]
31. Lecoultre, V.; Egli, L.; Carrel, G.; Theytaz, F.; Kreis, R.; Schneiter, P.; Boss, A.; Zwygart, K.; Le, K.A.; Bortolotti, M.; et al. Effects of fructose and glucose overfeeding on hepatic insulin sensitivity and intrahepatic lipids in healthy humans. *Obesity* **2013**, *21*, 782–785. [CrossRef] [PubMed]
32. Volynets, V.; Machann, J.; Küper, M.A.; Maier, I.B.; Spruss, A.; Königsrainer, A.; Bischoff, S.C.; Bergheim, I. A moderate weight reduction through dietary intervention decreases hepatic fat content in patients with non-alcoholic fatty liver disease (NAFLD): A pilot study. *Eur. J. Nutr.* **2013**, *52*, 527–535. [CrossRef] [PubMed]
33. Jegatheesan, P.; De Bandt, J.P. Fructose and NAFLD: The multifaceted aspects of fructose metabolism. *Nutrients* **2017**, *9*, E230. [CrossRef] [PubMed]
34. Malhi, H.; Kaufman, R.J. Endoplasmic reticulum stress in liver disease. *J. Hepatol.* **2011**, *54*, 795–809. [CrossRef] [PubMed]
35. Collison, K.S.; Saleh, S.M.; Bakheet, R.H.; Al-Rabiah, R.K.; Inglis, A.L.; Makhoul, N.J.; Maqbool, Z.M.; Zaidi, M.Z.; AI-Johi, M.A.; AI-Mohanna, F.A. Diabetes of the liver: The link between nonalcoholic fatty liver disease and HFCS-55. *Obesity* **2009**, *17*, 2003–2013. [CrossRef] [PubMed]
36. Stefan, N.; Häring, H.U. The role of hepatokines in metabolism. *Nat. Rev. Endocrinol.* **2013**, *9*, 144–152. [CrossRef] [PubMed]
37. Jung, T.W.; Lee, S.Y.; Hong, H.C.; Choi, H.Y.; Yoo, H.J.; Baik, S.H.; Choi, K.M. AMPK activator-mediated inhibition of endoplasmic reticulum stress ameliorates carrageenan-induced insulin resistance through the suppression of selenoprotein P in HepG2 hepatocytes. *Mol. Cell. Endocrinol.* **2014**, *382*, 66–73. [CrossRef] [PubMed]
38. Gatineau, E.; Savary-Auzeloux, I.; Migné, C.; Polakof, S.; Dardevet, D.; Mosoni, L. Chronic intake of sucrose accelerates sarcopenia in older male rats through alterations in insulin sensitivity and muscle protein synthesis. *J. Nutr.* **2015**, *145*, 923–930. [CrossRef] [PubMed]
39. Stanhope, K.L.; Schwarz, J.M.; Keim, N.L.; Griffen, S.C.; Bremer, A.A.; Graham, J.L.; et al. Consuming fructose-sweetened, not glucose-sweetened, beverages increases visceral adiposity and lipids and decreases insulin sensitivity in overweight/obese humans. *J. Clin. Investig.* **2009**, *119*, 1322–1334. [CrossRef] [PubMed]

40. Laclaustra, M.; Rodriguez-Artalejo, F.; Guallar-Castillon, P.; Banegas, J.R.; Graciani, A.; Garcia-Esquinas, E.; Ordovas, J.; Lopez-Garcia, E. Prospective association between added sugars and frailty in older adults. *Am. J. Clin. Nutr.* **2018**, *107*, 772–779. [CrossRef] [PubMed]
41. Jelenik, T.; Kaul, K.; Séquaris, G.; Flögel, U.; Phielix, E.; Kotzka, J.; Knebel, B.; Fahlbusch, P.; Horbelt, T.; Lehr, S.; et al. Mechanisms of insulin resistance in primary and secondary nonalcoholic fatty liver. *Diabetes* **2017**, *66*, 2241–2253. [CrossRef] [PubMed]
42. Koehler, E.; Swain, J.; Sanderson, S.; Krishnan, A.; Watt, K.; Charlton, M. Growth hormone, dehydroepiandrosterone and adiponectin levels in non-alcoholic steatohepatitis: An endocrine signature for advanced fibrosis in obese patients. *Liver Int.* **2012**, *32*, 279–286. [CrossRef] [PubMed]
43. Chishima, S.; Kogiso, T.; Matsushita, N.; Hashimoto, E.; Tokushige, K. The relationship between the growth hormone/insulin-like growth factor system and the histological features of nonalcoholic fatty liver disease. *Intern. Med.* **2017**, *56*, 473–480. [CrossRef] [PubMed]
44. Poggiogalle, E.; Lubrano, C.; Gnessi, L.; Mariani, S.; Lenzi, A.; Donini, L.M. Fatty liver index associates with relative sarcopenia and GH/ IGF-1 status in obese subjects. *PLoS ONE* **2016**, *11*, e0145811. [CrossRef] [PubMed]
45. Runchey, S.S.; Boyko, E.J.; Ioannou, G.N.; Utzschneider, K.M. Relationship between serum circulating insulin-like growth factor-1 and liver fat in the United States. *J. Gastroenterol. Hepatol.* **2014**, *29*, 589–596. [CrossRef] [PubMed]
46. Jegatheesan, P.; Surowska, A.; Campos, V.; Cros, J.; Stefanoni, N.; Rey, V.; Schneiter, P.; De Bandt, J.P.; Tappy, L. Dietary protein content modulates the amino-acid and IGF1 responses to sucrose overfeeding in humans. *Clin. Nutr.* **2017**, *36*, S285–S286. [CrossRef]
47. Cabrera, D.; Ruiz, A.; Cabello-Verrugio, C.; Brandan, E.; Estrada, L.; Pizarro, M.; Solis, N.; Torres, J.; Barrera, F.; Arrese, M. Diet-induced nonalcoholic fatty liver disease is associated with sarcopenia and decreased serum insulin-like growth factor-1. *Dig. Dis. Sci.* **2016**, *61*, 3190–3198. [CrossRef] [PubMed]
48. Marchand, A.; Tomkiewicz, C.; Magne, L.; Barouki, R.; Garlatti, M. Endoplasmic reticulum stress induction of insulin-like growth factor-binding protein-1 involves ATF4. *J. Biol. Chem.* **2006**, *281*, 19124–19133. [CrossRef] [PubMed]
49. Crossey, P.A.; Jones, J.S.; Miell, J.P. Dysregulation of the insulin/IGF binding protein-1 axis in transgenic mice is associated with hyperinsulinemia and glucose intolerance. *Diabetes* **2000**, *49*, 457–465. [CrossRef] [PubMed]
50. Theytaz, F.; Noguchi, Y.; Egli, L.; Campos, V.; Buehler, T.; Hodson, L.; Patterson, B.W.; Nishikata, N.; Kreis, R.; Mittendorfer, B.; et al. Effects of supplementation with essential amino acids on intrahepatic lipid concentrations during fructose overfeeding in humans. *Am. J. Clin. Nutr.* **2012**, *96*, 1008–1016. [CrossRef] [PubMed]
51. Gaggini, M.; Carli, F.; Rosso, C.; Buzzigoli, E.; Marietti, M.; Della Latta, V.; Ciociaro, D.; Abate, M.L.; Gambino, R.; Cassader, M.; et al. Altered amino acid concentrations in NAFLD: Impact of obesity and insulin resistance. *Hepatology* **2018**, *67*, 145–158. [CrossRef] [PubMed]
52. Meex, R.C.R.; Watt, M.J. Hepatokines: Linking nonalcoholic fatty liver disease and insulin resistance. *Nat. Rev. Endocrinol.* **2017**, *13*, 509–520. [CrossRef] [PubMed]
53. Meex, R.C.; Hoy, A.J.; Morris, A.; Brown, R.D.; Lo, J.C.Y.; Burke, M.; Goode, R.J.A.; Kingwell, B.A.; Kraakman, M.J.; Febbraio, M.A.; et al. Fetuin B is a secreted hepatocyte factor linking steatosis to impaired glucose metabolism. *Cell. Metab.* **2015**, *22*, 1078–1089. [CrossRef] [PubMed]
54. Musso, G.; Paschetta, E.; Gambino, R.; Cassader, M.; Molinaro, F. Interactions among bone, liver, and adipose tissue predisposing to diabesity and fatty liver. *Trends Mol. Med.* **2013**, *19*, 522–535. [CrossRef] [PubMed]
55. Ou, H.Y.; Wu, H.T.; Hung, H.C.; Yang, Y.C.; Wu, J.S.; Chang, C.J. Endoplasmic reticulum stress induces the expression of fetuin-A to develop insulin resistance. *Endocrinology* **2012**, *153*, 2974–2984. [CrossRef] [PubMed]
56. Srinivas, P.R.; Wagner, A.S.; Reddy, L.V.; Deutsch, D.D.; Leon, M.A.; Goustin, A.S.; Grunberger, G. Serum alpha 2-HS-glycoprotein is an inhibitor of the human insulin receptor at the tyrosine kinase level. *Mol. Endocrinol.* **1993**, *7*, 1445–1455. [PubMed]
57. Liu, J.; Xu, Y.; Hu, Y.; Wang, G. The role of fibroblast growth factor 21 in the pathogenesis of non-alcoholic fatty liver disease and implications for therapy. *Metabolism* **2015**, *64*, 380–390. [CrossRef] [PubMed]

58. Hong, S.H.; Ahmadian, M.; Yu, R.T.; Atkins, A.R.; Downes, M.; Evans, R.M. Nuclear receptors and metabolism: From feast to famine. *Diabetologia* **2014**, *57*, 860–867. [CrossRef] [PubMed]
59. Abdul-Wahed, A.; Guilmeau, S.; Postic, C. Sweet sixteenth for ChREBP: Established roles and future goals. *Cell. Metab.* **2017**, *26*, 324–341. [CrossRef] [PubMed]
60. Jiang, S.; Yan, C.; Fang, Q.; Shao, M.; Zhang, Y.; Liu, Y.; Deng, Y.; Shan, B.; Liu, J.; Li, H.; et al. Fibroblast growth factor 21 is regulated by the IRE1α-XBP1 branch of the unfolded protein response and counteracts endoplasmic reticulum stress-induced hepatic steatosis. *J. Biol. Chem.* **2014**, *289*, 29751–29765. [CrossRef] [PubMed]
61. Chukijrungroat, N.; Khamphaya, T.; Weerachayaphorn, J.; Songserm, T.; Saengsirisuwan, V. Hepatic FGF21 mediates sex differences in high-fat high-fructose diet-induced fatty liver. *Am. J. Physiol. Endocrinol. Metab.* **2017**, *313*, E203–E212. [CrossRef] [PubMed]
62. Staiger, H.; Keuper, M.; Berti, L.; Hrabe de Angelis, M.; Häring, H.U. Fibroblast Growth Factor 21-Metabolic role in mice and men. *Endocr. Rev.* **2017**, *38*, 468–488. [CrossRef] [PubMed]
63. Wu, H.T.; Ou, H.Y.; Hung, H.C.; Su, Y.C.; Lu, F.H.; Wu, J.S.; Yang, Y.C.; Wu, C.L.; Chang, C.J. A novel hepatokine, HFREP1, plays a crucial role in the development of insulin resistance and type 2 diabetes. *Diabetologia* **2016**, *59*, 1732–1742. [CrossRef] [PubMed]
64. Jung, T.W.; Chung, Y.H.; Kim, H.C.; Abd El-Aty, A.M.; Jeong, J.H. Hyperlipidemia-induced hepassocin in the liver contributes to insulin resistance in skeletal muscle. *Mol. Cell. Endocrinol.* **2018**, *470*, 26–33. [CrossRef] [PubMed]
65. Allaman, I.; Bélanger, M.; Magistretti, P.J. Methylglyoxal, the dark side of glycolysis. *Front. Neurosci.* **2015**, *9*, 23. [CrossRef] [PubMed]
66. Dhar, I.; Dhar, A.; Wu, L.; Desai, K. Arginine attenuates methylglyoxal- and high glucose-induced endothelial dysfunction and oxidative stress by an endothelial nitric-oxide synthase-independent mechanism. *J. Pharmacol. Exp. Ther.* **2012**, *342*, 196–204. [CrossRef] [PubMed]
67. Dhar, I.; Dhar, A.; Wu, L.; Desai, K.M. Increased methylglyoxal formation with upregulation of renin angiotensin system in fructose fed Sprague Dawley rats. *PLoS ONE* **2013**, *8*, e74212. [CrossRef] [PubMed]
68. Abdelmalek, M.F.; Lazo, M.; Horska, A.; Bonekamp, S.; Lipkin, E.W.; Balasubramanyam, A.; Bantle, J.P.; Johnson, R.J.; Diehl, A.M.; Clark, J.M.; et al. Higher dietary fructose is associated with impaired hepatic adenosine triphosphate homeostasis in obese individuals with type 2 diabetes. *Hepatology* **2012**, *56*, 952–960. [CrossRef] [PubMed]
69. Zhu, Y.; Hu, Y.; Huang, T.; Zhang, Y.; Li, Z.; Luo, C.; Luo, Y.; Yuan, H.; Hisatome, I.; Yamamoto, T.; et al. High uric acid directly inhibits insulin signalling and induces insulin resistance. *Biochem. Biophys. Res. Commun.* **2014**, *447*, 707–714. [CrossRef] [PubMed]
70. Fabbrini, E.; Serafini, M.; Colic Baric, I.; Hazen, S.L.; Klein, S. Effect of plasma uric acid on antioxidant capacity, oxidative stress, and insulin sensitivity in obese subjects. *Diabetes* **2014**, *63*, 976–981. [CrossRef] [PubMed]
71. Beavers, K.M.; Beavers, D.P.; Serra, M.C.; Bowden, R.G.; Wilson, R.L. Low relative skeletal muscle mass indicative of sarcopenia is associated with elevations in serum uric acid levels: Findings from NHANES III. *J. Nutr. Health Aging* **2009**, *13*, 177–182. [CrossRef] [PubMed]
72. Ticinesi, A.; Lauretani, F.; Milani, C.; Nouvenne, A.; Tana, C.; Del Rio, D.; Maggio, M.; Ventura, M.; Meschi, T. Aging gut microbiota at the cross-road between nutrition, physical frailty, and sarcopenia: Is there a gut-muscle axis? *Nutrients* **2017**, *9*, 1303. [CrossRef] [PubMed]

2

Nutritional Therapies in Congenital Disorders of Glycosylation (CDG)

Peter Witters [1,2,*], David Cassiman [3] and Eva Morava [1,2,4]

1 Metabolic Center, University Hospitals Leuven, B-3000 Leuven, Belgium; emoravakozicz@tulane.edu
2 Department of Development and Regeneration, Faculty of Medicine, KU Leuven, B-3000 Leuven, Belgium
3 Department of Gastroenterology-Hepatology and Metabolic Center, University Hospitals Leuven, B-3000 Leuven, Belgium; david.cassiman@kuleuven.be
4 Hayward Genetics Center, Tulane University School of Medicine, New Orleans, LA 70112, USA
* Correspondence: peter.witters@uzleuven.be

Abstract: Congenital disorders of glycosylation (CDG) are a group of more than 130 inborn errors of metabolism affecting *N*-linked, *O*-linked protein and lipid-linked glycosylation. The phenotype in CDG patients includes frequent liver involvement, especially the disorders belonging to the *N*-linked protein glycosylation group. There are only a few treatable CDG. Mannose-Phosphate Isomerase (MPI)-CDG was the first treatable CDG by high dose mannose supplements. Recently, with the successful use of D-galactose in Phosphoglucomutase 1 (PGM1)-CDG, other CDG types have been trialed on galactose and with an increasing number of potential nutritional therapies. Current mini review focuses on therapies in glycosylation disorders affecting liver function and dietary intervention in general in *N*-linked glycosylation disorders. We also emphasize now the importance of early screening for CDG in patients with mild hepatopathy but also in cholestasis.

Keywords: galactose; mannose; congenital disorders of glycosylation (CDG); treatment; glycosylation; diet

---

1. Introduction

Congenital disorders of glycosylation (CDG) are a family of diseases with the common denominator that they all affect the most important posttranslational modification of proteins, i.e., glycosylation [1]. They were initially described by Jaak Jaeken and currently compromise a group of more than 130 separate entities [1]. The most abundant type of CDG affect *N*-linked glycosylation. Most of these CDG are multisystemic diseases with hepatic involvement [2].

N-glycosylation is initiated with the activation of sugars in the cytoplasm of the cell. These phosphorylated sugars are subsequently transferred to the lipid dolichol, in the membrane of the endoplasmic reticulum (ER). This stepwise enzymatic assembly process leads to the formation of a glycan molecule. The base of this glycan consists of *N*-acetyl glucosamines (GlcNac), followed by several mannose (Man) residues. It is first assembled at the cytoplasmic surface and later inside the ER. Finally, the addition of glucose molecules is a signal to release the glycan from dolichol, followed by the attachment of the glycan to a protein. In the case of *N*-glycosylation, the glycan is linked to an amino group of an asparagine (N). The final steps of the glycosylation process take place in the Golgi apparatus with tailoring of the glycan molecule to its mature form by trimming away some of the mannose units and adding galactose and sialic acid [3,4].

While the assembly process in the ER is almost fully understood because it is conserved down to yeast and the consecutive building steps mirror each other, the process in the Golgi is very complicated as the success of the end product depends on several other factors outside the classic glycosylation steps. This glycosylation relies on the proper function of several transporters making the activated sugars available for synthesis. Defects in Golgi proteins that affect the trafficking and the transport of glycoproteins throughout the Golgi (functioning for example in the transport of protons and trace elements) can also lead to hypoglycosylation [3]. This is a rapidly growing family of newly described CDG [1,5].

The diagnosis of *N*-linked glycosylation disorders is made by serum transferrin isoelectric focusing, or mass spectrometry of transferrin isoforms. Depending on whether the defect is localized in the cytoplasm or endoplasmic reticulum (E.R.) or in the Golgi compartment, a different pattern can be observed, (type I and type II, respectively) [6].

In *O*-linked glycosylation, the glycan is linked to the OH-group of serine or threonine. *O*-linked glycan defects are often tissue specific. The mucin type of *O*-glycosylation is Golgi related and frequently associated with *N*-linked glycosylation defects. It can be screened by isoelectric focusing of serum apolipoprotein C-III, that is only *O*-glycosylated [3]. A well-known group of tissue specific *O*-glycosylation defects are the dystroglycanopathies [1,7].

Glycosylphosphatidylinositol (GPI)-anchored glycosylation defects is a growing group of genetic disorders clinically characterized by intellectual disability and biochemically by hyperphosphatasia. GPI anchors attach a number of proteins, including alkaline phosphatase, to membranes. Hyperphopsphatasia reflects the inability of the ectoenzyme (alkaline phosphatase) to anchor to the membrane and hence this will continue to circulate causing the hyperphosphatasia [3]. Lipid linked glycosylation is also important for the correct anchoring of T-cell antigens. The best known GPI-anchor defect, paroxysmal nocturnal hemoglobinuria, is a somatic disorder [4,7].

In CDG there is an important role of the dolichol phosphate mutase (DPM) complex. This complex is involved in the activation of mannose. Activated mannose is needed in all three glycosylation pathways *N*-linked, *O*-linked, and GPI-anchored [3]. The DPM complex has three subunits (DPM1, DPM2 and DPM3). Genetic defects in the DPM complex result in severe multisystem phenotypes, with biochemical anomalies of all three pathways (combined glycosylation defects) [3]. The phenotype consists of typical *N*-glycosylation symptoms, such as seizures, microcephaly, strabismus and developmental disability, but also eye anomalies and brain migration defects, seen in the dystroglycanopathies [8].

Liver disease is a feature of nearly all *N*-linked CDG. It mostly involves increased levels of transaminases (for example in the most prevalent CDG, PMM2-CDG). But sometimes it can manifest as hepatomegaly, cholestasis or liver failure. Histologically, liver fibrosis, ductal plate malformation, cirrhosis and steatosis have been observed. Especially the recently described CDG subtypes involving the Golgi can have liver disease, as their predominant feature (ATP6AP1-CDG, TMEM199-CDG and CCDC1115-CDG) [2,9–11]. In several *N*-linked CDG, liver transplantation has been necessary, due to progressive cirrhosis, for instance in MPI-CDG, or CCDC1115-CDG. Not only is transferrin, central to the diagnosis of *N*-linked CDG, produced by the liver, but so are a myriad of secreted and glycosylated proteins. For example, coagulation factors, except for factor VIII, are solely produced by the liver. In many CDG, there are disturbances of the coagulation profile. Usually this is due to a synthesis defect with decreased levels of factor IX, XI, protein C, antithrombin III and protein S, and also decreased glycosylation of these factors [12].

Dietary therapy is an important intervention in CDG [13]. Only a few CGD subtypes are "treatable". This article focuses on the different treatment options in *N*-linked glycosylation disorders with liver involvement.

2. Materials and Methods

The present literature review started with the search of the Medline database, using PubMed as search engine (last accessed October 2017). AND and OR operators were used in the database search to combine the keywords "therapy", "treatment", "supplement" or "diet" in combination with CDG or the two common full names for CDG: (a) carbohydrate-deficient glycoprotein syndrome(s) and (b) congenital disorder(s) of glycosylation. For the search algorithm see Supplementary File S1.

Papers were included in present review if they contained information on potential nutritional treatments in CDG that are known to affect the liver. Additionally, clinical trials were searched on www.ClincalTrials.gov using the same keywords.

3. Results

Two hundreds and forty-three articles matching these search terms were identified. Selection of the articles on *N*-glycosylation and describing nutritional therapy in at least 1 patient or a relevant animal model. Forty-nine articles were selected for further study. This information was complemented with the information presented at the World CDG-conference 2017 and the registered trials on Clinicaltrials.gov.

3.1. *Specific Dietary Therapies in Selected CDG Types*

Several CDG were found to be (at least partially) treatable by nutritional interventions such as mannose, galactose, etc. (Table 1).

Table 1. Specific dietary treatments in *N*-linked disorders of glycosylation.

	PMM2-CDG	MPI-CDG	PGM1-CDG	SLC 35A2-CDG	SLC39A8-CDG	TMEM165-CDG
Mannose	-	X	-	-	-	-
Galactose	-	-	X	X	X	X
Frequent complex carbohydrate feeding	+/—	+/—	X	-	-	-
Manganese	-	-	-	-	X	? *

Abbreviations: CDG: congenital disorders of glycosylation, PMM2: phosphomannomutase 2; MPI: Mannosephosphate Isomerase. * Manganese only trialed in vitro, cautious use is potentially useful as oral therapy. X Clinically trialed dietary supplement with positive biochemical and clinical effects. +/— This therapy has shown beneficiary effect in some of the patients.

3.2. *Mannose in PMM2-CDG (MIM # 212065)*

PMM2-CDG is the first described CDG and is due to phosphomannomutase-2 (PMM2) deficiency. It has two clinical presentations. The neurological subtype presents with cerebellar atrophy with ataxia, intellectual disability, seizures, retinopathy, stroke like episodes and peripheral neuropathy [14]. The more severe and potentially lethal multisystem phenotype, also has organ involvement such as hepato-gastrointestinal (chronic diarrhea, protein-losing enteropathy, liver failure, cirrhosis), cardiac and kidney disease [15]. Liver involvement (mainly hepatomegaly and raised transaminases) is present in up to 50% of patients [2].

Nutritional therapy has been considered and trialed in the past in these patients. In vitro, there was a clear improvement observed in the glycosylation pattern by treating patient fibroblast lines with mannose [16,17]. However, clinically, based on multiple clinical reports (but no structural therapy trials), there has been no confirmed clinical improvement, nor biochemical improvement at the level of the defective glycosylation, in patients [17,18].

As of now we have to conclude that mannose therapy is not effective in PMM2-CDG. Evaluating the reported laboratory data in PMM2 deficient patients is also difficult, since in older patients, transferrin isoforms may normalize spontaneously, and in many patients with PMM2-CDG there is a gradual improvement of transaminases over time [15], parallel with clinical stabilization. There is an absolute need for future nutritional therapeutic trials; ideally double blind randomized controlled trials, in PMM2-CDG.

3.3. *Mannose in MPI-CDG (MIM # 602579)*

MPI-CDG is longest known treatable CDG-type. It is characterized by bleeding diathesis, increased risk for thrombotic events, abnormal liver function, hyperinsulinism and chronic diarrhea.

Patients have a normal intellect. Transferrin analysis shows a type I pattern. On liver histology congenital hepatic fibrosis, microvesicular steatosis and fibrosis or cirrhosis has been documented.

Initial investigations showed successful restoration of glycosylation by mannose in vitro which was followed by compassionate use of mannose in MPI-CDG patients [19]. This is not surprising because mannose can be phosphorylated by the hexokinase so that the defective phophomannose isomerase (MPI) that converts fructose-6-phosphate to mannose-6-phosphate can be bypassed. The dose of 200 mg/kg 4–6 times/day was suggested to keep serum mannose levels high enough to alleviate endocrine abnormalities, coagulation defects and the chronic protein-losing enteropathy [19–21]. In some of the patients, a higher dosage was needed for full recovery. In a low percentage of patients high doses of mannose led to hemolysis and jaundice. It can also lead to seizures [22]. Coagulation abnormalities and hyperinsulinism usually improve within a few weeks of mannose supplements, both on intravenous and on oral therapy. Chronic diarrhea may recur in exceptional cases. Mannose therapy does not prevent further hepatic injury and about 1/3 of the patients develop liver cirrhosis, sometimes requiring liver transplantation [21,23]. Formal placebo-controlled clinical studies of oral or IV mannose in MPI-CDG patients have not been performed so far, so the data is anecdotal.

3.4. Galactose in PGM1-CDG (MIM # 614921)

PGM1-CDG is a combined disorder of glycogenolysis, glycolysis and glycosylation. Most patients are born with a midline defect of the palate, cardiomyopathy and multiple laboratory abnormalities including abnormal coagulation, endocrine parameters and liver function tests. Hypoglycemia is partially due to hyperinsulinism and the abnormal glycogenolysis in patients. Short stature is associated with feeding difficulties. Patients have normal intellect [24].

Phosphoglucomutase 1 (PGM1) deficiency is a unique glycosylation disorder showing a mixed type of glycosylation defect (type I/II). The most characteristic finding is decreased galactosylation additional to a global decrease in glycan synthesis. Based on the decreased number of galactose molecules in truncated glycans and the success of galactose supplements in vitro in patient fibroblasts, recently clinical trials were initiated to evaluate the success of galactose treatment in PGM1 patients [24]. Pilot studies showed an improvement in liver transaminases, coagulation factors (antithrombin III and factor XI) and in a variable degree of endocrine parameters. The frequency of rhabdomyolysis decreased, however, the treatment did not affect muscle weakness and creatine kinase (CK) levels [25,26]. A frequent complex carbohydrate rich diet remains necessary to keep blood glucose levels in the normal range in all patients. In three patients, transient tube feeding had been needed due to severe recurrent hypoglycemic episodes. The frequency of hypoglycemic episodes however did improve on D-galactose therapy.

3.5. Galactose in SLC35A2-CDG (UDP-Galactose Transporter) (MIM # 300896)

This CDG is due to a deficiency of the UDP-galactose transporter (solute carrier (SLC) 35A2) in the Golgi leading to a type II pattern on transferrin analysis. Clinically it manifests as an early infantile epilepsy with developmental delay, hypotonia, variable ocular anomalies, and brain malformations (cerebellar atrophy, delayed myelination and a thin corpus callosum) [27]. Many of the patients have a mosaic form of the mutation, not showing transferrin abnormalities. Non-mosaic patients have significant elevation of the transaminases.

In one patient, glycosylation could be nearly completely restored by galactose supplementation [28]. Although seizures tend to improve on galactose therapy, transaminases remain elevated (personal communication, European Metabolic Group conference 2016).

3.6. Galactose in SLC39A8-CDG (Manganese transporter) (MIM # 616721)

This type II CDG is a recently described multi-systemic neurodevelopmental disorder with phenotypes ranging from cranial synostosis, hypsarrhythmia and disproportionate dwarfism to strabismus, cerebellar atrophy, hypotonia, intellectual disability and recurrent infections [1]. Liver transaminases can be chronically mildly elevated. SLC39A8 is required for the manganese homeostasis in the Golgi, where manganese is a cofactor of the β-1,4-Galactosyltransferase. Unsurprisingly, manganese supplementation [29] and galactose supplementation [30,31] have been attempted. Galactose generally improves glycosylation and high dose manganese treats the epilepsy.

3.7. Galactose in TMEM165-CDG (MIM # 614727)

TMEM165-CDG, a type II CDG, combines impaired *N* and *O*-glycosylation and manifests with striking osseous changes as epiphyseal, metaphyseal, and diaphyseal dysplasia. Other features that accompany this peculiar skeletal phenotype are muscular hypotrophy, fat excess, partial growth hormone deficiency, and, in some patients, episodes of unexplained fever. Biochemically there is a mild to moderate increases of serum transaminases (particularly of aspartate transaminase (AST)), CK, and lactate dehydrogenase (LDH), as well as decreased coagulation factors VIII, IX, XI, and protein C [32,33].

Galactose therapy has very recently shown to be beneficial in patient fibroblasts improved glycosylation as well as biochemical parameters (blood coagulation) [5]. This could be due to an upregulation of manganese dependent transferases in the Golgi, such as B4GALT1 (β-1,4-Galactosyltransferase 1).

3.8. General Symptom Directed Dietary Therapy in CDG

Next to the specific treatment of several *N*-linked CDG, there are also nutritional treatments of certain syndromes that are often present in CDG.

For instance, hyperinsulism is a well-known feature of MPI-CDG, PGM1-CDG and PMM2-CDG. This can be treated by dietary interventions, such as using foods with a low glycemic index, nocturnal tube feeding and the use of uncooked corn-starch in children above 1 year of age [25]. Most patients need additional diazoxide therapy [25].

There is often a component of failure to thrive in CDG patients. In these patients complimentary feeding and tube feeding can be necessary. Moreover, an elementary diet can prove to be useful.

Protein losing enteropathy is a main feature of MPI-CDG but can also be present in the most prevalent CDG (PMM2-CDG). In some patients lymphangiectasia have been documented and a MCT diet has shown to be useful [12,34]. Somatostatin treatment is an additional non-nutritional intervention.

MAN1B1-CDG is the only known CDG (type II) that is known to be associated with obesity in addition to slight facial dysmorphism and psychomotor retardation [35]. In this CDG, caloric restriction can be necessary.

Similar to MELAS (mitochondrial encephalomyopathy, lactic acidosis, and stroke-like episodes) syndrome, L-arginine has been used to treat stroke-like episodes in CDG. L-arginine could improve NO production and hence vasodilation in these patients (personal communications, Prof P de Lonlay). However, no formal trials have been performed.

In CDG presenting with cholestasis (such as ALG8-CDG, COG6-CDG, COG7-CDG, CCDC115-CDG and ATP6AP1-CDG), nutritional interventions such as in other causes of cholestasis can be necessary [2]. These entail the supplementation of fat-soluble vitamins and MCT (medium-chain triglycerides) that are more easily absorbed in the absence of bile [36].

In pediatric neurology, the ketogenic diet has proven to be useful in controlling refractory seizures [37]. In CDG refractory seizure are rare, but the ketogenic diet could also be used. One issue complicating this is the occurrence of hyperinsulinism in some CDG often leading to hypoglycemia [15] while on the ketogenic diet as this contains a low amount of carbohydrates [37].

Dietary treatment of CDG has been mostly successful with the traditional method (fructose and lactose restrictions), however no clinical trial is available about the efficacy of this diet. Alcohol use worsens the liver phenotype in CDG significantly, and oppresses lipid linked oligosaccharide synthesis. The alcohol-related glycosylation abnormality is reversible.

4. Discussion

Congenital Disorders of Glycosylation are usually multisystem disorders, mostly affecting the central nervous system, in addition to diverse laboratory anomalies. *N*-linked glycosylation defects are always affecting liver function, leading to abnormal synthesis of secretory proteins, including albumin, hormone transporters, and coagulation and anticoagulation factors, partially due to abnormal synthetic function of the liver, but also due to a disturbed glycosylation and insufficient posttranslational regulation of important functional proteins [12]. Alpha 1 antitrypsin, ceruloplasmine and other liver proteins are frequently abnormal. Liver transaminase levels are almost always elevated, although spontaneous recovery is common. Hepatomegaly is uncommon and only a few *N*-linked disorders lead to cholestasis, fibrosis or cirrhosis [2,9].

Jaundice is rarely present. In fact, only two recently described disorders (CCDC115-CDG and ATP6VAP1-CDG) are cholestatic conditions. In addition, some patients had to undergo liver transplantation [9,10].

This is also the case for MPI-CDG, where a cryptogenic liver disease can progress to liver cirrhosis without overt symptoms, even on successful dietary therapy.

The biochemical background of dietary monosaccharide therapy in CDG is not completely understood. Mannose therapy has been for long the only treatment in Mannose-Phosphate Isomerase (MPI) deficiency. The background of the therapy is that the enzyme block in MPI-CDG does not allow producing sufficient amount of mannose-6-phosphate for the endoplasmic reticulum (ER) related glycosylation. Using a very high concentration of mannose, administered every 4 hours, could salvage this [20]. By this concentration mannose can be directly activated (phosphorylated) by hexokinase. This phosphorylation step requires a higher than physiologic concentration of mannose since the enzyme's natural substrate is glucose, and hexokinase is only moonlighting in this reaction under these conditions. Mannose supplements unfortunately do not solve the clinical problem in PMM2 deficiency where a lack of mannose-1-phosphate makes further mannose activation impossible [38]. Experimental treatments in fibroblasts using chemically disguised mannose-1-phosphate are ongoing [13].

The theory behind oral galactose treatment is different. In SLC35A2-CDG the galactose transporter appears to be upregulated by excess of galactose, which leads to an increase in galactose transport to the Golgi in vitro [28]. This mechanism is similar to that seen by defects of the fucose transporter SLC35A1 (SLC35A1-CDG), which also shows an improved function on oral fucose therapy, with improving glycosylation. In both cases, transferrin glycosylation increases significantly but also some of the clinical features improve [13].

Galactose mode of action is different in PGM1-CDG. The hypothesis is that increasing galactose concentrations in blood increase galactose-1-phosphate and UDP-galactose levels, which restore the altered balance within abnormal nucleotide sugar pools. This would improve hypogalactosylation in the Golgi. Interestingly, in some unknown way, galactose supports the ER related glycosylation as well in PGM1 deficiency, where it has been shown that lipid linked oligosaccharide synthesis is arrested, but recovers on in vitro galactose treatment [24–26]. Galactose might offer extra energy substrate for patients, since some of the adults with PGM1 deficiency also show an improvement of their muscle disease [39].

In TMEM165, galactose's positive effect is suspected secondary through B4GALT1, a Golgi enzyme, which is both manganese and galactose concentration sensitive. TMEM165 defect leads to abnormal manganese transport to the Golgi, affecting Golgi oligotransferases, which apparently improve their function with extra galactose, and increase galactosylation [5]. This is similar to galactose effect in SCLA39A8-CDG, providing manganese for the Golgi, and also for B4GALT1, where both manganese and galactose therapy restores glycosylation, however a cautiously administered high dose of oral manganese therapy is clinically more efficient [29].

Dietary intervention is an evolving and increasingly used therapy in CDG. More and more subtypes are trialed on monosaccharide supplementation, due to the relatively high safety, especially compared to experimental drug trials, and the ease of supplementation. Monosaccharides can be mixed with any type of food and usually have a pleasant, if any taste. Previous experience with monosaccharide therapy in individual cases showed that increasing the concentration of specific monosaccharides can lead to an increase in Golgi availability. This has been demonstrated by improvement in galactosylation on galactose therapy in SLC35A2-CDG [27,28]. Similar results were observed on fucose therapy in fucose transporter deficiency [40]. Based on these observations one should hypothesize a potential beneficial effect of sialic acid in SLC35A1-CDG, or of *N*-acetyl Glucosamine (GlcNAc) in SLC35A3-CDG as GlcNAc has been already used in the past safely in patients with different medical conditions, for example as supportive therapy in chronic osteoarthritis, as a health supplement. Oral sialic acid supplementation, however has not yet been proven to be efficient and its long acting form was recently withdrawn from clinical trials, due to not reaching any of the study end-points in GNE-CDG) [13]. The problem with the dietary use of sialic acid is that this molecule is not efficiently taken up by the cell and in the Golgi compartment as an oral therapy.

Additional dietary therapies could aim at increasing UDP concentrations in the cell, to have sufficient UDP available for the synthesis of UDP-sugars [24]. This novel approach has been successfully used in CAD-CDG [41]. This has not been systematically trialed in other CDGs. Other possible therapies include manganese supplementation in CDGs related to defective manganese transport, already shown to be effective in two cases of SLC39A8-CDG [29], and manganese can be probably a potential adjuvant therapy for TMEM165-CDG [5].

The question is, whether these dietary interventions are sufficient, and potentially the most efficient interventions in CDG? We learnt from the lesson on MPI-CDG, that mannose therapy is not only risky, when applied in higher doses, but also cannot prevent the progressive fibrotic liver disease in about one third of the patients [23]. Galactose therapy has beneficial effects in several CDGs but does not fully alleviate all clinical symptoms. The long term future of CDG therapy is most likely the use of activated monosaccharides instead of using single dietary sugars. In order to increase substrate concentrations, or supplement missing substrates, we should administer a more specific therapy by ingesting only a small amount of the active compound, compared to the currently used large amounts of simple sugars (in some cases 50 g/monosaccharide added to the diet daily). The efficacy of these novel potential drugs should be however carefully evaluated, for toxicity. The use of animal models is imperative instead of using cell culture models, since a successful cellular delivery of monosaccharides in fibroblasts does not mean that the oral supplementation would be effective [18,38].

5. Conclusions

In summary, in our current mini review we evaluated the different nutritional therapy options, associated with a positive effect on liver function in CDG. We believe this new type of nutritional therapy holds great promise for the future and over the last decade numerous CDG have been transformed to at least partially treatable disorders.

File S1: Search algorithm used in Pubmed (https://www.ncbi.nlm.nih.gov/pubmed/), accessed on 1 October 2017.

Acknowledgments: P.W. is supported by the clinical research fund, University Hospitals Leuven, Leuven, Belgium. E.M. and D.C. are recipients of the clinical investigatorship, FWO Flanders, Belgium.

Author Contributions: P.W., E.M. and D.C. conceived and designed the research; P.W., E.M. and D.C. analyzed the data; P.W., E.M. and D.C. wrote the paper.

Abbreviations

CDG	Congenital disorders of glycosylation
ER	Endoplasmic reticulum
GlcNac	*N*-acetyl glucosamines
Man	Mannose
GPI	Glycosylphosphatidylinositol
DPM	Dolichol phosphate mutase
PMM2	Phosphomannomutase-2
MPI	Phophomannose isomerase
PGM1	Phosphoglucomutase 1
CK	Creatine kinase
SLC	Solute carrier
AST	Aspartate transaminase
LDH	Lactate dehydrogenase
MELAS	Mitochondrial encephalomyopathy, lactic acidosis, and stroke-like episodes

References

1. Jaeken, J.; Peanne, R. What is new in CDG? *J. Inherit. Metab. Dis.* **2017**, *40*, 569–586. [CrossRef] [PubMed]
2. Marques-da-Silva, D.; Dos Reis Ferreira, V.; Monticelli, M.; Janeiro, P.; Videira, P.A.; Witters, P.; Jaeken, J.; Cassiman, D. Liver involvement in congenital disorders of glycosylation (CDG). A systematic review of the literature. *J. Inherit. Metab. Dis.* **2017**, *40*, 195–207. [CrossRef] [PubMed]
3. Witters, P.; Morava, E. Congenital disorders of glycosylation (CDG): Review. *eLS* **2016**, 1–6. [CrossRef]
4. Jaeken, J.; Hennet, T.; Matthijs, G.; Freeze, H.H. CDG nomenclature: Time for a change! *Biochim. Biophys. Acta* **2009**, *1792*, 825–826. [CrossRef] [PubMed]
5. Morelle, W.; Potelle, S.; Witters, P.; Wong, S.; Climer, L.; Lupashin, V.; Matthijs, G.; Gadomski, T.; Jaeken, J.; Cassiman, D.; et al. Galactose supplementation in patients with tmem165-CDG rescues the glycosylation defects. *J. Clin. Endocrinol. Metab.* **2017**, *102*, 1375–1386. [CrossRef] [PubMed]
6. Lefeber, D.J.; Morava, E.; Jaeken, J. How to find and diagnose a CDG due to defective *N*-glycosylation. *J. Inherit. Metab. Dis.* **2011**, *34*, 849–852. [CrossRef] [PubMed]
7. Freeze, H.H. Congenital disorders of glycosylation: CDG-I, CDG-II, and beyond. *Curr. Mol. Med.* **2007**, *7*, 389–396. [CrossRef] [PubMed]
8. Barone, R.; Aiello, C.; Race, V.; Morava, E.; Foulquier, F.; Riemersma, M.; Passarelli, C.; Concolino, D.; Carella, M.; Santorelli, F.; et al. DPM2-CDG: A muscular dystrophy-dystroglycanopathy syndrome with severe epilepsy. *Ann. Neurol.* **2012**, *72*, 550–558. [CrossRef] [PubMed]
9. Jansen, E.J.; Timal, S.; Ryan, M.; Ashikov, A.; van Scherpenzeel, M.; Graham, L.A.; Mandel, H.; Hoischen, A.; Iancu, T.C.; Raymond, K.; et al. ATP6AP1 deficiency causes an immunodeficiency with hepatopathy, cognitive impairment and abnormal protein glycosylation. *Nat. Commun.* **2016**, *7*, 11600. [CrossRef] [PubMed]
10. Jansen, J.C.; Cirak, S.; van Scherpenzeel, M.; Timal, S.; Reunert, J.; Rust, S.; Perez, B.; Vicogne, D.; Krawitz, P.; Wada, Y.; et al. CCDC115 deficiency causes a disorder of Golgi homeostasis with abnormal protein glycosylation. *Am. J. Hum. Genet.* **2016**, *98*, 310–321. [CrossRef] [PubMed]
11. Jansen, J.C.; Timal, S.; van Scherpenzeel, M.; Michelakakis, H.; Vicogne, D.; Ashikov, A.; Moraitou, M.; Hoischen, A.; Huijben, K.; Steenbergen, G.; et al. TMEM199 deficiency is a disorder of Golgi homeostasis characterized by elevated aminotransferases, alkaline phosphatase, and cholesterol and abnormal glycosylation. *Am. J. Hum. Genet.* **2016**, *98*, 322–330. [CrossRef] [PubMed]
12. Scott, K.; Gadomski, T.; Kozicz, T.; Morava, E. Congenital disorders of glycosylation: New defects and still counting. *J. Inherit. Metab. Dis.* **2014**, *37*, 609–617. [CrossRef] [PubMed]
13. Peanne, R.; de Lonlay, P.; Foulquier, F.; Kornak, U.; Lefeber, D.J.; Morava, E.; Perez, B.; Seta, N.; Thiel, C.; Van Schaftingen, E.; et al. Congenital disorders of glycosylation (CDG): Quo vadis? *Eur. J. Med. Genet.* **2017**. [CrossRef] [PubMed]
14. De Diego, V.; Martinez-Monseny, A.F.; Muchart, J.; Cuadras, D.; Montero, R.; Artuch, R.; Perez-Cerda, C.; Perez, B.; Perez-Duenas, B.; Poretti, A.; et al. Longitudinal volumetric and 2D assessment of cerebellar atrophy

in a large cohort of children with phosphomannomutase deficiency (PMM2-CDG). *J. Inherit. Metab. Dis.* **2017**. [CrossRef]

15. Schiff, M.; Roda, C.; Monin, M.L.; Arion, A.; Barth, M.; Bednarek, N.; Bidet, M.; Bloch, C.; Boddaert, N.; Borgel, D.; et al. Clinical, laboratory and molecular findings and long-term follow-up data in 96 french patients with PMM2-CDG (phosphomannomutase 2-congenital disorder of glycosylation) and review of the literature. *J. Med. Genet.* **2017**. [CrossRef] [PubMed]
16. Panneerselvam, K.; Freeze, H.H. Mannose corrects altered *N*-glycosylation in carbohydrate-deficient glycoprotein syndrome fibroblasts. *J. Clin. Investig.* **1996**, *97*, 1478–1487. [CrossRef] [PubMed]
17. Kjaergaard, S.; Kristiansson, B.; Stibler, H.; Freeze, H.H.; Schwartz, M.; Martinsson, T.; Skovby, F. Failure of short-term mannose therapy of patients with carbohydrate-deficient glycoprotein syndrome type 1A. *Acta Paediatr.* **1998**, *87*, 884–888. [CrossRef] [PubMed]
18. Mayatepek, E.; Kohlmuller, D. Mannose supplementation in carbohydrate-deficient glycoprotein syndrome type I and phosphomannomutase deficiency. *Eur. J. Pediatr.* **1998**, *157*, 605–606. [CrossRef] [PubMed]
19. Harms, H.K.; Zimmer, K.P.; Kurnik, K.; Bertele-Harms, R.M.; Weidinger, S.; Reiter, K. Oral mannose therapy persistently corrects the severe clinical symptoms and biochemical abnormalities of phosphomannose isomerase deficiency. *Acta Paediatr.* **2002**, *91*, 1065–1072. [CrossRef] [PubMed]
20. De Lonlay, P.; Seta, N. The clinical spectrum of phosphomannose isomerase deficiency, with an evaluation of mannose treatment for CDG-Ib. *Biochim. Biophys. Acta* **2009**, *1792*, 841–843. [CrossRef] [PubMed]
21. Mention, K.; Lacaille, F.; Valayannopoulos, V.; Romano, S.; Kuster, A.; Cretz, M.; Zaidan, H.; Galmiche, L.; Jaubert, F.; de Keyzer, Y.; et al. Development of liver disease despite mannose treatment in two patients with CDG-Ib. *Mol. Genet. Metab.* **2008**, *93*, 40–43. [CrossRef] [PubMed]
22. Schroeder, A.S.; Kappler, M.; Bonfert, M.; Borggraefe, I.; Schoen, C.; Reiter, K. Seizures and stupor during intravenous mannose therapy in a patient with CDG syndrome type 1b (MPI-CDG). *J. Inherit. Metab. Dis.* **2010**, *33* (Suppl. S3), S497–S502. [CrossRef] [PubMed]
23. Janssen, M.C.; de Kleine, R.H.; van den Berg, A.P.; Heijdra, Y.; van Scherpenzeel, M.; Lefeber, D.J.; Morava, E. Successful liver transplantation and long-term follow-up in a patient with MPI-CDG. *Pediatrics* **2014**, *134*, e279–e283. [CrossRef] [PubMed]
24. Tegtmeyer, L.C.; Rust, S.; van Scherpenzeel, M.; Ng, B.G.; Losfeld, M.E.; Timal, S.; Raymond, K.; He, P.; Ichikawa, M.; Veltman, J.; et al. Multiple phenotypes in phosphoglucomutase 1 deficiency. *N. Engl. J. Med.* **2014**, *370*, 533–542. [CrossRef] [PubMed]
25. Morava, E. Galactose supplementation in phosphoglucomutase-1 deficiency; review and outlook for a novel treatable CDG. *Mol. Genet. Metab.* **2014**, *112*, 275–279. [CrossRef] [PubMed]
26. Wong, S.Y.; Gadomski, T.; van Scherpenzeel, M.; Honzik, T.; Hansikova, H.; Holmefjord, K.S.B.; Mork, M.; Bowling, F.; Sykut-Cegielska, J.; Koch, D.; et al. Oral D-galactose supplementation in PGM1-CDG. *Genet. Med.* **2017**. [CrossRef] [PubMed]
27. Kodera, H.; Nakamura, K.; Osaka, H.; Maegaki, Y.; Haginoya, K.; Mizumoto, S.; Kato, M.; Okamoto, N.; Iai, M.; Kondo, Y.; et al. De novo mutations in SLC35A2 encoding a UDP-galactose transporter cause early-onset epileptic encephalopathy. *Hum. Mutat.* **2013**, *34*, 1708–1714. [CrossRef] [PubMed]
28. Dorre, K.; Olczak, M.; Wada, Y.; Sosicka, P.; Gruneberg, M.; Reunert, J.; Kurlemann, G.; Fiedler, B.; Biskup, S.; Hortnagel, K.; et al. A new case of UDP-galactose transporter deficiency (SLC35A2-CDG): Molecular basis, clinical phenotype, and therapeutic approach. *J. Inherit. Metab. Dis.* **2015**, *38*, 931–940. [CrossRef] [PubMed]
29. Park, J.H.; Hogrebe, M.; Fobker, M.; Brackmann, R.; Fiedler, B.; Reunert, J.; Rust, S.; Tsiakas, K.; Santer, R.; Gruneberg, M.; et al. SLC39A8 deficiency: Biochemical correction and major clinical improvement by manganese therapy. *Genet. Med.* **2017**. [CrossRef] [PubMed]
30. Park, J.H.; Hogrebe, M.; Gruneberg, M.; DuChesne, I.; von der Heiden, A.L.; Reunert, J.; Schlingmann, K.P.; Boycott, K.M.; Beaulieu, C.L.; Mhanni, A.A.; et al. SLC39A8 deficiency: A disorder of manganese transport and glycosylation. *Am. J. Hum. Genet.* **2015**, *97*, 894–903. [CrossRef] [PubMed]
31. Riley, L.G.; Cowley, M.J.; Gayevskiy, V.; Roscioli, T.; Thorburn, D.R.; Prelog, K.; Bahlo, M.; Sue, C.M.; Balasubramaniam, S.; Christodoulou, J. A SLC39A8 variant causes manganese deficiency, and glycosylation and mitochondrial disorders. *J. Inherit. Metab. Dis.* **2017**, *40*, 261–269. [CrossRef] [PubMed]
32. Foulquier, F.; Amyere, M.; Jaeken, J.; Zeevaert, R.; Schollen, E.; Race, V.; Bammens, R.; Morelle, W.; Rosnoblet, C.; Legrand, D.; et al. TMEM165 deficiency causes a congenital disorder of glycosylation. *Am. J. Hum. Genet.* **2012**, *91*, 15–26. [CrossRef] [PubMed]

33. Zeevaert, R.; de Zegher, F.; Sturiale, L.; Garozzo, D.; Smet, M.; Moens, M.; Matthijs, G.; Jaeken, J. Bone dysplasia as a key feature in three patients with a novel congenital disorder of glycosylation (CDG) type II due to a deep intronic splice mutation in tmem165. *JIMD Rep.* **2013**, *8*, 145–152. [PubMed]
34. Theodore, M.; Morava, E. Congenital disorders of glycosylation: Sweet news. *Curr. Opin. Pediatr.* **2011**, *23*, 581–587. [CrossRef] [PubMed]
35. Rymen, D.; Peanne, R.; Millon, M.B.; Race, V.; Sturiale, L.; Garozzo, D.; Mills, P.; Clayton, P.; Asteggiano, C.G.; Quelhas, D.; et al. MAN1B1 deficiency: An unexpected CDG-II. *PLoS Genet.* **2013**, *9*, e1003989. [CrossRef] [PubMed]
36. Los, E.L.; Lukovac, S.; Werner, A.; Dijkstra, T.; Verkade, H.J.; Rings, E.H. Nutrition for children with cholestatic liver disease. *Nestle Nutr. Workshop Ser. Pediatr. Program.* **2007**, *59*, 147–157. [PubMed]
37. Neal, E.G.; Chaffe, H.; Schwartz, R.H.; Lawson, M.S.; Edwards, N.; Fitzsimmons, G.; Whitney, A.; Cross, J.H. The ketogenic diet for the treatment of childhood epilepsy: A randomised controlled trial. *Lancet Neurol.* **2008**, *7*, 500–506. [CrossRef]
38. Freeze, H.H. Towards a therapy for phosphomannomutase 2 deficiency, the defect in CDG-IA patients. *Biochim. Biophys. Acta* **2009**, *1792*, 835–840. [CrossRef] [PubMed]
39. Schrapers, E.; Tegtmeyer, L.C.; Simic-Schleicher, G.; Debus, V.; Reunert, J.; Balbach, S.; Klingel, K.; Du Chesne, I.; Seelhofer, A.; Fobker, M.; et al. News on clinical details and treatment in PGM1-CDG. *JIMD Rep.* **2016**, *26*, 77–84. [PubMed]
40. Marquardt, T.; Luhn, K.; Srikrishna, G.; Freeze, H.H.; Harms, E.; Vestweber, D. Correction of leukocyte adhesion deficiency type II with oral fucose. *Blood* **1999**, *94*, 3976–3985. [PubMed]
41. Koch, J.; Mayr, J.A.; Alhaddad, B.; Rauscher, C.; Bierau, J.; Kovacs-Nagy, R.; Coene, K.L.; Bader, I.; Holzhacker, M.; Prokisch, H.; et al. CAD mutations and uridine-responsive epileptic encephalopathy. *Brain* **2017**, *140*, 279–286. [CrossRef] [PubMed]

3

Evaluation of a High Concentrate Omega-3 for Correcting the Omega-3 Fatty Acid Nutritional Deficiency in Non-Alcoholic Fatty Liver Disease (CONDIN)

Derek Tobin [1,*], Merethe Brevik-Andersen [2], Yan Qin [1], Jacqueline K. Innes [3] and Philip C. Calder [3,4]

1 BASF AS, NO-1327 Lysaker, Norway; Yan.Qin@basf.com
2 Formerly BASF AS, NO-1327 Lysaker, Norway; merethha@gmail.com
3 Human Development and Health Academic Unit, Faculty of Medicine, University of Southampton, Southampton SO16 6YD, UK; innesjackie@gmail.com (J.K.I.); P.C.Calder@soton.ac.uk (P.C.C.)
4 National Institute for Health Research Southampton Biomedical Research Centre, University Hospital Southampton NHS Foundation Trust and University of Southampton, Southampton SO16 6YD, UK
* Correspondence: Derek.Tobin@basf.com

Abstract: This randomized controlled trial investigated the safety and efficacy of MF4637, a high concentrate omega-3 fatty acid preparation, in correcting the omega-3 fatty acid nutritional deficiency in non-alcoholic fatty liver disease (NAFLD). The primary end point of the study was set as the change of red blood cell (RBC) eicosapentaenoic acid (EPA) and docosahexaenoic acid (DHA) by MF4637. Whether the omega-3 concentrate could lower liver fat was evaluated in a subset of patients. Furthermore, 176 subjects with NAFLD were randomized to receive the omega-3 concentrate ($n = 87$) or placebo ($n = 89$) for 24 weeks, in addition to following standard-of-care dietary guidelines. The omega-3 index, omega-6: omega-3 fatty acid ratio and quantitative measurements of RBC EPA and DHA were determined at baseline and study completion. Magnetic resonance imaging of liver fat was conducted in a subset of patients. Administration of high concentrate omega-3 for 24 weeks significantly increased the omega-3 index and absolute values of RBC EPA and DHA, and decreased the RBC omega-6: omega-3 fatty acid ratio ($p < 0.0001$). A significant reduction in liver fat content was reported in both groups.

Keywords: non-alcoholic fatty liver disease; NAFLD; omega-3 fatty acid; EPA; DHA; omega-3 index

---

1. Introduction

Non-alcoholic fatty liver disease (NAFLD) is the presence of hepatic steatosis (>5% liver fat assessed by imaging modalities or >5% of cells containing visible lipid droplets from histology) that is not related to significant alcohol consumption, hereditary disorders, viral infection or steatogenic medication [1]. Early NAFLD is typically reversible, but can develop in some 30% of cases into non-alcoholic steatohepatitis (NASH), presenting as hepatic steatosis with inflammation, ballooning and evidence of hepatocellular injury with or without fibrosis [1–3]. NAFLD is associated with metabolic risk factors such as obesity, diabetes and dyslipidemia, and its prevalence has risen sharply in line with the rising rates of obesity and diabetes [1,4,5]. In Western countries, NAFLD is the leading cause of liver disease [6]. NAFLD is estimated to affect 20–30% of the general population, with the prevalence increasing to approximately 75% of patients with obesity or diabetes, and 90–95% in the morbidly obese [6–9]. The estimated prevalence of NASH is lower, but significant, at 2–3% of the general population and one-third of the morbidly obese [1,7].

Identification of NAFLD patients in a clinical setting is commonly performed due to suspicion from raised liver enzymes and confirmation of hepatic steatosis by ultrasound. More recently, more advanced techniques such as Fibroscan (Echosens) and lipidomic analysis (OWL) have become available at specialised and general practitioner level. A validated algorithm for steatosis risk, called the fatty liver index (FLI), uses clinically available measurements to predict steatosis and to identify populations at risk of developing further liver-related morbidities [10].

NAFLD is increasingly considered as the hepatic manifestation of metabolic syndrome. The metabolic dysregulation occurring during metabolic syndrome often starts with excess peripheral fat and peripheral insulin resistance with hepatic steatosis and hepatic insulin resistance following as secondary events. Hepatic insulin resistance results in increased circulating glucose and very low density lipoproteins (VLDLs) [11]. The resulting hyperglycemia, hyper-triglyceridaemia and lowered HDL-cholesterol are all risk factors for the development of cardiovascular disease (CVD) [1,2,11,12]. In common with metabolic syndrome, NAFLD is associated with increased morbidity and mortality, particularly from CVD [1,2,12,13]. NASH also has the potential to develop into liver cirrhosis, from which 30–40% of patients will die of liver-related causes such as liver failure or hepatocellular carcinoma within a ten-year period [2,3,14]. Despite the increasing prevalence of NAFLD and its associated morbidity and mortality, there is currently no approved drug therapy for its treatment. The World Gastroenterology Organization (WGO) guidelines state that, in addition to pharmacological management of co-morbidities such as diabetes and dyslipidemia, weight loss and increased physical exercise are the most effective ways to reduce liver fat [6]. However, such lifestyle changes are typically difficult to sustain in the long term, creating a significant unmet need for this condition.

There is mounting evidence that long-chain polyunsaturated fatty acids (PUFAs), especially the marine omega-3 fatty acids eicosapentaenoic acid (EPA) and docosahexaenoic acid (DHA), are depleted in patients with NAFLD [15–19]. This may be due to several factors including impairment of the hepatic metabolic pathways responsible for the synthesis of EPA and DHA from their precursors, increased utilization due to lipid peroxidation caused by raised oxidative stress in NALFD, as well as reduced dietary intake [15,16,20,21]. Increased levels of omega-3 PUFAs and reduction of the omega-6: omega-3 ratio enables a shift in hepatic fat metabolism away from de novo lipogenesis and towards fatty acid oxidation and secretion, thereby potentially reducing steatosis in NAFLD [17,22–26]. In support of this, a recently published systematic review and meta-analysis of omega-3 fatty acids in NAFLD patients demonstrate statistically and clinically significant consistent reduction in steatosis with approximately 3 g EPA plus DHA daily [27]. Overall, existing data demonstrate that NAFLD patients have reduced levels of EPA and DHA compared to healthy individuals and that there are beneficial effects on liver steatosis from increased intake of omega-3 PUFAs at approximately 3 g/day.

The purpose of this study was to investigate the safety and the ability of an omega-3 fatty acid medical food (MF4637; BASF AS, Lysaker, Norway), to correct the omega-3 fatty acid nutritional deficiency present in NAFLD. The hypotheses being tested are that MF4637 will significantly improve the omega-3 index (EPA + DHA in red blood cells (RBCs)) and lower the RBC omega-6: omega-3 fatty acid ratio in patients with NAFLD. The potential for MF4637 to reduce hepatic fat content was evaluated using magnetic resonance imaging-proton density fat fraction (MRI-PDFF) in a subset of patients. Additional post hoc stratification was performed using the FLI.

2. Materials and Methods

2.1. Study Design

This was a randomized double-blind placebo-controlled study conducted at 21 investigative sites across the U.S. All procedures involving human participants were approved by Quorum Review IRB, Seattle, WA, USA. All participants provided written informed consent. The trial is registered with ID NCT02923804 at the U.S. National Library of Medicine's ClinicalTrials.gov website.

Participants were recruited based on the suspected diagnosis of NAFLD, confirmed either by diagnostic imaging performed within the previous year, or by abdominal ultrasound performed at screening. Eligibility was determined, after the informed consent process, at screening, which included review of medical history and current medications, measurement of vital signs (height, weight, blood pressure, heart rate and body mass index (BMI)), hemoglobin A1c (HbA1c), thyroid-stimulating hormone (TSH) and liver function testing. Following written informed consent, each participant was centrally randomized 1:1, stratifying by site, marine omega-3 fatty acid intake ($\geq$250 mg/day and <250 mg/day), diabetes and statin use, to receive either the omega-3 concentrate MF4637 or a placebo (olive oil) for 24 weeks. The duration of the study was determined by taking into account the delay of approximately 6 months required for stabilization of the incorporation of EPA and DHA demonstrated in healthy subjects [28] and an analysis of the literature on the use of omega-3 during NAFLD for periods ranging from 6 months to more than one year [27]. Randomization numbers corresponding to predetermined intervention were assigned in a sequential manner to each subject via an Interactive Voice/Web Response System. One hundred and seventy-six subjects were subsequently randomized to receive either MF4637 (n = 87) or placebo (n = 89) (Figure 1). The modified intention to treat population was defined as all subjects who took at least a 1-day dose of omega-3 fatty acids or placebo and underwent at least 1 post-randomization primary efficacy assessment.

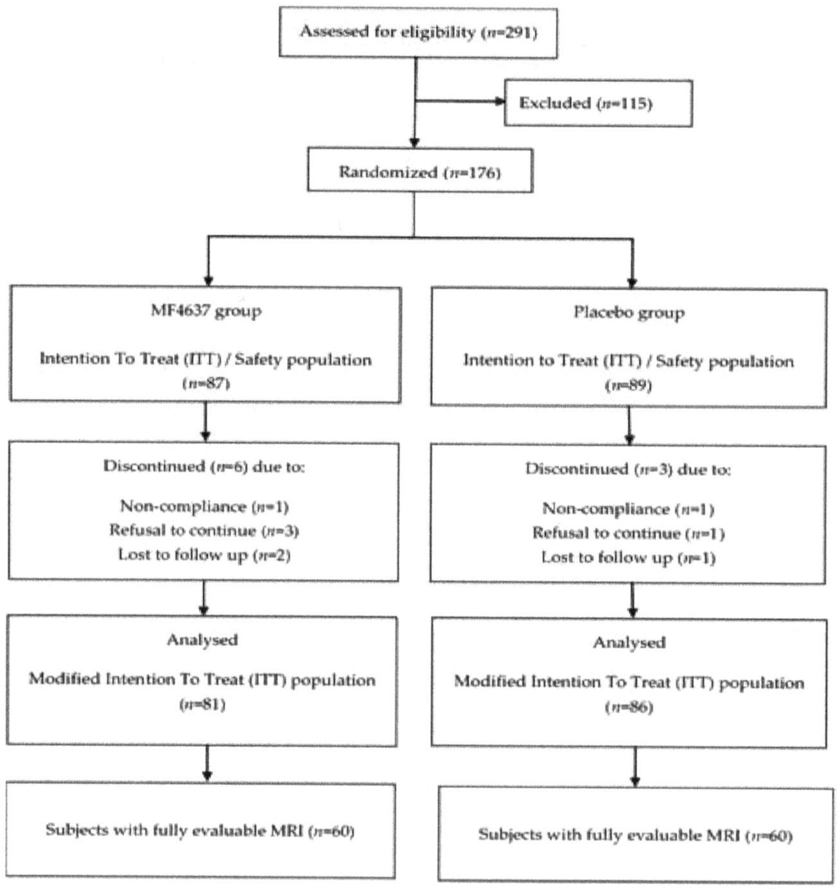

Figure 1. CONSORT flow chart of participant flow.

The omega-3 fatty acid medical food (MF4637; BASF AS, Lysaker, Norway) was provided as soft gel capsules, with each 1 g capsule containing marine-sourced EPA and DHA as ethyl esters (460 mg and 380 mg, respectively). Placebo capsules were identical in size and appearance to MF4637 and contained 1 g of olive oil. The investigational products were administered in a double-blinded fashion. Study participants were required to take three capsules per day of either MF4637 or placebo with food for 24 weeks. Thus, daily intakes of EPA and DHA in the MF4637 group were 1.38 g and 1.14 g, respectively. Compliance was measured via subject interview and unused capsule counts.

In addition to the investigational product, study participants were advised to reduce normal caloric intake as recommended by the American Association for the Study of Liver Disease (AASLD) standard-of-care guidelines for NAFLD [1], and to maintain stable physical activity levels throughout the study. To provide the American Heart Association (AHA) recommended dietary intake of omega-3 fatty acids [29], participants were required to consume two meals of omega-3 rich fish per week (from a choice of salmon, herring, whitefish, sardines, bluefish and trout) and to reduce foods rich in trans- and omega-6 fatty acids (fried foods and snacks, fast foods, bacon, turkey bacon, hams, nuts, peanut butter, sesame seeds, sunflower seeds, pumpkin seeds, vegetable oils and margarine (including soybean oil and corn oil), mayonnaise and salad dressing). Dietary intake was monitored regularly throughout the study via participant's food diaries.

At baseline (week 0), week 12 and study completion (week 24), weight, blood pressure, heart rate and BMI were recorded and blood samples collected to assess efficacy (Omega-3 index, RBC omega-6:omega-3 ratio and quantitative measurements of RBC EPA and DHA) and safety (vital signs, standard clinical biochemistry and hematology panels including liver function tests). Adverse events were monitored throughout the study. MRI-PDFF assessments of liver fat were performed at baseline (week 0) and study completion (week 24).

The primary endpoint of the trial was to test the effect of administration with concentrated EPA and DHA on the omega-3 index (RBC EPA + DHA). Secondary endpoints included quantitative measurement of RBC EPA and DHA and assessment of the RBC omega-6: omega-3 ratio. The potential for MF4637 to reduce hepatic fat content was evaluated as an exploratory outcome.

2.2. *Inclusion and Exclusion Criteria*

Selection of the NAFLD study population aimed to include subjects with hepatic steatosis, excluding those with a known previous diagnosis, at any time, of NASH indicating more advanced liver disease. Liver biopsy and histopathology are the only secure means of differentiating NASH from NAFL and therefore the study population may contain NASH patients. Inclusion criteria included age ≥18 years and a recent (<1 year) suspected clinical diagnosis of NAFLD including an imaging modality (e.g., ultrasound). If diagnosis was >1 year or an imaging test was absent, an abdominal ultrasound was performed at screening to confirm diagnosis of NAFLD. Other inclusion criteria included not smoking, BMI between 18–39.9 kg/m^2 and, if on statin medication, a history of >1 month on a stable dose. Exclusion criteria included a diagnosis of NASH; bilirubin >2 times the upper limit of normal; other causes of liver inflammation i.e., hepatitis A, B or C, HIV, cirrhosis, Wilson's disease, autoimmune hepatitis, hemochromatosis, alcoholic steatohepatitis, pancreatitis, or prescription medications known to cause liver toxicity or damage; history of bariatric surgery; significant weight loss (>5% body weight) or rapid weight loss (>1.6 kg/week) within six months of screening; cancer; significant cardiovascular disease including untreated hypertension and significant gastrointestinal, renal, pulmonary, hepatic, biliary or endocrine disease. Furthermore, subjects were excluded if there was significant alcohol consumption; use of any medicine or dietary supplement that may affect NAFLD or lipid metabolism (including omega-3 supplements); use of anti-coagulants; and pregnancy/breastfeeding or sensitivity to any of the study medications or excipients.

2.3. *Measurement of RBC EPA and DHA*

2.3.1. Quantitative Measurement of RBC EPA and DHA

Concentrations of total RBC EPA and DHA were measured quantitatively using UPLC-MS/MS. Method validation and all measurements were performed by Diteba Analytical and Bioanalytical Services, A Nutrasource Company (Mississauga, ON, Canada). Blood samples were collected into EDTA vacationer tubes, centrifuged, and plasma and white blood cells (buffy coat) removed.

The remaining RBCs were washed three times with saline, and 0.5 mL of the washed packed RBCs added to 1 mL of distilled water, to which was added 150 μL of EDTA/ascorbic acid. The sample was mixed well and stored at −80 °C until analyzed.

For the quantitative analytical methodology, a specific amount of standard curve solutions, matrix blanks, quality control samples and thawed study samples were acidified with HCl and internal standard was added to all tubes except for blanks. Samples were mixed well and incubated at 100 °C for 45 min, and then cooled to room temperature. Extraction solvent (hexane: dichloromethane: 2-propanol, in a 20:10:1 ratio) was added to each tube, which was mixed well and centrifuged. Capped tubes were submerged in a dry ice-acetone bath to freeze the aqueous layer, and the organic layer in each tube was transferred to another tube. This was evaporated to dryness at 45 °C; then, reconstitution solution was added, mixed thoroughly, and reconstituted samples were transferred into LC-MS vials for injection. The UPLC-MS/MS systems consisted of an Aquity Tandem Quadruple detector, auto-sample manager, binary solvent manager, column manager and Empower 3 data acquisition system. The UPLC column for optimum chromatographic conditions was an Aquity UPLC BEH, C18, 2.1 mm × 50 mm, 1.7 μm, assembled with a Waters in-line pre-column filter. The mobile phase was a 20:80 mixture of 5 mM ammonium acetate in water and acetonitrile. The injection volume was 5.0 mL, flow rate was 0.30 mL/min, run time was approximately 2.5 min, column temperature was ambient and sample temperature was 5 °C ± 2 °C. From the resulting chromatograms, EPA and DHA in each sample were calculated by calibration curve using peak area response ratio as response function. The quantitative method provided a range of 1 to 500 μg/mL for EPA, and 5 to 500 μg/mL for DHA.

2.3.2. Qualitative Measurement of RBC EPA and DHA

Qualitative measurement of EPA and DHA involved measuring the fatty acid profile of RBCs (consisting of a total of 30 fatty acids) using a gas chromatograph system with an auto sampler and FID detector (Diteba Analytical and Bioanalytical Services, Guelph, ON, Canada). Blood sample collection and processing was identical to that of quantitative analysis of RBC EPA and DHA. A specified amount (2 mL) of BF_3-MeOH was added to thawed RBC samples, mixed, flushed with N_2 gas and incubated for 10 min at 100 °C. After cooling, 250 μL of purified water and 750 μL of heptane were added to each tube and mixed well. Tubes were centrifuged at 4,000 rpm for 5 min and the top heptane layer was transferred to another tube and washed with purified water. The top (heptane) layer was transferred to another tube and evaporated to dryness under a stream of N_2 gas at 50 °C. Each tube was reconstituted with 10 μL of heptane, transferred to a GC vial and flushed with N_2 in preparation for injection. For this methodology, the column was a DB Wax, 30 m × 0.25 mm ID, 0.15 μm film or equivalent. The chromatic conditions were a GC with an FID detector, helium carrier gas, an initial oven temperature of 170 °C, increased at 3 °C/min to 200 °C, held for 3 min, increased at 2.5 °C/min to 225 °C, held for 5 min, then increased at 20 °C to 245 °C, and then held for 12 min. An external standard was injected three times and then reinjected for every 10 sample injections. From the three consecutive standard injections, an average response factor (RF) for each individual fatty acid was calculated, using the peak area of each individual fatty acid detected.

2.4. Assessment of Change in Liver Fat

Assessment of the change in hepatic fat fraction was measured via MRI-PDFF. For each subject, the MRI protocol included a localization sequence and a two-dimensional six-echo spoiled gradient-recalled-echo breath hold sequence. A three-plane localizer followed by a coronal breath-hold localizer was recommended for accurate axial slice prescription. If the scanner was not capable of acquiring six echoes simultaneously, multiple acquisitions with single-echo sequences were performed. From either the six-echo or six single-echo MRI series, the radiologist identified a circular region of interest (ROI) within each of the nine Cournand segments of the liver using the first echo of the series. The radiologist then identified regions with an approximately 2.5 cm diameter in each of the nine Cournand segments, except for segment 1 (the caudate), in which a region with a diameter of approximately 1.5 cm was identified. The ROI in the caudate was smaller since the caudate is generally too small to identify a region larger than 1.5 cm. The radiologist excluded blood vessels and the periphery of the liver when identifying the ROIs. A fat fraction map was calculated from the six-echo sequence using a multi-interference technique, which took into account the contribution from the individual resonances in the fat spectrum to the observed MRI signal to obtain an accurate estimate of fat. The whole liver hepatic fat fraction (HFF) was expressed as the mean fat fraction across all 9 user-defined ROIs in the liver.

2.5. Calculation of Fatty Liver Index (FLI) Score

Fatty liver index (FLI), an algorithm used to predict the presence of hepatic steatosis based on measured values for serum triglycerides (in mg/dL), serum GGT (in IU/L), BMI (in kg/m^2) and waist circumference (in cm), was calculated using the following equation [10]:

$$\text{FLI} = (\text{e } 0.953 \times \text{loge (triglycerides)} + 0.139 \times \text{BMI} + 0.718 \times \text{loge (GGT)} + 0.053 \times \text{waist circumference-15.745})/(1 + \text{e } 0.953 \times \text{loge (triglycerides)} + 0.139 \times \text{BMI} + 0.718 \times \text{loge (GGT)} + 0.053 \times \text{waist circumference-15.745}) \times 100. \quad (1)$$

2.6. Sample Size Calculations

It has been reported that the omega-3 index is 0.5% higher in healthy subjects compared to those with some form of liver dysfunction, leading to the assumption that a minimum increase of 0.5% in RBC EPA + DHA may be necessary to achieve nutritional sufficiency in NAFLD patients [30,31]. A conservative between-intervention difference for RBC EPA + DHA, measured as a change from baseline score between standard of care and standard of care plus MF4637, was set at 1.0% [32] and the standard deviation at 2.0 with a correlation of 0.5 and equal allocation of subjects across the two intervention groups, yielding 64 subjects per intervention arm for a total of 128. To address the uncertainty of the estimates of intervention effectiveness from the emerging literature, an adaptive blinded mid-course sample size re-estimation procedure was originally planned for the point at which approximately 30% of the subjects had completed one post-baseline visit (i.e., to Week 12) and had provided the RBC EPA + DHA results (for baseline and Week 12). The sample size re-estimation was performed by one unblinded study statistician. When 30% of the subjects had provided the Week 24 RBC DHA and EPA data, and the data were considered "lockable" by data management, the data file was exported to a limited access subdirectory, the effect size (change from baseline in plasma level) estimated and the conditional power (CP) were calculated. Because the CP was between 41% and 90%, the number of subjects per intervention arm was increased, in order to recover the targeted power of 90%. Given that the interim analysis was performed at 30% of the initial sample size, and the targeted power was 90%, the minimum conditional power cut-off value (CP min) was set at 41%. The procedure was performed, as per the Charter, and the recommendation was to increase the sample size to 75 subjects per intervention (i.e., 150 subjects). The actual number of participants recruited to the study was 176.

2.7. Statistical Analysis

The primary outcome (RBC EPA + DHA) was analyzed using a repeated analysis of covariance (ANCOVA) with the stratification factors as covariates, in order to compare the changes in the combined EPA + DHA outcome between the two intervention groups (MF4637 group and placebo) across the study. Stratification factors were baseline omega-3 intake, diabetes status and statin use. Additional outcomes were analyzed using the same ANCOVA model applied to the primary outcome: RBC EPA, RBC DHA and the omega-6: omega-3 ratio. All programming was performed in SAS version 9.2 (SAS Institute, Cary, NC, USA) or higher under the Windows Server 2008R2 operating system.

A regression analysis for absolute RBC EPA + DHA and change in liver fat for the MF4637 group and placebo was planned without testing of statistical significance. Similarly, regression analysis of changes in omega-3 index against baseline omega-3 index was performed. Post hoc analysis of the change in liver fat for intervention and placebo groups after stratification using the baseline Fatty Liver Index was tested using ANCOVA.

3. Results

Of the 176 participants that underwent randomization, safety was assessed for 87 subjects in the intervention group and 89 in the placebo group (Figure 1). Of those participants randomized, 167 (81 in the MF4637 group and 86 in the placebo group) were included in the modified intention to treat (mITT) primary outcome analysis.

Baseline anthropometric and biochemical variables of participants randomized to the placebo and MF4637 groups are detailed in Table 1. Of note is the higher mean fasting insulin concentration in the placebo group, which, together with the comparable mean fasting glucose concentration, suggests a likelihood that the placebo group was more insulin resistant than the MF4637 group at study entry.

Table 1. Baseline anthropometric and biochemical variables of participants randomized to placebo and MF4637 groups.

Variables	Placebo [1]	MF4637 [2]	*p*-Value *
Age, years	55.1 (10.9)	55.3 (13.3)	0.93
Sex, M/F	44/42	36/45	0.39
Weight, kg	90.1 (18.8)	88.4 (18.4)	0.55
Waist circumference, cm	105.9 (13.1)	106.3 (13.2)	0.87
Hip circumference, cm	110.5 (12.1)	110.9 (11.8)	0.85
Waist to hip ratio	0.96 (0.09)	0.96 (0.08)	0.95
BMI, kg/m^2	32.4 (5.0)	32.1 (4.8)	0.59
Systolic blood pressure, mm Hg	127.0 (10.7)	128.0 (11.9)	0.64
Diastolic blood pressure, mm Hg	80.3 (7.2)	79.8 (7.6)	0.33
Heart rate, beats/min	74.7 (8.7)	73.2 (9.1)	0.25
Statin use, %	34.9	30.9	0.58
Diabetes, %	39.5	35.0	0.97
Fasting glucose, mg/dL	120.1 (48.5) [2]	119.4 (38.1) [3]	0.97
Fasting insulin, µIU/mL	30.2 (41.3)	20.8 (18.2) [4]	0.04
HbA1c, %	6.5 (1.5) [5]	6.3 (1.4) [6]	0.20
Triglycerides, mg/dL	199.1 (123.0) [7]	192.0 (125.1) [4]	0.70
BUN, mg/dL	14.7 (4.9) [7]	15.4 (5.0) [4]	0.24
Creatinine, mg/dL	0.8 (0.2) [7]	0.3 (0.2) [4]	0.83
TSH µIU/mL	1.9 (1.0) [7]	1.7 (0.9) [8]	0.17
Hs-CRP, mg/L	6.4 (9.2) [7]	8.1 (17.5)	0.61
Albumin, g/dL	4.29 (0.3) [7]	4.29 (0.3) [4]	0.91
ALT, IU/L	35.6 (24.0)	37.5 (39.0)	0.40
AST, IU/L	25.8 (12.2)	27.1 (20.3)	0.79
ALP, IU/L	81.5 (31.0)	85.5 (45.3)	0.62
GGT, IU/L	47.1 (49.0)	62.2 (151.4)	0.78
Bilirubin, mg/dL	0.5 (0.2)	0.5 (0.3)	0.91

[1] Data for n = 86 participants unless otherwise specified. [2] Data for n = 81 participants unless otherwise specified. [3] Data for n = 75 participants. [4] Data for n = 80 participants. [5] Data for n = 83 participants. [6] Data for n = 79 participants. [7] Data for n = 85 participants. [8] Data for n = 78 participants. Values expressed as Mean (SD). Abbreviations: ALP, alkaline phosphatase; ALT, alanine aminotransferase; AST, aspartate aminotransferase; BMI, body mass index; BUN, blood urea nitrogen; GGT, gamma-glutamyl transferase; HbA1c, glycated haemoglobin; hs-CRP, high-sensitivity C-reactive protein; TSH, thyroid stimulating hormone. * All statistical tests performed were t-tests except for chi-square tests for the following variables: Sex; Statin use and Diabetes, and Wilcoxon two-sample tests for the following variables: Fasting glucose; HbA1c; ALP and GGT.

Table 2 details the main anthropometric and biochemical variables for participants randomized to the placebo and MF4637 groups at baseline and after 24 weeks of intervention. The overall weight of subjects in either intervention group remained unchanged from study start to study end. Triglyceride levels at baseline were similar in both groups and would be clinically regarded as borderline raised. At the end of the study, a statistically significant reduction in triglycerides was only seen in the MF4637 group. Interestingly, the liver enzymes ALT, AST and GGT showed statistical reductions at the end of study in the placebo group and not in the MF4637 group. This implies an overall improvement in liver function without weight loss.

Compliance regarding the investigational products was 89% in the MF4637 group and 91% in the placebo group. There were no serious adverse events related to study interventions reported during the 24-week study. Mild incidences of eructation ($n = 1$), dysgeusia ($n = 1$), abdominal bloating ($n = 1$) and increased blood triglycerides ($n = 1$) together with a moderate case of diarrhea ($n = 1$) were reported in the MF4637 group and suspected to be related. One participant in the MF4637 group and two participants in the placebo group discontinued the study due to adverse events.

Table 2. Anthropometric and biochemical variables of participants randomized to placebo and MF4637 groups at baseline and study completion.

Variables	Placebo [1]			MF4637 [2]			Two-Sample Test for Change from Baseline *p*-Value [#]
	Baseline	End of Study	*p*-Value *	Baseline	End of Study	*p*-Value *	
Age, years	55.1 (10.9)			55.3 (13.3)			
Sex, M/F	44/42			36/45			
Weight, kg	90.1 (18.8)	89.5 (18.5)	0.84	88.4 (18.4)	89.0 (18.8)	0.082	0.23
Waist circumference, cm	105.9 (13.1)	104.7 (13.9)	0.005	106.3 (13.2)	105.5 (12.2)	0.72	0.18
Hip circumference, cm	110.5 (12.1)	110.0 (11.7)	0.31	110.9 (11.8)	110.4 (11.9)	0.81	0.42
Waist to hip ratio	0.96 (0.1)	0.95 (0.1)	0.081	0.96 (0.08)	0.96 (0.1)	0.66	0.58
BMI, kg/m^2	32.4 (5.0)	32.3 (4.8)	0.74	32.1 (4.8)	32.3 (5.0)	0.078	0.18
SBP, mm Hg	127.0 (10.7)	128.8 (15.0)	0.23	128.0 (11.9)	126.6 (10.6)	0.29	0.11
DBP, mm Hg	80.3 (7.2)	79.9 (9.9)	0.25	79.8 (7.6)	77.8 (8.4)	0.032	0.53
Heart rate, beats/min	74.7 (8.7)	74.1 (8.2)	0.59	73.2 (9.1)	74.2 (9.8)	0.17	0.17
Statin use, %	34.9			30.9			
Diabetes, %	39.5			35.0			
Fasting glucose, mg/dL	120.1 (48.5) [3]	125.4 (56.8) [3]	0.39	119.4 (38.1) [3]	127.5 (55.2) [3]	0.0616	0.38
Fasting insulin, μIU/mL	30.2 (41.3) [4]	30.1 (35.8) [4]	0.51	20.8 (18.2) [5]	24.0 (24.3) [5]	0.21	0.63
HbA1c, %	6.5 (1.5) [6]	6.6 (1.7) [6]	0.67	6.3 (1.4) [7]	6.3 (1.4) [7]	0.83	0.87
Triglycerides, mg/dL	199.1 (123.0) [2]	185.7 (118.0) [2]	0.52	192.0 (125.1) [5]	157.8 (84.2) [5]	0.0008	0.053
BUN, mg/dL	14.7 (4.9) [2]	15.0 (4.5) [2]	0.88	15.4 (5.0) [5]	16.2 (4.9) [5]	0.25	0.46
Creatinine, mg/dL	0.8 (0.2) [2]	0.82 (0.2) [2]	0.51	0.3 (0.2) [5]	0.84 (0.2) [5]	0.26	0.19
TSH μIU/mL	1.9 (1.0) [2]	2.5 (2.7) [2]	0.025	1.7 (0.9) [7]	1.8 (0.9) [7]	0.043	0.86
Hs-CRP, mg/L	6.4 (9.2) [2]	5.5 (5.8) [2]	0.46	8.1 (17.5) [8]	6.7 (10.9) [8]	0.75	0.82
Albumin, g/dL	4.29 (0.3) [2]	4.3 (0.3) [2]	0.69	4.29 (0.3) [5]	4.3 (0.3) [5]	0.62	0.91
ALT, IU/L	35.6 (24.0)	29.8 (21.2)	0.005	37.5 (39.0)	38.1 (37.7)	0.48	0.015
AST, IU/L	25.8 (12.2)	23.9 (13.5)	0.036	27.1 (20.3)	28.7 (24.6)	0.37	0.036
ALP, IU/L	81.5 (31.0)	76.3 (21.5)	0.01	85.5 (45.3)	83.2 (40.3)	0.09	0.73
GGT, IU/L	47.1 (49.0)	37.1 (32.2)	<.0001	62.2 (151.4)	57.1 (108.7)	0.37	0.058
Bilirubin, mg/dL	0.5 (0.2)	0.47 (0.2)	0.70	0.5 (0.3)	0.5 (0.2)	0.88	0.72

[1] Data for $n = 86$ participants unless otherwise specified. [2] Data for $n = 81$ participants unless otherwise specified. [3] Data for $n = 72$ participants. [4] Data for $n = 82$ participants. [5] Data for $n = 78$ participants. [6] Data for $n = 74$ participants. [7] Data for $n = 76$ participants. [8] Data for $n = 79$ participants. Values are expressed as Mean (SD). Abbreviations: ALP, alkaline phosphatase; ALT, alanine aminotransferase; AST, aspartate aminotransferase; BMI, body mass index; BUN, blood urea nitrogen; DBP, diastolic blood pressure; GGT, gamma-glutamyl transferase; HbA1c, glycated haemoglobin; hs-CRP, high-sensitivity C-reactive protein; SBP, systolic blood pressure.* Within-group differences were assessed using paired *t*-tests or Wilcoxon signed rank tests. [#] Intergroup differences were assessed using two-sample *t*-tests or two-sample Wilcoxon tests.

3.1. *Effect of Intervention on Omega-3 Index*

The baseline omega-3 index was similar for placebo and intervention groups. Compared to placebo, the mean omega-3 index increased significantly from 4.8% to 8.0% at study completion in the MF4637 group, representing a mean 3.2% change from baseline ($p < 0.0001$) (Table 3). In the placebo group, the omega-3 index increased slightly from 4.9% at baseline to 5.3% at study completion, representing a mean change of 0.4%. Regression analysis of the data for participants in the MF4637 group suggests that the change in omega-3 index was inversely related to the baseline omega-3 index, with lower baseline values resulting in greater increases by the end of the 24-week intervention (data not shown [33]).

Table 3. RBC fatty acid content at baseline and after 12- and 24-week intervention with placebo or MF4637.

	Placebo (n = 86)				MF4637 (n = 81)				
	Baseline	T = 12 weeks	T = 24 weeks	Change from Baseline	Baseline	T = 12 weeks	T = 24 weeks	Change from Baseline	p-Value [1]
RBC omega-3 index, %	4.9 (1.2)	5.8 (1.3)	5.3 (1.1)	0.4 (1.0)	4.8 (1.1)	8.7 (2.3)	8.0 (2.6)	3.2 (2.7)	<0.0001
RBC EPA + DHA, μg/mL	32.3 (26.4)	34.9 (21.0)	33.1 (20.5)	1.2 (14.9)	29.6 (17.5)	51.5 (38.9)	52.9 (40.7)	21.2 (28.7)	<0.0001
RBC EPA, %	0.54 (0.3)	0.54 (0.2)	0.54 (0.2)	0.002 (0.3)	0.53 (0.2)	1.6 (0.9)	1.4 (0.9)	0.9 (1.0)	<0.0001
RBC EPA, μg/mL	3.8 (6.6)	3.7 (2.6)	4.1 (5.7)	0.4 (7.0)	3.0 (2.6)	10.4 (10.7)	10.6 (12.0)	7.1 (10.5)	<0.0001
RBC DHA, %	4.3 (1.1)	5.2 (1.2)	4.8 (1.0)	0.4 (0.9)	4.3 (1.0)	7.1 (1.5)	6.6 (1.8)	2.3 (1.9)	<0.0001
RBC DHA, μg/mL	28.5 (21.0)	31.2 (18.6)	29.0 (16.2)	0.7 (10.7)	26.6 (15.3)	41.0 (28.8)	42.4 (29.8)	14.1 (19.5)	<0.0001
RBC omega-6: omega-3	4.9 (1.1)	4.5 (0.9)	4.7 (0.8)	−0.2 (0.7)	4.9 (1.2)	3.0 (0.9)	3.3 (1.5)	−1.6 (1.8)	<0.0001

[1] p-value is for the mean percentage change from baseline to 24 weeks between placebo and MF4637 groups using ANCOVA. Values are expressed as Mean (SD). Abbreviations: RBC, red blood cell; DHA, docosahexaenoic acid; EPA, eicosapentaenoic acid; T: Time.

3.2. *Effect of Intervention on RBC EPA + DHA, EPA and DHA Values*

Absolute RBC EPA + DHA increased on average from 29.6 μg/mL at baseline to 52.9 μg/mL at study completion (representing a significant increase of 21.2 μg/mL) in the MF4637 group, compared to a 1.2 μg/mL increase from baseline in the placebo group (significance between groups, $p < 0.0001$) (Table 3). In terms of absolute values of EPA and DHA separately, RBC EPA increased by a significant 7.1 μg/mL to 10.6 μg/mL at study completion in the MF4637 group versus a 0.4 μg/mL increase in the placebo group ($p < 0.0001$) (Table 3). RBC DHA increased by more than EPA, with a mean of 14.1 μg/mL increase to 42.4 μg/mL in the MF4637 group versus a 0.7 μg/mL increase in the placebo group ($p < 0.0001$) (Table 3).

Regarding the percentage of individual EPA and DHA as a proportion of total RBC fatty acids, both parameters increased significantly in the MF4637 group compared to placebo (Table 3). Specifically, RBC EPA as a percentage of total fatty acids increased by a significant 0.9% to 1.4% in the MF4637 group compared to a 0.002% increase in the placebo group ($p < 0.0001$). RBC DHA as a percentage of total fatty acids increased by a greater proportion than EPA, resulting in a 2.3% increase to 6.6% in the MF4637 group versus 0.4% increase in the placebo group ($p < 0.0001$).

3.3. *Effect of Intervention on RBC Omega-6: Omega-3 Ratio*

RBC omega-6: omega-3 ratio was not different between the two groups at baseline. Following administration of MF4637 for 24 weeks, the RBC omega-6: omega-3 ratio decreased by a mean of 1.6 from 4.9 at baseline to 3.3 at study completion, compared to a 0.2 decrease to 4.7 in the placebo group ($p < 0.0001$) (Table 3).

3.4. *Effect of Intervention on Liver Fat*

In the mITT analysis of liver fat content, 120 participants (60 in each trial arm) completed both the baseline and end of study MRI-PDFF assessment. In this population, baseline liver fat was 17.4% in the placebo group and 14.4% in the MF4637 group ($p = 0.0689$). Both the MF4637 and placebo groups demonstrated a decrease in liver fat percentage (26% and 28%, respectively), (Table 4). As such, there was no statistically significant difference in the decrease in liver fat between the groups.

Table 4. MRI-PDFF liver fat percentage at baseline and after 24-week intervention with placebo or MF4637.

	Placebo [1]				MF4637 [1]				p-Value
	T = 0 weeks	T = 24 weeks	Change from Baseline		T = 0 weeks	T = 24 weeks	Change from Baseline		
			Absolute	Relative			Absolute	Relative	
Liver fat, %	17.4 (10.4)	12.6 (8.0)	−4.4 (6.9)	−27.6	14.4 (10.1)	10.7 (7.6)	−2.8 (5.8)	−25.7	0.1838

[1] As assessed for modified ITT population (Placebo, $n = 60$; MF4637, $n = 60$). Values expressed as Mean (SD); T: Time.

3.5. Relationship between RBC EPA + DHA Enrichment and Liver Fat Content

Regression analysis of the data by intervention group suggests that the change from baseline in liver fat percentage was inversely related to the change in absolute RBC EPA + DHA values in the MF4637 group. Thus, the largest decreases in liver fat were observed in participants with the greatest increases in absolute RBC EPA + DHA (Figure 2). Hence, whilst there was no significant difference between MF4637 and placebo with regard to overall reduction of liver fat, there was an association between increasing RBC EPA+DHA enrichment and decreasing percentage liver fat content.

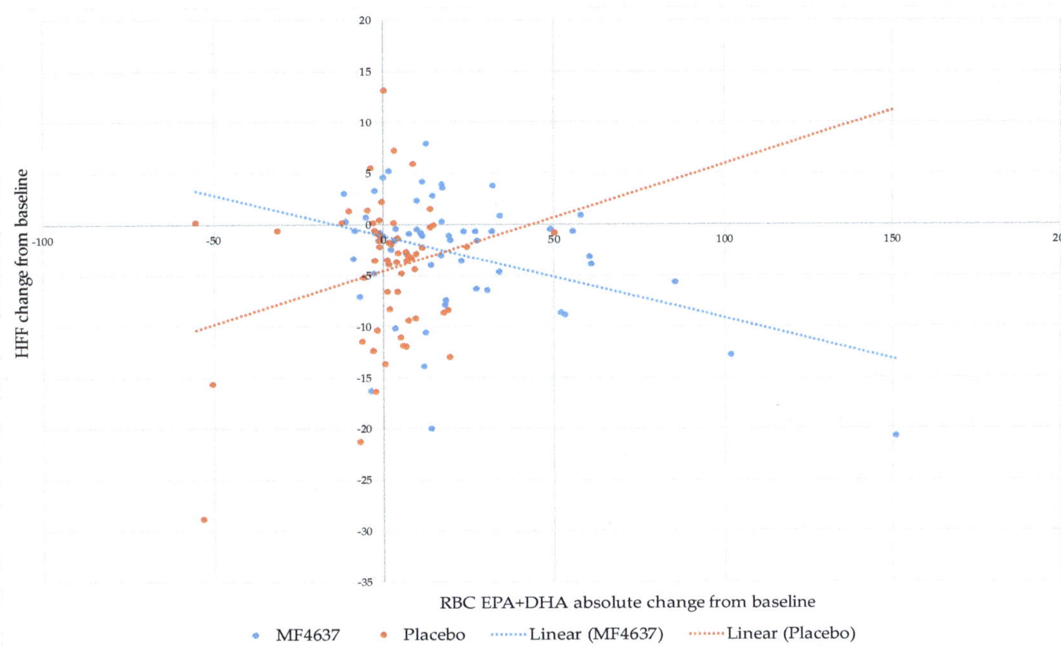

Figure 2. Relationship between change in absolute RBC EPA + DHA and change in liver fat.

3.6. Relationship between Baseline Fatty Liver Index (FLI) and Change in Liver Fat Content

Post hoc analysis of the MF4637 group utilizing ANCOVA with baseline fatty liver index (FLI) as covariate found that, in those patients with higher baseline FLI scores (indicative of more probable fatty liver), there was a greater reduction in liver fat compared to placebo (Table 5). Following 24 weeks of intervention with MF4637, patients with baseline FLI ≥ 40 ($n = 17$) had a placebo corrected, statistically significant 44% relative decrease in liver fat content ($p = 0.009$). This equates to a 7.45% absolute decrease in placebo corrected liver fat content for the MF4637 group.

Table 5. Change in MRI-PDFF liver fat percentage after 24-week intervention with MF4637 stratified by baseline FLI score.

		Baseline HFF Mean (SD)	Study End HFF Mean (SD)	Change in MRI-PDFF Liver Fat Percentage (%)			
				Absolute Change	p-Value [1]	Relative Change	p-Value [1]
FLI <30 [2]	Placebo	15.6 (11.2)	11.2 (7.8)	2.25 (1.39)	0.11	2.7 (11.3)	0.81
	Omega-3	12.5 (8.6)	10.3 (7.7)				
FLI ≥30 [3]	Placebo	20.6 (9.4)	16.0 (7.9)	−2.47 (2.53)	0.34	−9.3 (15.3)	0.55
	Omega-3	19.3 (11.1)	13.5 (7.0)				
FLI ≥40 [4]	Placebo	20.2 (9.5)	16.3 (8.4)	−7.45 (2.81)	0.02	−44.1 (14.6)	0.009
	Omega-3	20.7 (10.4)	10.6 (5.2)				

[1] *p*-value is for the mean percentage change from baseline to 24 weeks (placebo corrected) using ANCOVA. [2] Data for $n = 89$ participants ($n = 43$ placebo; $n = 46$ MF4637). [3] Data for $n = 28$ participants ($n = 16$ placebo; $n = 12$ MF4637).[4] Data for $n = 17$ participants ($n = 12$ placebo; $n = 5$ MF4637). Values expressed as Mean (SD). Abbreviations: FLI, Fatty Liver Index; HFF, Hepatic Fat Fraction.

3.7. Relationship between RBC EPA + DHA Enrichment and Liver Enzymes AST and ALT

At study entry, the mean baseline concentrations of the liver enzymes AST and ALT were within the normal range for both the placebo and MF4637 groups. This is not surprising considering that liver enzymes may be normal in up to 80% of NAFLD patients [34]. Similar to the relationship between RBC EPA + DHA enrichment and change in liver fat discussed above, a non-statistical inverse association was also found between the change in absolute RBC EPA + DHA and change in the concentrations of the liver enzymes AST and ALT in the intervention group. Thus, with increasing change in absolute RBC EPA + DHA, there were greater decreases in both AST and ALT concentrations (data not shown). However, there were significant reductions in AST, ALT and GGT in the placebo group (unrelated to omega-3 measurements), suggesting that multiple factors may be impacting the clinical outcome of the study groups.

3.8. Effect of Intervention on Plasma Triglycerides

At study completion, plasma triglycerides (Table 2) decreased by a statistically significant 18% from baseline values in the intervention group ($p = 0.0008$) compared to a 7% reduction in triglycerides from baseline values in the placebo group ($p = 0.52$; for placebo adjusted effect of M4637 $p = 0.053$). The baseline levels for triglycerides were only moderately increased compared to normality and would clinically be defined as "borderline high".

4. Discussion

This study demonstrates that intervention with high concentrate omega-3 for 24 weeks significantly raises the omega-3 index and decreases the omega-6: omega-3 fatty acid ratio in adults with NAFLD. Furthermore, the EPA and DHA enrichment achieved with intervention was significantly greater than that obtained by dietary recommendation alone. This is of importance, considering the depleted omega-3 status of NAFLD patients [15–19] and the current lack of therapeutic options for the treatment of NAFLD other than lifestyle recommendation [6]. Furthermore, the metabolic efficacy of the high concentrate omega-3 was confirmed through its significant lowering of plasma triglyceride levels compared to baseline levels.

When assessing the mITT population from whom baseline and post-intervention data from MRI-PDFF were available, intervention with both a high concentrate omega-3 and placebo caused a significant reduction in hepatic steatosis that was significant within each of the groups. There may be several reasons for the liver fat-lowering effect observed in the placebo group. All study participants were required to follow the standard-of-care dietary recommendations for the management of NAFLD. This included adherence to a diet with reduced caloric intake, and increased omega-3 and reduced omega-6 and trans-fatty acid consumption. Hence, participants in the placebo group may have achieved a decrease in liver fat percentage from the effects of these dietary recommendations alone, particularly from increased omega-3 fatty acid intake from the diet. However, it should be remembered that the intervention group had a greater increase in omega-3 index than placebo, suggesting a minimal influence from dietary changes. Similar findings of liver fat improvement in the placebo group have been reported in several other studies. These studies propose that MRI-PDFF volatility in early NAFLD subjects may contribute to data variability [35].

Of general note in the current study is the relatively low baseline liver fat by MRI-PDFF (mean 17% and 14% in placebo and intervention groups, respectively), which, together with relatively low baseline AST and ALT levels, indicate an early stage of NAFLD in this study population. Early stages of NAFLD are characterized by changeable liver fat content that can be affected by factors such as high-fat meals. This is in contrast to advanced NAFLD, in which the liver fat is likely to be more stable and less influenced by such factors.

A further confounding factor may be the high number (over one-third) of diabetic participants, and the number of subjects taking metformin and thiazolidinedione during the trial. From the mean baseline fasting insulin and glucose concentrations, the placebo group is also likely to have been more insulin resistant than the intervention group at study entry. These factors may have had some effect on liver fat metabolism. Indeed, on stratification of the data by diabetes status, those with diabetes had a greater reduction in liver fat from baseline (mean decrease of 4.9% in MF4637 group versus 6.3% decrease in placebo group) compared to those that did not have diabetes (mean decrease of 1.6% in MF4637 group versus 3.3% decrease in placebo group). To date, there have been very few trials conducted in the diabetic NAFLD population. One limitation of this study is the lack of additional lifestyle background information on variables that may act as confounders; these include smoking habits, annual income, academic background, and level of physical activity both at baseline and at the end of the study.

A number of individual studies and several meta-analyses have reported favorable outcomes with omega-3 fatty acid intervention in patients with NAFLD [27,36,37]. Despite a high degree of heterogeneity in patient population, study duration, dose and form of omega-3 fatty acids, a recent meta-analysis concluded that omega-3 fatty acids are associated with significant improvements in liver fat content and the liver enzymes ALT and GGT when taking approximately 3 g/day of EPA and DHA [27]. The positive effect of omega-3 fatty acids on liver fat was also confirmed in an earlier meta-analysis [37]. Surprisingly, only four of the eight trials performed to date included some form of measurement of EPA and DHA enrichment following intervention [38–41]. A strength of the current study is the measurement of both omega-3 fatty acids and omega-6: omega-3 fatty acid ratio, as well as the quantification of individual EPA and DHA in RBCs at baseline and study completion. This has enabled additional regression analyses to be performed, which suggest an inverse relationship between change in absolute RBC EPA + DHA and change in liver fat content and liver enzyme concentrations, although these data are exploratory and not supported by statistical analysis. Similar findings were reported in a study of high dose omega-3 in NAFLD patients where beneficial effects on liver fat content correlated with DHA content in RBCs [40]. Another strength of the current study was the use of MRI-PDFF to accurately assess change in liver fat content, which is the most accurate assessment method besides highly invasive liver biopsy [42].

A limitation of this study was the finding of a relatively low level of hepatic steatosis in participants, which restricted the potential for more significant effects to be observed on liver-related outcomes.

Post hoc use of the FLI to stratify patients showed an association between higher FLI scores and greater decrease in hepatic fat in the omega-3 intervention group. FLI scores below 30 are predictive of a liver without steatosis [10]. The high number of subjects with FLI < 30 confirms that this study recruited a relatively healthy population. However, highly statistically significant improvements in hepatic fat content were seen in those with a baseline FLI > 40, suggesting that this patient group can receive beneficial effects of intervention compared to placebo. Such a use of FLI is in accordance with the aims of its developers who propose that the "potential clinical uses of FLI include the selection of subjects to be referred for ultrasonography and the identification of (NAFLD) patients for intensified lifestyle counselling" [10]. Stratification by MRI-PDFF assessed steatosis levels was unable to identify omega-3 "responders"; however, the FLI score was able to do this. In this case, we can consider the study population as a population enriched for the presence of hepatic steatosis. The FLI score is composed, in part, of measurements of triglycerides and the liver enzyme GGT. Increased triglycerides in the liver is the cause of steatosis and increased liver enzymes are a consequence of liver damage. Plasma triglycerides are sensitive to omega-3 fatty acid intervention. In a meta-analysis, omega-3 fatty acids were shown to decrease liver enzymes (in particular GGT) in NAFLD patients, providing evidence that omega-3 intervention has a beneficial effect on liver cell physiology [27]. As such, the FLI may represent an easily available and economic set of biomarkers of relevance for identifying omega-3 sensitive patients and future studies may consider using this tool a priori for patient selection/stratification purposes.

5. Conclusions

The current randomized placebo-controlled study supports the use of omega-3 supplementation to increase the omega-3 index in NAFLD patients, significantly greater than that obtained by dietary recommendation alone. This study is therefore in line with recently published research which encourages NAFLD patients to increase their intakes of *n*-3 LC-PUFAs and confirms their beneficial effect [27]. The liver fat content of patients was significantly reduced amongst both placebo and intervention arms, thereby masking any effects omega-3 may have had on the fat content of the liver. Limitations and suggestions for future study design are discussed. In a post-hoc analysis significant placebo adjusted reductions in liver fat were seen in sub-populations with a high FLI score. This economic and easily available test may provide a simple means of identifying omega-3 responsive patients.

Author Contributions: D.T., M.B.A., Y.Q. and P.C.C. designed the study; D.T., M.B.A. and Y.Q. administered and oversaw the study; D.T., M.B.A., Y.Q. and P.C.C. interpreted data; J.K.I. drafted the manuscript; D.T., Y.Q. and P.C.C. reviewed and edited the manuscript; all authors approved the final version of the manuscript.

References

1. Chalasani, N.; Younossi, Z.; Lavine, J.E.; Diehl, A.M.; Brunt, E.M.; Cusi, K.; Charlton, M.; Sanyal, A.J. The diagnosis and management of non-alcoholic fatty liver disease: Practice Guideline by the American Association for the Study of Liver Diseases, American College of Gastroenterology, and the American Gastroenterological Association. *Hepatology* **2012**, *55*, 2005–2023. [CrossRef] [PubMed]
2. Levene, A.P.; Goldin, R.D. The epidemiology, pathogenesis and histopathology of fatty liver disease. *Histopathology* **2012**, *61*, 141–152. [CrossRef] [PubMed]
3. McCullough, A.J. The clinical features, diagnosis and natural history of nonalcoholic fatty liver disease. *Clin. Liver Dis.* **2004**, *8*, 521–533. [CrossRef] [PubMed]
4. Dowman, J.K.; Tomlinson, J.W.; Newsome, P.N. Pathogenesis of non-alcoholic fatty liver disease. *Q. J. Med.* **2010**, *103*, 71–83. [CrossRef] [PubMed]
5. Bedogni, G.; Miglioli, L.; Masutti, F.; Tiribelli, C.; Marchesini, G.; Bellentani, S. Prevalence of and risk factors for nonalcoholic fatty liver disease: The dionysos nutrition and liver study. *Hepatology* **2005**, *42*, 44–52. [CrossRef] [PubMed]
6. LaBrecque, D.; Abbas, Z.; Anania, F.; Ferenci, P.; Khan, A.; Goh, K.; Hamid, S.; Isakov, V.; Lizarzabal, M.; Penaranda, M.; et al. World Gastroenterology Organisation Global Guidelines: Nonalcoholic fatty liver disease and nonalcoholic steatohepatitis. *J. Clin. Gastroenterol.* **2014**, *48*, 467–473. [CrossRef] [PubMed]
7. Neuschwander-Tetri, B.A.; Caldwell, S.H. Nonalcoholic steatohepatitis: Summary of an AASLD single topic conference. *Hepatology* **2003**, *37*, 1202–1219. [CrossRef] [PubMed]

8. Machado, M.; Marques-Vidal, P.; Cortez-Pinto, H. Hepatic histology in obese patients undergoing bariatric surgery. *J. Hepatol.* **2006**, *45*, 600–606. [CrossRef] [PubMed]
9. Targher, G.; Bertolini, L.; Padovani, R.; Rodella, S.; Tessari, R.; Zenari, L.; Day, C.; Arcaro, G. Prevalence of nonalcoholic fatty liver disease and its association with cardiovascular disease among Type 2 diabetic patients. *Diabetes Care* **2007**, *30*, 1212–1218. [CrossRef] [PubMed]
10. Bedogni, G.; Bellentani, S.; Miglioli, L.; Masutti, F.; Passalacqua, M.; Castiglione, A.; Tiribelli, C. The Fatty Liver Index: A simple and accurate predictor of hepatic steatosis in the general population. *BMC Gastroenterol.* **2006**, *6*, 1–7. [CrossRef] [PubMed]
11. Kotronen, A.; Yki-Järvinen, H. Fatty liver: A novel component of the metabolic syndrome. *Arterioscler. Thromb. Vasc. Biol.* **2008**, *28*, 27–38. [CrossRef] [PubMed]
12. Vuppalanchi, R.; Chalasani, N. Nonalcoholic fatty liver disease and nonalcoholic steatohepatitis: Selected practical issues in their evaluation and management. *Hepatology* **2009**, *49*, 306–317. [CrossRef] [PubMed]
13. Ekstedt, M.; Franzén, L.E.; Mathiesen, U.L.; Thorelius, L.; Holmqvist, M.; Bodemar, G.; Kechagias, S. Long-term follow-up of patients with NAFLD and elevated liver enzymes. *Hepatology* **2006**, *44*, 865–873. [CrossRef] [PubMed]
14. Chitturi, S.; Abeygunasekera, S.; Farrell, G. NASH and insulin resistance: Insulin hypersecretion and specific association with the insulin resistance syndrome. *Hepatology* **2002**, *2*, 373–379. [CrossRef] [PubMed]
15. Allard, J.P.; Aghdassi, E.; Mohammed, S.; Raman, M.; Avand, G.; Arendt, B.M.; Jalali, P.; Kandasamy, T.; Prayitno, N.; Sherman, M.; et al. Nutritional assessment and hepatic fatty acid composition in non-alcoholic fatty liver disease (NAFLD): A cross-sectional study. *J. Hepatol.* **2008**, *48*, 300–307. [CrossRef] [PubMed]
16. Araya, J.; Rodrigo, R.; Videla, L.; Thielemann, L.; Orellana, M.; Pettinelli, P.; Poniachik, J. Increase in long-chain polyunsaturated fatty acid *n*-6/*n*-3 ratio in relation to hepatic steatosis in patients with non-alcoholic fatty liver disease. *Clin. Sci.* **2004**, *106*, 635–643. [CrossRef] [PubMed]
17. Pettinelli, P.; del Pozo, T.; Araya, J.; Rodrigo, R.; Araya, A.V.; Smok, G.; Csendes, A.; Gutierrez, L.; Rojas, J.; Korn, O.; et al. Enhancement in liver SREBP-1c/PPAR-α ratio and steatosis in obese patients: Correlations with insulin resistance and *n*-3 long-chain polyunsaturated fatty acid depletion. *Biochim. Biophys. Acta-Mol. Basis. Dis.* **2009**, *1792*, 1080–1086. [CrossRef] [PubMed]
18. Elizondo, A.; Araya, J.; Rodrigo, R.; Poniachik, J.; Csendes, A.; Maluenda, F.; Díaz, J.C.; Signorini, C.; Sgherri, C.; Comporti, M.; et al. A polyunsaturated fatty acid pattern in liver and erythrocyte phospholipids from obese patients. *Obesity* **2007**, *15*, 24–31. [CrossRef] [PubMed]
19. Rose, M.; Veysey, M.; Lucock, M.; Niblett, S.; King, K.; Baines, S.; Garg, M.L. Association between erythrocyte omega-3 polyunsaturated fatty acid levels and fatty liver index in older people is sex dependent. *J. Nutr. Intermed. Metab.* **2016**, *5*, 78–85. [CrossRef]
20. Toshimitsu, K.; Matsuura, B.; Ohkubo, I.; Niiya, T.; Furukawa, S.; Hiasa, Y.; Kawamura, M.; Ebihara, K.; Onji, M. Dietary habits and nutrient intake in non-alcoholic steatohepatitis. *Nutrition* **2007**, *23*, 46–52. [CrossRef] [PubMed]
21. Cortez-Pinto, H.; Jesus, L.; Barros, H.; Lopes, C.; Moura, M.C.; Camilo, M.E. How different is the dietary pattern in non-alcoholic steatohepatitis patients? *Clin. Nutr.* **2006**, *25*, 816–823. [CrossRef] [PubMed]
22. Clarke, S.D. Molecular mechanism for polyunsaturated fatty acid regulation of gene transcription. *Am. J. Physiol.* **2001**, *281*, 865–869. [CrossRef] [PubMed]
23. Bouzianas, D.G.; Bouziana, S.D.; Hatzitolios, A.I. Potential treatment of human nonalcoholic fatty liver disease with long-chain omega-3 polyunsaturated fatty acids. *Nutr. Rev.* **2013**, *71*, 753–771. [CrossRef] [PubMed]
24. Hodson, L.; Bhatia, L.; Scorletti, E.; Smith, D.E.; Jackson, N.C.; Shojaee-Moradie, F.; Umpleby, M.; Calder, P.C.; Byrne, C.D. Docosahexaenoic acid enrichment in NAFLD is associated with improvements in hepatic metabolism and hepatic insulin sensitivity: A pilot study. *Eur. J. Clin. Nutr.* **2017**, *71*, 973–979. [CrossRef] [PubMed]
25. Chen, L.; Wang, Y.; Xu, Q.; Chen, S.-S. Omega-3 fatty acids as a treatment for non-alcoholic fatty liver disease in children: A systematic review and meta-analysis of randomized controlled trials. *Clin. Nutr.* **2018**, *37*, 516–521. [CrossRef] [PubMed]
26. De Castro, G.S.; Calder, P.C. Non-alcoholic fatty liver disease and its treatment with n-3 polyunsaturated fatty acids. *Clin. Nutr.* **2017**. [CrossRef] [PubMed]

27. Musa-Veloso, K.; Venditti, C.; Lee, H.; Darch, M.; Floyd, S.; West, S.; Simon, R. Systematic review and meta-analysis of controlled intervention studies on the effectiveness of long chain omega-3 fatty acids in patients with non-alcoholic fatty liver disease. *Nutr. Rev.* **2018**, *76*, 581–602. [CrossRef] [PubMed]
28. Katan, M.B.; Deslypere, J.P.; van Birgelen, A.P.; Penders, M.; Zegwaard, M. Kinetics of the incorporation of dietary fatty acids into serum cholesteryl esters, erythrocyte membranes, and adipose tissue: An 18-month controlled study. *J. Lipid Res.* **1997**, *38*, 2012–2022. [PubMed]
29. Krauss, R.; Eckel, R.; Howard, B.; Appel, L.J.; Daniels, S.R.; Deckelbaum, R.J.; Erdman, J.W.; Kris-etherton, P.; Goldberg, I.J.; Kotchen, T.A.; et al. AHA dietary guidelines. *Circulation* **2000**, *102*, 2284–2299. [CrossRef] [PubMed]
30. Jørgensen, M.; Ott, P.; Michaelsen, K.; Porsgaard, T.; Jensen, F.; Lanng, S. Long-chain PUFA in granulocytes, mononuclear cells, and RBC in patients with cystic fibrosis: Relation to liver disease. *J. Pediatr. Gastroenterol. Nutr.* **2012**, *55*, 76–81. [CrossRef] [PubMed]
31. Petit, J.M.; Guiu, B.; Duvillard, L.; Jooste, V.; Brindisi, M.C.; Athias, A.; Bouillet, B.; Habchi, M.; Cottet, V.; Gambert, P.; et al. Increased erythrocytes n-3 and n-6 polyunsaturated fatty acids is significantly associated with a lower prevalence of steatosis in patients with type 2 diabetes. *Clin. Nutr.* **2012**, *31*, 520–525. [CrossRef] [PubMed]
32. Arterburn, L.M.; Hall, E.B.; Oken, H. Distribution, interconversion, and dose response of n-3 fatty acids in humans. *Am. J. Clin. Nutr.* **2006**, *83*, 1467S–1476S. [CrossRef] [PubMed]
33. Tobin, D. BASF AS, Norway. CONDIN study. Unpublished work. 2018.
34. Browning, L.M.; Walker, C.G.; Mander, A.P.; West, A.L.; Madden, J.; Gambell, J.M.; Young, S.; Wang, L.; Jebb, S.A.; Calder, P.C. Incorporation of eicosapentaenoic and docosahexaenoic acids into lipid pools when given as supplements providing doses equivalent to typical intakes of oily fish. *Am. J. Clin. Nutr.* **2012**, *96*, 748–758. [CrossRef] [PubMed]
35. Chalasani, N.; Vuppalanchi, R.; Rinella, M.; Middleton, M.S.; Siddiqui, M.S.; Barritt, A.S.; Kolterman, O.; Flores, O.; Alonso, C.; Iruarrizaga-Lejarreta, M.; et al. Randomised clinical trial: A leucine-metformin-sildenafil combination (NS-0200) vs placebo in patients with non-alcoholic fatty liver disease. *Aliment. Pharmacol. Ther.* **2018**, *47*, 1639–1651. [CrossRef] [PubMed]
36. He, X.-X.; Wu, X.-L.; Chen, R.-P.; Chen, C.; Liu, X.-G.; Wu, B.-J.; Huang, Z.-M. Effectiveness of omega-3 polyunsaturated fatty acids in non-alcoholic fatty liver disease: A meta-analysis of randomized controlled trials. *PLoS One* **2016**, *11*, e0162368. [CrossRef] [PubMed]
37. Parker, H.M.; Johnson, N.A.; Burdon, C.A.; Cohn, J.S.; Connor, H.T.O.; George, J. Omega-3 supplementation and non-alcoholic fatty liver disease: A systematic review and meta-analysis. *J. Hepatol.* **2012**, *56*, 944–951. [CrossRef] [PubMed]
38. Capanni, M.; Calella, F.; Biagini, M.R.; Genise, S.; Raimondi, L.; Bedogni, G.; Svegliati-Baroni, G.; Sofi, F.; Milani, S.; Abbate, R.; et al. Prolonged *n*-3 polyunsaturated fatty acid supplementation ameliorates hepatic steatosis in patients with non-alcoholic fatty liver disease: A. pilot study. *Aliment. Pharmacol. Ther.* **2006**, *23*, 1143–1151. [CrossRef] [PubMed]
39. Qin, Y.; Zhou, Y.; Chen, S.H.; Zhao, X.L.; Ran, L.; Zeng, X.L.; Wu, Y.; Chen, J.L.; Kang, C.; Shu, F.R.; et al. Fish oil supplements lower serum lipids and glucose in correlation with a reduction in plasma fibroblast growth factor 21 and prostaglandin E2 in nonalcoholic fatty liver disease associated with hyperlipidemia: A randomized clinical trial. *PLoS ONE* **2015**, *10*, 1–13. [CrossRef] [PubMed]
40. Scorletti, E.; Bhatia, L.; Mccormick, K.G.; Clough, G.F.; Nash, K.; Hodson, L.; Moyses, H.E.; Calder, P.C.; Byrne, C.D. Effects of purified eicosapentaenoic and docosahexaenoic acids in nonalcoholic fatty liver disease: Results from the WELCOME study. *Hepatology* **2014**, *60*, 1211–1221. [CrossRef] [PubMed]
41. Vega, G.; Chandalia, M.; Szczepaniak, L.; Grundy, S. Effects of N-3 fatty acids on hepatic triglyceride content in humans. *J. Investig. Med.* **2008**, *56*, 780–785. [CrossRef] [PubMed]
42. Dulai, P.; Sirlin, C.; Loomba, R. MRI and MRE for non-invasive quantitative assessment of hepatic steatosis and fibrosis in NAFLD and NASH: Clinical trials to clinical practice. *J. Hepatol.* **2016**, *65*, 1006–1016. [CrossRef] [PubMed]

4

Folate and B12 Levels Correlate with Histological Severity in NASH Patients

Mahmud Mahamid [1,2,†], Naim Mahroum [3,†], Nicola Luigi Bragazzi [4], Kasem Shalaata [2,5], Yarden Yavne [3], Mohammad Adawi [6], Howard Amital [3] and Abdulla Watad [3,*]

1. Endoscopy Unit, Nazareth Hospital EMMS, 16100 Nazareth, Israel; mahmudmahamid@yahoo.com
2. Azrieli Faculty of Medicine, Bar-Ilan University, 13195 Safed, Israel; sh.kasem@hotmail.com
3. Department of Medicine 'B', Sheba Medical Center, Tel-Hashomer, Israel, Sackler Faculty of Medicine, Tel-Aviv University, 52621 Tel-Aviv, Israel; naim.mahroum@gmail.com (N.M.); yavneyarden@gmail.com (Y.Y.); Howard.Amital@sheba.health.gov.il (H.A.)
4. School of Public Health, Department of Health Sciences, University of Genoa, 16132 Genoa, Italy; robertobragazzi@gmail.com
5. Internal Medicine Department, Nazareth Hospital EMMS, 16100 Nazareth, Israel
6. Ziv and Padeh Medical centers, 13195 Safed, Israel; Limak@012.net.il

* Correspondence: watad.abdulla@gmail.com

† These authors contributed equally to this work.

Abstract: Background: The correlation between abnormal vitamin serum levels and chronic liver disease has been previously described in literature. However, the association between the severity of folate serum levels (B9), vitamin B12 and nonalcoholic steatohepatitis (NASH) has not been widely evaluated. Therefore, the aim of this study was to investigate the existence of such a correlation in a cohort of NASH patients. Methods: All patients aged 18 years and older who were diagnosed with biopsy-proven NASH at the EMMS hospital in Nazareth during the years 2015–2017 were enrolled in this study. Data regarding demographic, clinical and laboratory parameters was collected. Patients with other liver diseases were excluded. Results: Eighty-three NASH patients were enrolled during the study period. The mean age was 41 ± 11 years and the majority of patients were male. Mean values of folate and B12 were 9.85 ± 10.90 ng/mL and 387.53 ± 205.50 pg/mL, respectively. Half of the patients were presented with a grade 1 steatosis (43.4%), a grade 2 fibrosis (50.6%) and a grade 3 activity score (55.4%). The fibrosis grade was significantly correlated with low folate levels on multivariate analysis (p-value < 0.01). Similarly, low B12 levels were significantly associated with a higher fibrosis grade and NASH activity (p-value < 0.001 and p-value < 0.05 respectively). Conclusion: Our study demonstrated a statistically significant correlation between low levels of folate and vitamin B12 with the histological severity of NASH. These findings could have diagnostic and therapeutic implications for patient management and follow-up.

Keywords: nonalcoholic fatty liver disease; NAFLD; nonalcoholic steatohepatitis; NASH; vitamin B9; folate; vitamin B12

1. Introduction

Nonalcoholic fatty liver disease (NAFLD) is defined as the presence of liver steatosis, as demonstrated on imaging or histology, in patients who ingest less than 20 mg of alcohol per day [1,2]. It is the most prevalent liver disease worldwide, with an estimated global prevalence of 25.24% (95% confidence interval (CI) 22.10–28.65), of which the highest rates are found in the Middle East and South America [3,4]. Different metabolic co-morbidities are often associated with NAFLD, including central obesity, insulin resistance, type 2 diabetes mellitus, hyperlipidemia, hypertension, and metabolic syndrome [4,5].

NAFLD is a wide spectrum of disorders ranging from a simple form of steatosis to a progressive form known as nonalcoholic steatohepatitis (NASH), which is characterized by hepatocellular injury and inflammation [6]. Furthermore, NAFLD is considered to be an important cause of cryptogenic cirrhosis [7]. According to a recently published meta-analysis, the mean annual rate of fibrosis progression in NASH is 0.09 (95% CI 0.06–0.12), whilst the overall fibrosis progression proportion is 40.76% (95% CI 34.69–47.13) [4]. Treatment of NASH continues to be challenging for physicians as there is no approved effective pharmacotherapy for this disorder and life style modification remains the mainstay of therapy for these patients [2,8,9].

Vitamin deficiency/hypovitaminosis is a general term for a wide-spread condition which has reached epidemic proportions in developing and developed countries alike, mainly due to lifestyle and dietary habits. Although sub-clinical hypovitaminosis can occur in well-nourished subjects, it is most often the result of limited dietary intake or vitamin malabsorption [9,10]. Several studies have shown that chronic liver diseases are associated with lower levels of vitamins such as vitamin D, E, B6, and A [11–14]. Moreover, a trial therapeutic combination of vitamins E and A as a treatment for NASH was found to minimize oxidative stress damage and to curb cirrhosis formation processes [15].

Despite the indications in the literature regarding the association between chronic liver diseases and hypovitaminosis, little is known about a specific correlation between hypovitaminosis and NASH severity. Thus, in this study we sought to investigate potential correlations between folate and B12 serum levels with NASH severity, as defined in terms of the fibrosis grade and activity, in a geographical area characterized by a significant epidemiological burden of NASH. We chose to focus on these vitamins because the relationship between their serum levels and fibrosis severity has been scarcely reported. More specifically, we expected to find a negative correlation, in analogy with what was found for other vitamins.

2. Material and Methods

2.1. Ethical Approval

The current study received ethical approval from the local hospital ethical committee and was conducted according to the Helsinki declaration and its subsequent amendments. The data was coded in order to preserve the anonymity of the patients. Informed consent was waived because of the non-interventional design of the study.

2.2. Patients Selection

All patients diagnosed with biopsy-proven NASH at the EMMS Nazareth Hospital (located in Nazareth, Israel) between the years 2015 to 2017 were considered potentially eligible and enrolled in the study. Furthermore, patients were included in the present study if (i) age > 18 years old; and (ii) they had no history of alcohol abuse (their weekly ethanol consumption was less than 210 gm).

Patients with other hepatic pathology or autoimmune phenotypes (such as alcoholic liver disease, drug-induced liver injury, autoimmune hepatitis, viral hepatitis, cholestatic liver disease and metabolic/genetic liver disease) were excluded using specific clinical, laboratory, radiological and/or histological criteria/tests (serology of viral hepatitis A, B, and C, autoimmune markers including ANA, anti-LKM, anti-smooth mussels protein electrophoresis, immune electrophoresis, metabolic markers such as serum ceruloplasmin, 24-h urine collection for copper, ferritin, iron, transferrin saturation, TSH, HbA1c and alpha-1 antitrypsin).

Extracted data included socio-demographic variables (such as age and gender), body mass index (BMI), fat volume, histopathological biopsy results, serum levels of alanine transaminase (ALT), aspartate transaminase (AST), low-density lipoprotein cholesterol (LDL), high-density lipoprotein cholesterol (HDL), triglycerides, insulin and insulin resistance index (HOMA-IR), glycated hemoglobin (hemoglobin A1c or HbA1c), C-reactive protein (CRP), folate, and vitamin B12.

A hepatopathologist reviewed all of the liver biopsies and utilized the SAF scoring system (encompassing an assessment of steatosis (S), activity (A) and fibrosis (F)) scoring system for the grading and staging of steatohepatitis developed and validated by Bedossa and collaborators [16]. The staging, according to this scoring system, is as follows: steatosis: Stage 1—lipid droplets in ~30% of hepatocytes, Stage 2—steatosis in 60% of hepatocytes and Stage 3—steatosis in >80% of hepatocytes; fibrosis: Stage 0—no fibrosis, Stage 1—zone 3 perisinusoidal fibrosis, Stage 2—as before with portal fibrosis, Stage 3—as before with bridging fibrosis, and Stage 4—cirrhosis; activity score: A0—no activity, A1—mild activity, A2—moderate activity, A3 ($A \geq 3$)—severe activity).

2.3. Statistical Analysis

Before commencing any statistical processing and analysis, the data was visually inspected and assessed for outliers. Continuous variables were computed as the mean with standard deviation (SD), whereas categorical variables were expressed as percentages. Univariate and multivariate regression analyses were conducted using the vitamin levels as dependent variables. Rank correlation analysis was performed; both Spearman's *rho* and Kendall's tau coefficients were computed. Spearman's *rho* coefficient was interpreted using the following rule of thumb (in absolute value): 0.00–0.19—very weak correlation, 0.20–0.39—weak correlation, 0.40–0.59—moderate correlation, 0.60–0.79—strong correlation, and 0.80–1.0—very strong correlation. Chi-squared test and analysis of variance (ANOVA)-one way were also performed.

All statistical analyses were performed with the commercial software Statistical Package for Social Science (SPSS version 24.0, IBM, Chicago, IL, USA). ROC analysis was performed with the commercial software MedCalc Statistical Software version 17.9.7 (MedCalc Software bvba, Ostend, Belgium; http://www.medcalc.org; 2017). A p-value of less than 0.05 was considered statistically significant.

3. Results

Eighty-three NASH patients were enrolled in this study. The mean age of the study population was 41.12 (SD ± 11.18) years. The majority of participants were male (61.4%). The mean serum levels of folate and vitamin B12 amongst the study population were 9.85 ± 10.90 ng/mL and 387.53 ± 205.50 pg/mL, respectively. Roughly half of the patients were presented with a grade 1 steatosis (43.4%), grade 2 fibrosis (50.6%) and a grade 3 activity score (55.4%). Further details regarding the study population can be seen in Table 1.

Table 1. Descriptive statistics of the population studied.

Variables	Values
Age (years)	41.12 ± 11.18; 42 (18–74)
Gender	
Male	51 (61.4%)
Female	32 (38.6%)
BMI (kg/m^2)	28.86 ± 2.83; 29 (22–40)
Fat volume	55.66 ± 24.60; 60 (10–90)
ALT (units)	80.61 ± 31.33; 78 (11–212)
AST (units)	48.81 ± 14.99; 45 (24–85)
CRP (mg/dL)	3.80 ± 2.44; 3.6 (0–13)
HDL (mg/dL)	37.69 ± 8.63; 36 (16–58)
LDL (mg/dL)	132.36 ± 24.01; 139 (68–187)
TG (mg/dL)	153.12 ± 36.63; 152 (69–274)
Insulin (IU/ML)	24.71 ± 5.21; 26 (12–36.2)
HbA1c (%)	5.38 ± 0.63; 5.4 (2–6.2)
HOMA-IR	2.88 ± 1.06; 2.8 (1.2–5.9)
B12 (pg/mL)	387.53 ± 205.50; 321 (123–823)
Folate (ng/mL)	9.85 ± 10.90; 8.9 (2.2–105)

Table 1. *Cont.*

Variables	Values
Steatosis (S0–S3)	
S1	36 (43.4%)
S2	24 (28.9%)
S3	23 (27.7%)
Fibrosis (F0–F4)	
Grade 0	11 (13.3%)
Grade 1	20 (24.1%)
Grade 2	42 (50.6%)
Grade 3	7 (8.4%)
Grade 4	3 (3.6%)
Activity (A0–A4)	
Grade 2	36 (43.4%)
Grade 3	46 (55.4%)
Grade 4	1 (1.2%)

Abbreviations: BMI, body mass index; ALT, alanine transaminase; AST, aspartate aminotransferase; CRP, C-reactive protein; HDL, high-density lipoproteins; LDL, low-density lipoproteins; TG, triglycerides; HOMA-IR, homeostatic model assessment-Insulin resistance (HOMA-IR).

A statistically significant association was found between lower levels of folate and fibrosis grade on univariate regression analysis (p-value < 0.01). Older age, CRP levels, HOMA-IR, fibrosis grade and NASH disease activity grade were all significantly correlated with lower levels of vitamin B12 (Table 2).

Table 2. Univariate regression analysis for each vitamin studied in the present investigation.

Variable	Folate (ng/mL)	B12 (pg/mL)
Age (years)	0.002 ± 0.108	−4.846 ± 1.971 *
Gender	2.730 ± 2.454	−2.138 ± 46.629
BMI (kg/m^2)	0.085 ± 0.428	0.764 ± 8.062
Fat volume	0.008 ± 0.049	0.755 ± 0.924
ALT (units)	−0.034 ± 0.038	−1.291 ± 0.715
AST (units)	−0.090 ± 0.080	−1.972 ± 1.507
CRP (mg/dL)	−0.056 ± 0.500	−20.007 ± 9.072 *
HDL (mg/dL)	−0.105 ± 0.140	3.765 ± 2.612
LDL (mg/dL)	0.077 ± 0.050	−0.136 ± 0.951
TG (mg/dL)	0.032 ± 0.033	−0.722 ± 0.618
Insulin (IU/mL)	−0.431 ± 0.227	−7.564 ± 4.300
HbA1c (%)	−1.004 ± 1.908	−62.653 ± 35.350
HOMA-IR	−1.714 ± 1.127	−45.663 ± 20.947 *
Steatosis	−0.773 ± 1.450	30.421 ± 27.186
Fibrosis	−3.665 ± 1.218 **	−160.835 ± 16.351 ***
Activity	−3.196 ± 2.298	−131.579 ± 41.334 **

Abbreviations: BMI, body mass index; ALT, alanine transaminase; AST, aspartate aminotransferase; CRP, C-reactive protein; HDL, high-density lipoproteins; LDL, low-density lipoproteins; TG, triglycerides; HOMA-IR, homeostatic model assessment-insulin resistance (HOMA-IR). * statistically significant with p-value < 0.05; ** statistically significant with p-value < 0.01; *** statistically significant with p-value < 0.001.

When confounders such as obesity and insulin resistance were taken into account on multivariate analysis, fibrosis was found to be significantly associated with folate serum levels (standardized beta coefficient −0.353, p = 0.009). On rank correlation analysis, the link between folate levels and fibrosis grade was of statistical significance (Spearman's *rho* −0.608 (95%CI from −0.728 to −0.451), p-value < 0.001, strong correlation; Kendall's tau −0.487 (95%CI from −0.603 to −0.335), p-value < 0.001). Fibrosis was also significantly correlated with vitamin B12 levels, on both the regression (standardized beta coefficient −0.623, p-value = 0.000) and on rank correlation analysis (Spearman's *rho* −0.737 (95%CI from −0.822 to −0.620), p-value < 0.001, strong correlation; Kendall's tau −0.606 (95%CI from −0.688 to −0.489), p-value < 0.001). Activity was also associated with vitamin B12 levels (standardized beta coefficient −0.183, p-value = 0.039), even though the correlation found was very weak (Spearman's *rho* −0.288 [95%CI from −0.474 to −0.0770), *p*-value = 0.0083; Kendall's tau −0.237 (95%CI from −0.416 to −0.020), *p*-value = 0.0015). The analyses are presented in Table 3.

Table 3. Multivariate regressions for each vitamin.

Variables	Non-Standardized Coefficients		Standardized Coefficients	T	Sig.
	B	Standard Deviation	Beta		
			Folate (B9)		
(Constant)	6.959	21.122		0.329	0.743
Age (years)	0.188	0.128	0.193	1.469	0.147
Gender	5.101	2.710	0.229	1.882	0.064
BMI (kg/m^2)	0.382	0.480	0.099	0.795	0.429
AST (units)	−0.087	0.095	−0.119	−0.914	0.364
ALT (units)	−0.003	0.107	−0.004	−0.031	0.975
TG (mg/dL)	0.024	0.035	0.079	0.680	0.499
HDL (mg/dL)	−0.147	0.148	−0.116	−0.996	0.323
LDL (mg/dL)	0.034	0.053	0.074	0.637	0.526
CRP (mg/dL)	0.519	0.567	0.116	0.915	0.364
HbA1c (%)	−0.065	2.113	−0.004	−0.031	0.976
Insulin (IU/mL)	−0.304	0.324	−0.145	−0.938	0.352
HOMA-IR	−0.742	1.697	−0.072	−0.438	0.663
Fibrosis	−4.079	1.513	−0.353	−2.695	0.009 **
Activity	−0.595	2.575	−0.028	−0.231	0.818
Steatosis	−6.073	3.461	−0.464	−1.755	0.084
Fat volume	0.188	0.120	0.424	1.566	0.122
			Vitamin B12		
(Constant)	1264.063	280.796		4.502	0.000 ***
Age (years)	−0.814	1.705	−0.044	−0.478	0.634
Gender	−9.612	36.033	−0.023	−0.267	0.790
BMI (kg/m^2)	−5.805	6.384	−0.080	−0.909	0.366
AST (units)	−0.586	1.260	−0.043	−0.465	0.643
ALT (units)	−2.413	1.416	−0.137	−1.704	0.093
TG (mg/dL)	−0.451	0.460	−0.080	−0.981	0.330
HDL (mg/dL)	3.060	1.961	0.129	1.561	0.123
LDL (mg/dL	0.547	0.702	0.064	0.780	0.438
CRP (mg/dL)	−5.564	7.537	−0.066	−0.738	0.463
HbA1c (%)	−31.261	28.088	−0.096	−1.113	0.270
Insulin (IU/mL)	1.503	4.304	0.038	0.349	0.728
HOMA-IR	−4.149	22.558	−0.021	−0.184	0.855
Fibrosis	−135.886	20.118	−0.623	−6.754	0.000 ***
Activity	−72.172	34.236	−0.183	−2.108	0.039 *
Steatosis	66.491	46.012	0.270	1.445	0.153
Fat volume	−1.966	1.594	−0.235	−1.233	0.222

Abbreviations: BMI, body mass index; ALT, alanine transaminase; AST, aspartate aminotransferase; CRP, C-reactive protein; HDL, high-density lipoproteins; LDL, low-density lipoproteins; TG, triglycerides; HOMA-IR, homeostatic model assessment-Insulin resistance (HOMA-IR). * statistically significant with *p*-value < 0.05; ** statistically significant with *p*-value < 0.01; *** statistically significant with *p*-value < 0.001.

4. Discussion

Information regarding the relationship between folate and vitamin B12 status and the histological severity of NASH is scarce in the literature. In this study, both folate and vitamin B12 serum levels were found to be significantly correlated with the liver fibrosis grade, whereas vitamin B12 status was also associated with NASH degree of activity.

To date, the correlation between vitamin levels and chronic liver diseases has been investigated in several studies, although most of the data focused on vitamin D status [17–19]. Dasarathy et al. [20] compared plasma vitamin D concentration levels between 81 NAFLD/NASH patients, 67 individuals with hepatic steatosis and 39 healthy controls. Vitamin D serum levels were found to be significantly lower in NAFLD/NASH patients, with a negative correlation between vitamin D status and NAFLD activity scores. Low concentrations of vitamin D were additionally associated with greater severity of steatosis, hepatocyte ballooning, and fibrosis, although only the association with the severity of hepatocyte ballooning remained statistically significant after it was adjusted for confounders. Furthermore, plasma vitamin D and insulin concentrations were independent predictors of the NAFLD activity score on biopsy, while a higher fat mass was found to correlate with the low vitamin D levels in NAFLD patients. An additional study, which examined 46 morbidly obese patients with diabetes mellitus and metabolic syndrome, of which 72% had NASH [21], discovered a relationship between a higher fibrosis stage and higher levels of HOMA-IR and vitamin D. On the other hand, according to a study by Brill and colleagues [22], although subjects with NASH had higher insulin resistance than individuals without NASH, plasma vitamin D concentration was similar between both groups. However, despite these controversies concerning the role of vitamin D in NASH, other vitamins, such as folate and vitamin B12, have been overlooked in the extant literature.

Various studies have demonstrated that obese subjects have lower folate serum levels in comparison with normal-range BMI subjects [23,24]. Furthermore, obesity is a well-known risk factor for NAFLD [25]. Therefore, it has been suggested that folate deficiency may have a pathogenic role in NAFLD. This leads to a more severe form of the disease, mainly in metabolic syndrome and diabetes mellitus type 2 patients [26]. Moreover, Sid et al. [26] highlighted the importance of folate in the progression of NAFLD, thus raising the possibility that supplementary folate may be a treatment option. These findings are consistent with our results, in which a correlation between lower folate levels and a higher histological grading of NASH was revealed.

In a cohort of Chinese patients with NAFLD, low serum concentration of folate was identified as an independent risk factor for NAFLD [27]. Furthermore, it was demonstrated that inclusion of serum folate levels in the current NAFLD prediction score has led to a significant improvement in NAFLD prediction [27]. However, in an open-label pilot study [28], ten NASH patients with a median fibrosis stage 2 were treated with 1 mg/day of folic acid for 6 months. No significant effects in terms of biochemical improvement could be detected. Furthermore, folate deficiency was observed only in a cirrhotic patient. Therefore, it is clear that the controversy in the literature regarding the complex interplay between folate and non-alcoholic fatty liver disease and steatohepatitis has yet to be resolved. However, unveiling the pathogenetic process underlying the association between folate and NAFLD may provide important insights into the diagnosis and prediction of NASH, thus enabling treatment initiation in a timely and effective manner.

Another important finding of this study was the role of low vitamin B12 levels as an independent predictor of NASH histological severity, in terms of disease activity and fibrosis grade. These results corroborated the outcomes of previous studies, which, for instance, demonstrated that NAFLD patients have lower serum levels of vitamin B12 in comparison to controls, which correlated with a higher grade of steatohepatitis [29]. In another study [30], higher levels of homocysteine were observed in 71 NAFLD patients, which correlated negatively with folate and B12 concentrations.

However, in a study by Polyzos et al. [31], no difference in serum vitamin B12 and folate levels was detected in 30 NAFLD patients in comparison with 24 healthy controls. Additionally, no correlation was found between the levels of both vitamins and the severity of liver disease, in terms of steatosis grade and fibrosis stage. These results were in contrast with the findings of another study which reported that B12 could be used as a biomarker in a sample of 116 patients with chronic hepatitis C [32]. Serum B12 levels positively correlated with AST, ALT, baseline viral load, stage of fibrosis, and favorable interferon-λ3/4 rs12979860 genotypes. However, they were found to be inversely correlated with sustained virological response, as well as with rapid virological response.

Moreover, Goel et al. [33] found higher serum levels of vitamin B12 in patients with cryptogenic cirrhosis when compared to patients with idiopathic non-cirrhotic intrahepatic portal hypertension (NCIPH), therefore suggesting that B12 levels may be used as a differentiating marker between the two pathologies. Similarly, levels of vitamin B12 were also found to be significantly higher in patients with alcoholic liver cirrhosis than in matching healthy individuals [34]. Nevertheless, when taking into account the relevance of these results to the findings in our study, it should be noted that the majority (96%) of NASH patients in our study did not have cirrhosis. Therefore, it could be surmised that while low levels of vitamin B12 may predict the development of a severe form of NASH, high levels may indicate the commencement of end stage liver disease.

The relationship between serum vitamin B12 levels and insulin resistance has been widely addressed in the literature, yet remains controversial. Our study found that levels of vitamin B12 are inversely correlated with HOMA-IR, which is a known risk factor for NAFLD development [35]. This illustrates the probability that low serum levels of vitamin B12 might play a pathogenic part in NAFLD development. Similar findings regarding the ability of low levels of vitamin B12 and folate to predict insulin resistance were reported by Li et al. [36], however it should be noted that this study was conducted on obese subjects. Despite these compelling results, other studies did not detect a link between low vitamin B12 levels and insulin resistance or metabolic syndrome, whereas a correlation was found with obesity and being overweight [37]. Gammon et al. [38] reached an identical conclusion when assessing the relationship between insulin resistance and vitamin B12 levels in a vegetarian population.

Our study has several limitations which ought to be properly addressed. The major drawback is the cross-sectional study design which, due to its very nature, does not enable the deduction of causal inferences with regard to the relationship between vitamin status and NASH in terms of development and pathophysiology. Another limitation is the lack of data concerning patient co-morbidities and drugs regimens.

5. Conclusions

NASH is a chronic liver condition which imposes a dramatic burden, both in epidemiological and clinical terms. Our study demonstrated that low levels of folate (B9) and vitamin B12 can be used as independent predictors of the histological severity of NASH. Thus, these findings may have practical implications in the follow-up and prognosis assessment of NASH patients. Further studies regarding the pathological role of low folate and B12 levels in NASH development are warranted.

Author Contributions: M.M., N.M. and A.W. directed the study; M.M., A.W. and H.A. conceived and designed the study; M.M. and K.S. collected the data; N.L.B. analyzed the data; K.S., Y.Y., M.A. and N.M. wrote the paper.

References

1. Abd El-Kader, S.M.; El-Den Ashmawy, E.M.S. Non-alcoholic fatty liver disease: The diagnosis and management. *World J. Hepatol.* **2015**, *7*, 846–858. [CrossRef] [PubMed]
2. Tolman, K.G.; Dalpiaz, A.S. Treatment of non-alcoholic fatty liver disease. *Ther. Clin. Risk Manag.* **2007**, *3*, 1153–1163. [PubMed]
3. Bedossa, P. Pathology of non-alcoholic fatty liver disease. *Liver Int. Off. J. Int. Assoc. Study Liver* **2017**, *37*, 85–89. [CrossRef] [PubMed]
4. Younossi, Z.M.; Koenig, A.B.; Abdelatif, D.; Fazel, Y.; Henry, L.; Wymer, M. Global epidemiology of nonalcoholic fatty liver disease-Meta-analytic assessment of prevalence, incidence, and outcomes. *Hepatology* **2016**, *64*, 73–84. [CrossRef] [PubMed]
5. Milic, S.; Mikolasevic, I.; Krznaric-Zrnic, I.; Stanic, M.; Poropat, G.; Stimac, D.; Vlahovic-Palcevski, V.; Orlic, L. Nonalcoholic steatohepatitis: Emerging targeted therapies to optimize treatment options. *Drug Des. Dev. Ther.* **2015**, *9*, 4835–4845. [CrossRef] [PubMed]
6. Takahashi, Y.; Fukusato, T. Histopathology of nonalcoholic fatty liver disease/nonalcoholic steatohepatitis. *World J. Gastroenterol.* **2014**, *20*, 15539–15548. [CrossRef] [PubMed]
7. Aithal, G.P.; Ramsay, L.; Daly, A.K.; Sonchit, N.; Leathart, J.B.; Alexander, G.; Kenna, J.G.; Caldwell, J.; Day, C.P. Hepatic adducts, circulating antibodies, and cytokine polymorphisms in patients with diclofenac hepatotoxicity. *Hepatology* **2004**, *39*, 1430–1440. [CrossRef] [PubMed]
8. Hardy, T.; Anstee, Q.M.; Day, C.P. Nonalcoholic fatty liver disease: New treatments. *Curr. Opin. Gastroenterol.* **2015**, *31*, 175–183. [CrossRef] [PubMed]
9. Barchetta, I.; Cimini, F.A.; Cavallo, M.G. Vitamin D Supplementation and Non-Alcoholic Fatty Liver Disease: Present and Future. *Nutrients* **2017**, *9*, 1015. [CrossRef] [PubMed]

10. McKinney, T.J.; Patel, J.J.; Benns, M.V.; Nash, N.A.; Miller, K.R. Vitamin D Status and supplementation in the critically Ill. *Curr. Gastroenterol. Rep.* **2016**, *18*, 18. [CrossRef] [PubMed]
11. Stokes, C.S.; Volmer, D.A.; Grunhage, F.; Lammert, F. Vitamin D in chronic liver disease. *Liver Int. Off. J. Int. Assoc. Study Liver* **2013**, *33*, 338–352. [CrossRef] [PubMed]
12. Di Sario, A.; Candelaresi, C.; Omenetti, A.; Benedetti, A. Vitamin E in chronic liver diseases and liver fibrosis. *Vitam. Horm.* **2007**, *76*, 551–573. [PubMed]
13. Rossouw, J.E.; Labadarios, D.; McConnell, J.B.; Davis, M.; Williams, R. Plasma pyridoxal phosphate levels in fulminant hepatic failure and the effects of parenteral supplementation. *Scand. J. Gastroenterol.* **1977**, *12*, 123–127. [PubMed]
14. Venu, M.; Martin, E.; Saeian, K.; Gawrieh, S. High prevalence of Vitamin A deficiency and Vitamin D deficiency in patients evaluated for liver transplantation. *Liver Transplant.* **2013**, *19*, 627–633. [CrossRef] [PubMed]
15. Kawanaka, M.; Nishino, K.; Nakamura, J.; Suehiro, M.; Goto, D.; Urata, N.; Oka, T.; Kawamoto, H.; Nakamura, H.; Yodoi, J.; et al. Treatment of nonalcoholic steatohepatitis with Vitamins E and C: A pilot study. *Hepatic Med. Evid. Res.* **2013**, *5*, 11–16. [CrossRef] [PubMed]
16. Bedossa, P.; Poitou, C.; Veyrie, N.; Bouillot, J.L.; Basdevant, A.; Paradis, V.; Tordjman, J.; Clement, K. Histopathological algorithm and scoring system for evaluation of liver lesions in morbidly obese patients. *Hepatology* **2012**, *56*, 1751–1759. [CrossRef] [PubMed]
17. Iruzubieta, P.; Terán, Á.; Crespo, J.; Fábrega, E. Vitamin D deficiency in chronic liver disease. *World J. Hepatol.* **2014**, *6*, 901–915. [CrossRef] [PubMed]
18. Chen, E.-Q.; Shi, Y.; Tang, H. New insight of Vitamin D in chronic liver diseases. *Hepatobiliary Pancreat. Dis. Int.* **2014**, *13*, 580–585. [CrossRef]
19. Chaves, G.V.; Peres, W.A.; Goncalves, J.C.; Ramalho, A. Vitamin A and retinol-binding protein deficiency among chronic liver disease patients. *Nutrition* **2015**, *31*, 664–668. [CrossRef] [PubMed]
20. Dasarathy, J.; Periyalwar, P.; Allampati, S.; Bhinder, V.; Hawkins, C.; Brandt, P.; Khiyami, A.; McCullough, A.J.; Dasarathy, S. Hypovitaminosis D is associated with increased whole body fat mass and greater severity of non-alcoholic fatty liver disease. *Liver Int. Off. J. Int. Assoc. Study Liver* **2014**, *34*, e118–e127. [CrossRef] [PubMed]
21. Luger, M.; Kruschitz, R.; Kienbacher, C.; Traussnigg, S.; Langer, F.B.; Schindler, K.; Wurger, T.; Wrba, F.; Trauner, M.; Prager, G.; et al. Prevalence of Liver Fibrosis and its Association with Non-invasive Fibrosis and Metabolic Markers in Morbidly Obese Patients with Vitamin D Deficiency. *Obes. Surg.* **2016**, *26*, 2425–2432. [CrossRef] [PubMed]
22. Bril, F.; Maximos, M.; Portillo-Sanchez, P.; Biernacki, D.; Lomonaco, R.; Subbarayan, S.; Correa, M.; Lo, M.; Suman, A.; Cusi, K. Relationship of Vitamin D with insulin resistance and disease severity in non-alcoholic steatohepatitis. *J. Hepatol.* **2015**, *62*, 405–411. [CrossRef] [PubMed]
23. Casanueva, E.; Drijanski, A.; Fernández-Gaxiola, A.C.; Meza, C.; Pfeffer, F. Folate deficiency is associated with obesity and anemia in Mexican urban women. *Nutr. Res.* **2000**, *20*, 1389–1394. [CrossRef]
24. Hirsch, S.; Poniachick, J.; Avendano, M.; Csendes, A.; Burdiles, P.; Smok, G.; Diaz, J.C.; de la Maza, M.P. Serum folate and homocysteine levels in obese females with non-alcoholic fatty liver. *Nutrition* **2005**, *21*, 137–141. [CrossRef] [PubMed]
25. Fabbrini, E.; Sullivan, S.; Klein, S. Obesity and Nonalcoholic Fatty Liver Disease: Biochemical, Metabolic and Clinical Implications. *Hepatology* **2010**, *51*, 679–689. [CrossRef] [PubMed]
26. Sid, V.; Siow, Y.L.; O, K. Role of folate in nonalcoholic fatty liver disease. *Can. J. Physiol. Pharmacol.* **2017**, *95*, 1141–1148. [CrossRef] [PubMed]
27. Xia, M.F.; Bian, H.; Zhu, X.P.; Yan, H.M.; Chang, X.X.; Zhang, L.S.; Lin, H.D.; Hu, X.Q.; Gao, X. Serum folic acid levels are associated with the presence and severity of liver steatosis in Chinese adults. *Clin. Nutr.* **2017**. [CrossRef] [PubMed]
28. Charatcharoenwitthaya, P.; Levy, C.; Angulo, P.; Keach, J.; Jorgensen, R.; Lindor, K.D. Open-label pilot study of folic acid in patients with nonalcoholic steatohepatitis. *Liver Int. Off. J Int. Assoc. Study Liver* **2007**, *27*, 220–226. [CrossRef] [PubMed]
29. Koplay, M.; Gulcan, E.; Ozkan, F. Association between serum Vitamin B12 levels and the degree of steatosis in patients with nonalcoholic fatty liver disease. *J. Investig. Med.* **2011**, *59*, 1137–1140. [CrossRef] [PubMed]

30. Gulsen, M.; Yesilova, Z.; Bagci, S.; Uygun, A.; Ozcan, A.; Ercin, C.N.; Erdil, A.; Sanisoglu, S.Y.; Cakir, E.; Ates, Y.; et al. Elevated plasma homocysteine concentrations as a predictor of steatohepatitis in patients with non-alcoholic fatty liver disease. *J. Gastroenterol. Hepatol.* **2005**, *20*, 1448–1455. [CrossRef] [PubMed]
31. Polyzos, S.A.; Kountouras, J.; Patsiaoura, K.; Katsiki, E.; Zafeiriadou, E.; Zavos, C.; Deretzi, G.; Tsiaousi, E.; Slavakis, A. Serum Vitamin B12 and folate levels in patients with non-alcoholic fatty liver disease. *Int. J. Food Sci. Nutr.* **2012**, *63*, 659–666. [CrossRef] [PubMed]
32. Mechie, N.C.; Goralzcyk, A.D.; Reinhardt, L.; Mihm, S.; Amanzada, A. Association of serum Vitamin B12 levels with stage of liver fibrosis and treatment outcome in patients with chronic hepatitis C virus genotype 1 infection: A retrospective study. *BMC Res. Notes* **2015**, *8*, 260. [CrossRef] [PubMed]
33. Goel, A.; Ramakrishna, B.; Muliyil, J.; Madhu, K.; Sajith, K.G.; Zachariah, U.; Ramachandran, J.; Keshava, S.N.; Selvakumar, R.; Chandy, G.M.; et al. Use of serum Vitamin B12 level as a marker to differentiate idiopathic noncirrhotic intrahepatic portal hypertension from cryptogenic cirrhosis. *Dig. Dis. Sci.* **2013**, *58*, 179–187. [CrossRef] [PubMed]
34. Kazimierska, E.; Czestochowska, E. Serum homocysteine, Vitamin B12 and folic acid concentrations in patients with alcoholic liver cirrhosis. *Polski Merkur. Lek.* **2003**, *15*, 140–143.
35. Gaggini, M.; Morelli, M.; Buzzigoli, E.; DeFronzo, R.A.; Bugianesi, E.; Gastaldelli, A. Non-Alcoholic Fatty Liver Disease (NAFLD) and Its Connection with Insulin Resistance, Dyslipidemia, Atherosclerosis and Coronary Heart Disease. *Nutrients* **2013**, *5*, 1544–1560. [CrossRef] [PubMed]
36. Li, Z.; Gueant-Rodriguez, R.M.; Quilliot, D.; Sirveaux, M.A.; Meyre, D.; Gueant, J.L.; Brunaud, L. Folate and Vitamin B12 status is associated with insulin resistance and metabolic syndrome in morbid obesity. *Clin. Nutr.* **2017**. [CrossRef] [PubMed]
37. Baltaci, D.; Kutlucan, A.; Turker, Y.; Yilmaz, A.; Karacam, S.; Deler, H.; Ucgun, T.; Kara, I.H. Association of Vitamin B12 with obesity, overweight, insulin resistance and metabolic syndrome, and body fat composition; primary care-based study. *Med. Glas.* **2013**, *10*, 203–210.
38. Gammon, C.S.; von Hurst, P.R.; Coad, J.; Kruger, R.; Stonehouse, W. Vegetarianism, Vitamin B12 status, and insulin resistance in a group of predominantly overweight/obese South Asian women. *Nutrition* **2012**, *28*, 20–24. [CrossRef] [PubMed]

5

Optimizing the Nutritional Support of Adult Patients in the Setting of Cirrhosis

Brandon J. Perumpail [1], Andrew A. Li [2], George Cholankeril [2], Radhika Kumari [2] and Aijaz Ahmed [2,*]

1 Department of Medicine, Drexel University College of Medicine, Philadelphia, PA 19129, USA; bjp63@drexel.edu

2 Division of Gastroenterology and Hepatology, Stanford University School of Medicine, Stanford, CA 94305, USA; andrewli@stanford.edu (A.A.L.); georgetc@stanford.edu (G.C.); rkumari@stanford.edu (R.K.)

* Correspondence: aijazahmed@stanford.edu

Abstract: Aim: The aim of this work is to develop a pragmatic approach in the assessment and management strategies of patients with cirrhosis in order to optimize the outcomes in this patient population. Method: A systematic review of literature was conducted through 8 July 2017 on the PubMed Database looking for key terms, such as malnutrition, nutrition, assessment, treatment, and cirrhosis. Articles and studies looking at associations between nutrition and cirrhosis were reviewed. Results: An assessment of malnutrition should be conducted in two stages: the first, to identify patients at risk for malnutrition based on the severity of liver disease, and the second, to perform a complete multidisciplinary nutritional evaluation of these patients. Optimal management of malnutrition should focus on meeting recommended daily goals for caloric intake and inclusion of various nutrients in the diet. The nutritional goals should be pursued by encouraging and increasing oral intake or using other measures, such as oral supplementation, enteral nutrition, or parenteral nutrition. Conclusions: Although these strategies to improve nutritional support have been well established, current literature on the topic is limited in scope. Further research should be implemented to test if this enhanced approach is effective.

Keywords: nutrition; cirrhosis; end-stage liver disease; Child-Turcotte-Pugh; malnutrition; dietary intervention; improved oral intake

---

1. Introduction

Malnutrition has become increasingly common in end-stage liver disease [1]. The prevalence of malnutrition has been reported in a significant proportion of patients with cirrhosis and ranges from 10% to 100%, contingent on severity of hepatic decompensation in the setting of cirrhosis [2,3]. However, even with this high occurrence, malnutrition is still under-diagnosed and ineffectively treated [4]. More specifically, many patients who are awaiting liver transplantation develop various nutritional deficiencies [1]. Malnutrition is a predictor of morbidity and mortality in patients with cirrhosis [3]. Malnutrition related to liver disease has been linked to a risk of infections, complications associated with surgery, poor candidacy for liver transplantation, and a prolonged length of stay in the hospital or intensive care unit [2,5]. Routine screening of patients with end-stage liver disease for malnutrition can facilitate prompt diagnosis leading to timely initiation of treatment and improved outcomes [6,7].

2. Malnutrition in End-Stage Liver Disease

In the presence of cirrhosis, malnutrition is diagnosed and defined as a deficiency in nutrients [8]. Under normal post-prandial conditions, ingested carbohydrates are metabolized by the liver and stored as glycogen. Subsequently, during the normal fasting period glycogen can be broken down (glycogenolysis) to glucose (gluconeogenesis) to maintain stable blood glucose levels (glucose homeostasis). Patients with cirrhosis have a compromised ability to store glycogen and blunted gluconeogenesis. Therefore, cirrhotic patients may enter a starvation state between dinner and breakfast, stimulating lipid oxidation, thus shifting from carbohydrate to fat as the main source of energy metabolism. A complex interaction of many factors are involved in increasing the risk of malnutrition in cirrhosis [9]. Poor calorie intake is a common contributor in these patients, which often stems from a lack of appetite or anorexia. The molecular mechanisms involved in malnutrition in the cirrhotic state are not fully understood and include zinc deficiency, early satiety resulting from an increased amount of leptin and tumor necrosis factor-alpha in the blood, etc. [8,9]. In addition, many patients may develop a poor appetite due to ascites or hepatic encephalopathy [10]. The resulting dietary restriction of salt may make food unpalatable, further escalating poor nutritional status [11]. Another cause of malnutrition is impaired absorption and digestion resulting from a host of factors, such as decreased bile-salt, bacterial overgrowth, and portal hypertension [8]. Finally, hypermetabolism leads to malnutrition through increased energy expenditure and is an independent predictor of both transplant-free and post-transplant survival [8,10,12]. This is mainly caused by changes in nutrient utilization due to the lack of available carbohydrates for energy, which places the body in a state of starvation, especially overnight [12]. Infection and ascites also contribute to the hypermetabolic state [10]. In the setting of cirrhosis, protein-energy malnutrition (PEM) is noted in up to two-thirds of affected individuals and correlates with Child-Turcotte-Pugh classification. PEM is associated with poor survival in this patient population. The contributing factors to PEM include hypermetabolism, poor caloric intake, malabsorption, increased intestinal permeability leading to protein loss, and decreased hepatic protein synthesis. In addition, PEM leads to muscle wasting manifested by a reduction in skeletal muscle volume and strength (secondary sarcopenia related to cirrhosis). Secondary sarcopenia associated with cirrhosis is an independent predictor of poor survival. Furthermore, certain disease-specific issues impacting the management of malnutrition must be individualized. For example, alcohol abuse associated with low socio-economic status and poor psycho-social support may pose a complex challenge in the management of malnutrition.

In order to fully address the issue of malnutrition in end-stage liver disease, improvement must be made in promptly diagnosing patients in need for nutritional support.

3. Improved Assessment of Malnutrition

A systematic approach to screen for malnutrition in cirrhotic patients must be established to more directly address the growing problem of malnutrition. During the initial evaluation (stage 1 assessment), cirrhotic patients with immediate need for nutritional support must be identified. Subsequently, these selected patients must undergo a standardized evaluation (stage 2 assessment) leading to individualized patient care with a focus to optimize the nutritional status. This two-stage approach is summarized in Figure 1.

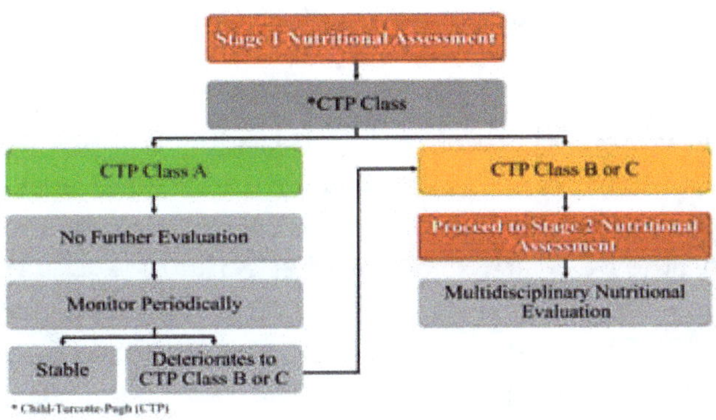

Figure 1. Two-stage approach to nutritional assessment in cirrhosis.

3.1. Stage 1 Assessment for Malnutrition: Define Immediate-Need Populations

The goal of a two-stage approach is to maximize the allocation of time and resources to those who need it the most to improve overall outcomes. Not every patient needs an immediate full evaluation (stage 2 assessment) for malnutrition; patients who are the most at risk should be targeted first and assessed. Malnutrition severity is strongly associated with the severity of hepatic decompensation (liver failure) in the setting of cirrhosis [3,13]. A Chinese study evaluating malnutrition in patients with chronic liver disease found that patients with the highest rate of nutritional risk were also those with the greatest degree of liver failure (patients in Child-Turcotte-Pugh (CTP) classes B and C) [13]. The two-stage approach uses the association between malnutrition and severity of liver failure to identify the patient population in immediate need of nutritional assessment using the CTP scoring system. This classification, created by Child and Turcotte in 1964 and later adjusted in 1973 by Pugh, is a commonly-used tool for measuring the severity of liver failure in cirrhotic patients and to estimate the risk of surgical procedures [14–16]. The CTP system scores 1–3 points, with one being the most normal and three being the most abnormal, in five different categories (albumin, bilirubin, prothrombin prolongation time, and hepatic encephalopathy) to grade patients into three classes: A (5–6 points), B (7–9 points), and C (10–15 points), with classes B and C being the most severe [17]. This constitutes the 'stage 1 assessment' and identifies patients with cirrhosis at the highest risk of malnutrition, namely CTP classes B and C [13]. Another study evaluated of cirrhotic patients for malnutrition categorized by the three CTP classes and noted malnourishment in more than half the patients in the CTP class B and C groups, 77.3% and 94.4% respectively, while less than half of the patients in CTP class A developed malnutrition [3]. In a study that compared the Subjective Global Assessment (SGA) of patients' nutrition with their CPT class, only patients in class B and C were indicated to have levels of malnutrition ranging from moderate to severe [11]. Thus, cirrhotic patients with CTP class B and C have been shown to be the most likely to develop malnutrition and require comprehensive 'stage 2 assessment' for poor nutritional status.

3.2. Stage 2 Assessment for Malnutrition: Multidisciplinary Nutritional Assessment

A more thorough and comprehensive evaluation of the nutritional status can be achieved and a focused individualized approach can be pursued. This not only allows for proper apportionment of resources and time, but also provides a more targeted approach in which patients can be prioritized based on the severity of malnutrition. A study evaluating protein depletion in patients with cirrhosis concluded that the utilization of multiple nutritional assessment tools were crucial in making an accurate assessment of severity of malnutrition [18]. End-stage liver disease is a confounding factor that affects the results of multiple nutritional assessment tools and, thus, there has to be confirmation across many techniques to diagnose malnutrition [5]. For example, weight and albumin concentrations could be unreliable measurements alone due to other complications from cirrhosis, such as ascites or low protein synthesis, respectively [10,18,19]. Other cross-sectional studies looking at nutritional assessment techniques found that the use of a variety of techniques, such as the SGA, biochemical tests, and anthropometry, lead to a better understanding of nutritional status [2,20–22]. A variety of tests should be used to evaluate different aspects and severity of nutrition rather than any single nutritional screening tool, thus creating a multidisciplinary approach shown in Figure 2 [1,19].

A standard nutritional evaluation often used in hospitals is the SGA [23]. It is an attractive test due to its accuracy while also being cheap, non-invasive, and simple to execute [23]. Multiple studies compare the SGA results with other nutritional measurement tools and have found it to provide consistent results, validating the SGA's precision and specificity [2,22,24]. It was also studied in the context of liver transplantation and was shown to predict complications during transplantation, as well as post-operative outcomes [5]. The SGA is a questionnaire with two main components, history and physical examination [25]. The history portion asks questions regarding previous weight changes over time, recent alterations of food intake, recent functionality, and symptoms affecting intake [25]. The physical examination measures fat loss, muscle wasting, and the presence of edema and ascites [25].

A score is calculated based on the evaluation and the patient is assigned to one of three stages—Stage A, well nourished; Stage B, moderately malnourished; or Stage C, severely malnourished, with each stage having a list of features characterizing the multiple categories assessed [25].

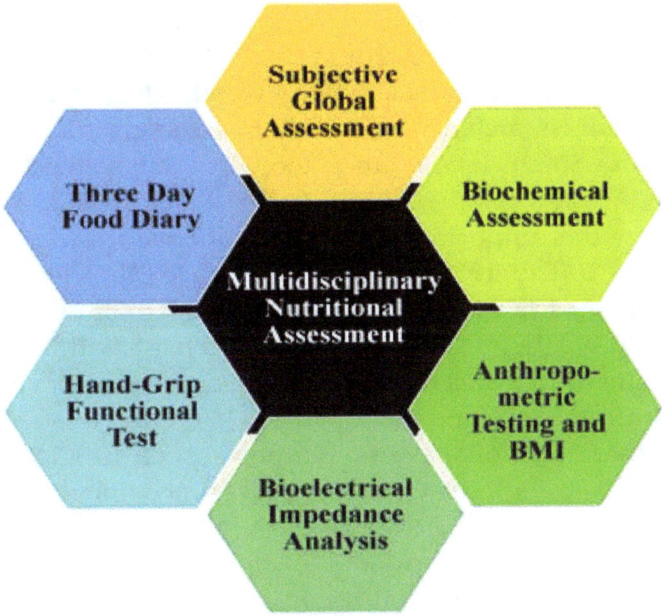

Figure 2. Multidisciplinary nutritional assessment.

A biochemical assessment for markers of malnutrition is commonly used for monitoring nutrition [1]. The test should include many factors, such as hemoglobin, albumin, white blood cell count, retinol-binding protein, transferrin, liver function exams, glucose, cholesterol, urea nitrogen, C-reactive protein, pre-albumin, nitrogen balance, creatinine, sodium, magnesium, zinc, potassium, and others [19,20]. Serum albumin is a common tool used to measure nutritional status and can help categorize the level of malnutrition [20]. However, one issue is that albumin also declines due to hepatic damage, making it an unreliable marker [19,26]. Pre-albumin and transferrin are impacted by malnutrition and hepatic damage similarly, but respond faster and, therefore, could also be used as early indications of malnutrition [26]. Retinol binding protein (RBP) relies on the presence of other nutrients, such as vitamin A and zinc, in order to carry out its function. Thus, micronutrient deficiency due to malnutrition would affect the blood levels of RBP as well [27]. Nitrogen balance is a good measure of dietary protein intake and protein metabolism [28]. Deficiency occurs when protein metabolism is greater than protein intake, as indicated by a negative nitrogen balance [28].

Furthermore, anthropometric testing and body mass index (BMI) are necessary tools when assessing nutritional body composition [29]. Anthropometric testing measures height, weight, mid-arm circumference, mid-arm muscle circumference, triceps skin fold thickness, and biceps skin fold thickness [20,21]. BMI and anthropometric measures can be used to assess skeletal muscle mass and adipose deposit levels [30–32]. A recent study found that thigh muscle thickness when used with BMI can be an important tool in identifying sarcopenia and malnutrition [31]. A potential problem with BMI is that edema and ascites could increase the measured weight and make BMI inaccurate; however, dry BMI can be measured by using corrective factors for dry weight that account for the level of edema. Five, ten, or fifteen percent are subtracted from the measured weight for mild, moderate, or severe ascites, and an extra 5% would be subtracted if edema is present [30,31]. Another way to account for ascites is to use the established BMI standards for ascites where BMI below or equal to 22 with no ascites, a BMI of 23 kg/m [2] with mild ascites, or a BMI of 25 kg/m [2] with tension ascites is considered a state of malnutrition [33]. Another useful tool to measure body composition is bioelectrical impedance analysis (BIA) [33–35]. BIA is swift, simple, and non-invasive, which makes it an attractive new technique that is gaining interest [35–37]. It conducts an electric current through the body and calculates its electric impedance, which is made up of two components—resistance, which measures body water, and reactance, which measures body cell mass (BCM). Based on this information, measurements about body composition can be estimated, such as BCM, BCM%, extracellular mass, mass that is not from body fat, body fat mass, phase angle, and total body water [34,37,38]. This information can be utilized to understand various aspects of body composition and determine how they change over time with intervention [33]. For example, BIA can calculate body water, which could be indicative of edema or ascites [33]. Furthermore, recent research has found that phase angle is a better predictor of nutritional status in cirrhosis than anthropomethric evaluation tools and can even be used for early diagnosis of malnutrition [35].

Functional testing is another important evaluation when assessing nutrition; this allows for a means of testing the strength and ability of the skeletal muscle [2]. A longitudinal study found that although muscle strength and muscle mass both deteriorate with malnutrition, the former declines at a much quicker rate [39]. Additionally, muscle strength can decrease without a loss in muscle mass [39]. Hand-grip strength is a tool used to assess muscle strength and has been validated as an independent method of identifying malnutrition and muscle capability [40]. Moreover, a comparative study found that when tested against other nutritional assessment tools, such as SGA, BMI, and anthropometric measurements, the hand-grip strength test had the highest accuracy for detecting the presence of nutritional compromise in the context of liver disease [41]. Another study found that not only does hand-grip strength correlate with nutritional level, it also predicts hospital outcomes, such as post-operative complications, length of hospitalization, risk of re-hospitalization, and physical ability.

The final portion of the assessment is an evaluation of dietary intake [2]. The best method to record this is through a three-day food diary with specific instructions given to the patient on how to complete the diary so that accurate information on food consumption can be documented [2]. Many studies have validated the three-day food diary as an effective measure of dietary intake and it has been shown to be more accurate than other methods such as the food frequency questionnaire and 24-h recall [42,43]. The food diary helps physicians and dieticians understand the different food habits, dietary choices, and overall consumption levels (calories and protein content) of the patient over time so that they can assess nutrition in an individualized manner [44]. The use of multiple tools and tests to evaluate the patient's nutritional status creates a well-rounded image of the patient's health so that an assessment of malnutrition are both thorough and specific. An initial assessment stage that filters patients based on severity of hepatic decompensation in the setting of cirrhosis allows only the malnourished or most at-risk for malnutrition to proceed to the next stage. Furthermore, this individualized approach results in pragmatic utilization and allocation of restricted resources.

4. Treatment Options for Malnourished Patients

Malnutrition in the setting of cirrhosis has been noted as a reliable indicator of quality of life and key predictor of inpatient outcomes (morbidity and mortality) [3]. Studies have indicated that these outcomes can be improved by optimizing the nutritional status of a patient with cirrhosis [7]. Unfortunately, malnutrition remains an alarmingly prevalent problem, especially in patients with cirrhosis [3,45]. Therefore, it is very important to develop an objective and standardized initial and follow-up evaluation pathway/management protocol to assess the nutritional status of patients with cirrhosis. In particular, patients with hepatic decompensation/liver failure awaiting liver transplantation require an ongoing evaluation of their nutritional status in the era of donor organ shortage and longer waiting times on transplant waitlists.

4.1. Proper Dietary Recommendations and Education

In patients with cirrhosis, the recommendation for different macromolecules has changed over time and health care practitioners need to be aware of these changes so that patients are properly managed [12]. Gastroenterology and hepatology fellowships do not always offer a comprehensive training in nutritional assessment and treatment; therefore, physicians may not always know the best methods available for diagnosing or treating patients who face malnourishment [9]. The most important aspect of malnourishment management is ensuring that the patient's rehabilitative diet has the correct amount of each essential nutrient or macromolecule according to the current regulations [12]. Furthermore, diet plays a substantial role in cirrhosis and the related severity of hepatic decompensation/liver failure. Inadequate diets have been associated with further progression of liver disease and increased risk of cirrhosis. However, proper diet alterations have been noted to not only prevent disease progression, but also to reduce the severity of liver failure [46,47]. The recommendation for malnourished patients with cirrhosis is 35–40 kcal/kg/day to promote anabolism [33,48]. Protein deficiency is a significant problem in malnutrition which can be addressed through an intake of 1.2–1.5 g/kg/day [48,49]. Furthermore, hepatic damage causes an increase in aromatic amino acids (AAA) and decreases branched-chain amino acids (BCAA) which can lead to hepatic encephalopathy and other neurological complications [29]. Studies have found that increasing the BCAA to AAA ratio through improved dietary BCAA intake has led to normalization and increased survival [12,50]. The guideline for carbohydrates is 50–70% of daily calories [51]. However, simple sugars, especially fructose, should be avoided as much as possible [6]. The recommendation for lipids is 10–20% of calories with the majority being monounsaturated and polyunsaturated fatty acids [6,11]. Special considerations have to be taken for hepatic encephalopathy and ascites [33]. In hepatic encephalopathy, there should be an increased emphasis on BCAAs and fiber with decreased ammonia [33]. Previous recommendations for hepatic encephalopathy included decreased protein intake, but more recent data have shown that this practice is outdated and incorrect [6,9,10]. Patients with ascites should be on a low-sodium diet (less than or equal to 2 g/day) and should also have water restriction when edema is present or if hyponatremia occurs [33]. Ensuring patients meet these requirements, organized in Table 1, is the first step in optimizing nutritional support in patients with end-stage liver disease. In patients with cirrhosis associated with nonalcoholic steatohepatitis caloric restriction, but not protein restriction, can be recommended. Furthermore, patients with fluid retention must be educated to restrict their sodium intake to less than 2 g per day and fluid intake of 2 L per day.

Table 1. Nutritional recommendations for malnutrition in cirrhosis.

Nutritional Recommendations for Malnutrition in Cirrhosis	
Daily Calories	35–40 kcal/kg/day
Proteins	1.2–1.5 g/kg/day with increased BCAAs
Carbohydrates	50–70% of daily calories with decreased simple sugars—especially fructose
Lipids	10–20% of daily calories with increased MUFAs and PUFAs
Special Considerations	
Hepatic Encephalopathy	Maintain protein intake, increase BCAAs and decreased ammonia intake
Ascites	Low-sodium diet ($\leq$2 g/day) and water restriction when necessary

4.2. *Techniques to Promote Oral Intake*

In general, adequate oral intake has been a difficult task for many patients facing malnutrition related to cirrhosis and other chronic ailments [52]. Patients with malnutrition are unable to maintain their daily caloric targets and requirements for nutrients despite institution of reinforced diet plans [52]. Many studies have reported that patients with malnutrition have significant amounts of calories wasted with each partially-ingested meal [53,54]. One study questioned patients after meals at the hospital in an attempt to understand the reasoning behind incomplete meal intake and suspected that meal sensory perception affected eating capability despite hunger [55]. Patients responded regarding various aspects of their meal experience (appearance, aroma, taste, texture, temperature, and food variety) and requested that more attention be paid to provide a more individualized eating experience [55]. These factors should be continuously re-evaluated to reflect the preferences of the patients as their appetite changes based on the severity of hepatic decompensation [55]. In addition to this study, others have shown that meal presentation and appearance impacts the desire to eat; patients ate more from a neatly-arranged plate rather than a disorganized one [54,55]. Additionally, overwhelming odors from food discouraged eating [55]. For example, when feeling nauseous, patients desired meals that had neutral tastes [55]. Often softer foods that were easier to ingest were associated with increased intake [55,56]. A hot meal versus a cold meal was more likely to be ingested [55]. Another study assessing issues with oral intake showed that interruptions during meal times by nurses, physicians, or tests led to missed meals that were never served later; patients were also unaware of the options available for extra snacks between meals [53]. This suggests that patients should have scheduled meal times that are protected and nursing staff should ensure that the patients eat during the dedicated meal period without interruption, plus improving patient awareness regarding additional accessible snacks can increase caloric intake [53]. Studies to improve intake noted that smaller meals, increased meal frequency, and fortified nutrition within these meals were effective in instituting increased nutritional support [57]. Furthermore, studies in the setting of cirrhosis found that 4–6 meals high in carbohydrates with an evening snack fortified with BCAAs prevented hypoglycemia and led to increased nutrition due to reduced catabolism overnight [8]. Another important factor found in studies was the level of nursing education [58]. Poulsen and colleagues [58] noticed increased nutrition and oral intake in patients when nurses were given a short class on nutritional care to provide individualized nutritional support. Figure 3 summarizes the various interventions that can be used to promote oral intake and improve nutritional status of patients with cirrhosis.

Methods to Improve Oral Intake

- Improved Meal Sensory Perception
- Uninterrupted Meals
- Increased Patient Information
- Increased Meal Frequency
- Smaller Meal Size
- Fortified Meal Nutrition
- Increased Nutritional Education of Healthcare Staff

Figure 3. Methods to improve oral intake.

4.3. Alternative Feeding Methods

Although oral intake of food is the preferred route of nutrition, factors, such as patient weakness or inability to eat, may necessitate pursuit of alternative methods for nutrient delivery [10,59]. Oral supplements should be used in an individualized approach to fulfill any specific nutrient deficiencies a patient may have [10,59]. A clinical trial noted that patients given oral supplements between meals met the recommended nutritional intakes [59]. Other options for patients unable to handle oral intake are enteral nutrition through a nasogastric tube and, if necessary, parenteral nutrition [10]. Both of these have been shown to be effective in various studies assessing malnutrition [10,60]. Complications of cirrhosis and end-stage liver disease associated with gut microbiota dysfunction, such as hepatic encephalopathy, are effectively managed with prebiotics, probiotics and synbiotics. Optimal management of hepatic encephalopathy and favorable gut microbiota may lead to improved nutritional status in patients with cirrhosis. Herbal remedies and supplements should be avoided with cirrhosis due to increased risk of hepatotoxicity with marginal hepatic reserve.

5. Conclusions

Malnutrition is a growing problem, especially in cirrhotic patients with end-stage liver disease. The enhancement of methods to assess and treat malnutrition is the key to optimizing patient outcomes. Assessment of malnutrition should be done in two stages, the first to identify patients at risk for malnutrition based on cirrhosis and the second to run a complete multidisciplinary nutritional evaluation on these patients. Treatments for malnutrition should make sure patients reach the recommended daily caloric and nutrient goals by increasing oral intake or by using other measures, such as oral supplementation, enteral nutrition, or parenteral nutrition. Further prospective data are needed from dedicated studies to optimize the nutritional status and outcomes in patients with cirrhosis improved through proper nutritional support of patients with advanced liver disease [7]. Therefore, standardized protocols to screen for malnutrition associated with cirrhosis and timely intervention with nutritional support is a pivotal step in reducing the risk of morbidity and mortality.

Author Contributions: All authors designed the project. First prepared the manuscript. Manuscript was reviewed and edited by all authors. The last author (senior author) supervised the project.

References

1. Lim, H.S.; Kim, H.C.; Park, Y.H.; Kim, S.K. Evaluation of Malnutrition Risk after Liver Transplantation Using the Nutritional Screening Tools. *Clin. Nutr. Res.* **2015**, *4*, 242–249. [CrossRef] [PubMed]
2. Marr, K.J.; Shaheen, A.A.; Lam, L.; Stapleton, M.; Burak, K.; Raman, M. Nutritional status and the performance of multiple bedside tools for nutrition assessment among patients waiting for liver transplantation: A Canadian experience. *Clin. Nutr. ESPEN* **2017**, *17*, 68–74. [CrossRef] [PubMed]
3. Maharshi, S.; Sharma, B.C.; Srivastava, S. Malnutrition in cirrhosis increases morbidity and mortality. *J. Gastroenterol. Hepatol.* **2015**, *30*, 1507–1513. [CrossRef] [PubMed]
4. Cheung, K.; Lee, S.S.; Raman, M. Prevalence and mechanisms of malnutrition in patients with advanced liver disease, and nutrition management strategies. *Clin. Gastroenterol. Hepatol.* **2012**, *10*, 117–125. [CrossRef] [PubMed]
5. Stephenson, G.R.; Moretti, E.W.; El-Moalem, H.; Clavien, P.A.; Tuttle-Newhall, J.E. Malnutrition in liver transplant patients: Preoperative subjective global assessment is predictive of outcome after liver transplantation. *Transplantation* **2001**, *72*, 666–670. [CrossRef] [PubMed]
6. McClain, C.J. Nutrition in patients with cirrhosis. *Gastroenterol. Hepatol.* **2016**, *12*, 507–510.
7. Alberda, C.; Gramlich, L.; Jones, N.; Jeejeebhoy, K.; Day, A.G.; Dhaliwal, R.; Heyland, D.K. The relationship between nutritional intake and clinical outcomes in critically ill patients: Results of an international multicenter observational study. *Intensive Care Med.* **2009**, *35*, 1728–1737. [CrossRef] [PubMed]
8. Ye, Q.; Yin, W.; Zhang, L.; Xiao, H.; Qi, Y.; Liu, S.; Qian, B.; Wang, F.; Han, T. The value of grip test, lysophosphatidlycholines, glycerophosphocholine, ornithine, glucuronic acid decrement in assessment of nutritional and metabolic characteristics in hepatitis B cirrhosis. *PLoS ONE* **2017**, *12*, e0175165. [CrossRef] [PubMed]
9. Patton, H.M. Nutritional assessment of patients with chronic liver disease. *Gastroenterol. Hepatol.* **2012**, *8*, 687–690.
10. Patel, J.J.; McClain, C.J.; Sarav, M.; Hamilton-Reeves, J.; Hurt, R.T. Protein requirements for critically Ill patients with renal and liver failure. *Nutr. Clin. Pract.* **2017**, *32* (Suppl. 1), 101S–111S. [CrossRef] [PubMed]
11. Teiusanu, A.; Andrei, M.; Arbanas, T.; Nicolaie, T.; Diculescu, M. Nutritional status in cirrhotic patients. *Maedica* **2012**, *7*, 284–289. [PubMed]
12. Eghtesad, S. Malnutrition in liver cirrhosis: The influence of protein and sodium. *Middle East J. Dig. Dis.* **2013**, *5*, 65–75. [PubMed]
13. Shi, S.; Han, J.; Yan, M.; Wang, K.; Yu, H.; Meng, Q. Nutritional risk assessment in patients with chronic liver disease. *Zhonghua Gan Zang Bing Za Zhi* **2014**, *22*, 536–539. [PubMed]
14. Child, C.G.; Turcotte, J.G. Surgery and portal hypertension. *Major Probl. Clin. Surg.* **1964**, *1*, 1–85. [PubMed]

15. Pugh, R.N.; Murray-Lyon, I.M.; Dawson, J.L.; Pietroni, M.C.; Williams, R. Transection of the oesophagus for bleeding oesophageal varices. *Br. J. Surg.* **1973**, *60*, 646–649. [CrossRef] [PubMed]
16. Zhou, C.; Hou, C.; Cheng, D.; Tang, W.; Lv, W. Predictive accuracy comparison of MELD and Child-Turcotte-Pugh scores for survival in patients underwent TIPS placement: A systematic meta-analytic review. *Int. J. Clin. Exp. Med.* **2015**, *8*, 13464–13472. [PubMed]
17. Raszeja-Wyszomirska, J.; Wasilewicz, M.P.; Wunsch, E.; Szymanik, B.; Jarosz, K.; Wójcicki, M.; Milkiewicz, P. Assessment of a modified Child-Pugh-Turcotte score to predict early mortality after liver transplantation. *Transplant. Proc.* **2009**, *41*, 3114–3116. [CrossRef] [PubMed]
18. Prijatmoko, D.; Strauss, B.J.; Lambert, J.R.; Sievert, W.; Stroud, D.B.; Wahlqvist, M.L.; Katz, B.; Colman, J.; Jones, P.; Korman, M.G. Early detection of protein depletion in alcoholic cirrhosis: Role of body composition analysis. *Gastroenterology* **1993**, *105*, 1839–1845. [CrossRef]
19. Bharadwaj, S.; Ginoya, S.; Tandon, P.; Gohel, T.D.; Guirguis, J.; Vallabh, H.; Jevenn, A.; Hanouneh, I. Malnutrition: Laboratory markers vs nutritional assessment. *Gastroenterol. Rep.* **2016**, *4*, 272–280. [CrossRef] [PubMed]
20. Tai, M.L.; Goh, K.L.; Mohd-Taib, S.H.; Rampal, S.; Mahadeva, S. Anthropometric, biochemical and clinical assessment of malnutrition in Malaysian patients with advanced cirrhosis. *Nutr. J.* **2010**, *9*, 27. [CrossRef] [PubMed]
21. Nunes, F.F.; Bassani, L.; Fernandes, S.A.; Deutrich, M.E.; Pivatto, B.C.; Marroni, C.A. Food consumption of cirrhotic patients, comparison with the nutritional status and disease staging. *Arq. Gastroenterol.* **2016**, *53*, 250–256. [CrossRef] [PubMed]
22. Filipovic, B.F.; Gajic, M.; Milinic, N.; Milovanović, B.; Filipović, B.R.; Cvetković, M.; Sibalić, N. Comparison of two nutritional assessment methods in gastroenterology patients. *World J. Gastroenterol.* **2010**, *16*, 1999–2004. [CrossRef] [PubMed]
23. Da Silva Fink, J.; Daniel de Mello, P.; Daniel de Mello, E. Subjective global assessment of nutritional status—A systematic review of the literature. *Clin. Nutr.* **2015**, *34*, 785–792. [CrossRef] [PubMed]
24. Mourao, F.; Amado, D.; Ravasco, P.; Vidal, P.M.; Camilo, M.E. Nutritional risk and status assessment in surgical patients: A challenge amidst plenty. *Nutr. Hosp.* **2004**, *19*, 83–88. [PubMed]
25. Detsky, A.S.; McLaughlin, J.R.; Baker, J.P.; Johnston, N.; Whittaker, S.; Mendelson, R.A.; Jeejeebhoy, K.N. What is subjective global assessment of nutritional status? *JPEN J. Parenter. Enteral Nutr.* **1987**, *11*, 8–13. [CrossRef] [PubMed]
26. Fuhrman, M.P.; Charney, P.; Mueller, C.M. Hepatic proteins and nutrition assessment. *J. Am. Diet. Assoc.* **2004**, *104*, 1258–1264. [CrossRef] [PubMed]
27. Chaves, G.V.; Peres, W.A.; Goncalves, J.C.; Ramalho, A. Vitamin A and retinol-binding protein deficiency among chronic liver disease patients. *Nutrition* **2015**, *31*, 664–668. [CrossRef] [PubMed]
28. Rand, W.M.; Pellett, P.L.; Young, V.R. Meta-analysis of nitrogen balance studies for estimating protein requirements in healthy adults. *Am. J. Clin. Nutr.* **2003**, *77*, 109–127. [PubMed]
29. Johnson, T.M.; Overgard, E.B.; Cohen, A.E.; DiBaise, J.K. Nutrition assessment and management in advanced liver disease. *Nutr. Clin. Pract.* **2013**, *28*, 15–29. [CrossRef] [PubMed]
30. Tandon, P.; Ney, M.; Irwin, I.; Ma, M.M.; Gramlich, L.; Bain, V.G.; Esfandiari, N.; Baracos, V.; Montano-Loza, A.J.; Myers, R.P. Severe muscle depletion in patients on the liver transplant wait list: Its prevalence and independent prognostic value. *Liver Transpl.* **2012**, *18*, 1209–1216. [CrossRef] [PubMed]
31. Tandon, P.; Low, G.; Mourtzakis, M.; Zenith, L.; Myers, R.P.; Abraldes, J.G.; Shaheen, A.A.; Qamar, H.; Mansoor, N.; Carbonneau, M.; et al. A model to identify sarcopenia in patients with cirrhosis. *Clin. Gastroenterol. Hepatol.* **2016**, *14*, 1473–1480. [CrossRef] [PubMed]
32. Ponziani, F.R.; Gasbarrini, A. Sarcopenia in patients with advanced liver disease. *Curr. Protein Pept. Sci.* **2017**. [CrossRef] [PubMed]
33. Moctezuma-Velazquez, C.; Garcia-Juarez, I.; Soto-Solis, R.; Hernandez-Cortes, J.; Torre, A. Nutritional assessment and treatment of patients with liver cirrhosis. *Nutrition* **2013**, *29*, 1279–1285. [CrossRef] [PubMed]
34. Verney, J.; Metz, L.; Chaplais, E.; Cardenoux, C.; Pereira, B.; Thivel, D. Bioelectrical impedance is an accurate method to assess body composition in obese but not severely obese adolescents. *Nutr. Res.* **2016**, *36*, 663–670. [CrossRef] [PubMed]
35. Fernandes, S.A.; de Mattos, A.A.; Tovo, C.V.; Marroni, C.A. Nutritional evaluation in cirrhosis: Emphasis on the phase angle. *World J. Hepatol.* **2016**, *8*, 1205–1211. [CrossRef] [PubMed]

36. Dehghan, M.; Merchant, A.T. Is bioelectrical impedance accurate for use in large epidemiological studies? *Nutr. J.* **2008**, *7*, 26. [CrossRef] [PubMed]
37. Walter-Kroker, A.; Kroker, A.; Mattiucci-Guehlke, M.; Glaab, T. A practical guide to bioelectrical impedance analysis using the example of chronic obstructive pulmonary disease. *Nutr. J.* **2011**, *10*, 35. [CrossRef] [PubMed]
38. Lee, Y.; Kwon, O.; Shin, C.S.; Lee, S.M. Use of bioelectrical impedance analysis for the assessment of nutritional status in critically ill patients. *Clin. Nutr. Res.* **2015**, *4*, 32–40. [CrossRef] [PubMed]
39. Goodpaster, B.H.; Park, S.W.; Harris, T.B.; Kritchevsky, S.B.; Nevitt, M.; Schwartz, A.V.; Simonsick, E.M.; Tylavsky, F.A.; Visser, M.; Newman, A.B. The loss of skeletal muscle strength, mass, and quality in older adults: The health, aging and body composition study. *J. Gerontol. A Biol. Sci. Med. Sci.* **2006**, *61*, 1059–1064. [CrossRef] [PubMed]
40. Flood, A.; Chung, A.; Parker, H.; Kearns, V.; O'Sullivan, T.A. The use of hand grip strength as a predictor of nutrition status in hospital patients. *Clin. Nutr.* **2014**, *33*, 106–114. [CrossRef] [PubMed]
41. Sharma, P.; Rauf, A.; Matin, A.; Agarwal, R.; Tyagi, P.; Arora, A. Handgrip strength as an important bed side tool to assess malnutrition in patient with liver disease. *J. Clin. Exp. Hepatol.* **2017**, *7*, 16–22. [CrossRef] [PubMed]
42. Crawford, P.B.; Obarzanek, E.; Morrison, J.; Sabry, Z.I. Comparative advantage of 3-day food records over 24-h recall and 5-day food frequency validated by observation of 9- and 10-year-old girls. *J. Am. Diet. Assoc.* **1994**, *94*, 626–630. [CrossRef]
43. Yang, Y.J.; Kim, M.K.; Hwang, S.H.; Ahn, Y.; Shim, J.E.; Kim, D.H. Relative validities of 3-day food records and the food frequency questionnaire. *Nutr. Res. Pract.* **2010**, *4*, 142–148. [CrossRef] [PubMed]
44. Ortega, R.M.; Perez-Rodrigo, C.; Lopez-Sobaler, A.M. Dietary assessment methods: Dietary records. *Nutr. Hosp.* **2015**, *31* (Suppl. 3), 38–45. [PubMed]
45. Rojas-Loureiro, G.; Servin-Caamano, A.; Perez-Reyes, E.; Servin-Abad, L.; Higuera-de la Tijera, F. Malnutrition negatively impacts the quality of life of patients with cirrhosis: An observational study. *World J. Hepatol.* **2017**, *9*, 263–269. [CrossRef] [PubMed]
46. Pimentel, C.F.; Lai, M. Nutrition interventions for chronic liver diseases and nonalcoholic fatty liver disease. *Med. Clin. N. Am.* **2016**, *100*, 1303–1327. [CrossRef] [PubMed]
47. Kim, W. Treatment options in non-alcoholic fatty liver disease. *Korean J. Gastroenterol.* **2017**, *69*, 353–358. [CrossRef] [PubMed]
48. Chao, A.; Waitzberg, D.; de Jesus, R.P.; Bueno, A.A.; Kha, V.; Allen, K.; Kappus, M.; Medici, V. Malnutrition and nutritional support in alcoholic liver Disease: A review. *Curr. Gastroenterol. Rep.* **2016**, *18*, 65. [CrossRef] [PubMed]
49. Putadechakum, S.; Klangjareonchai, T.; Soponsaritsuk, A.; Roongpisuthipong, C. Nutritional status assessment in cirrhotic patients after protein supplementation. *ISRN Gastroenterol.* **2012**, *2012*, 690402. [CrossRef] [PubMed]
50. Hanai, T.; Shiraki, M.; Nishimura, K.; Ohnishi, S.; Imai, K.; Suetsugu, A.; Takai, K.; Shimizu, M.; Moriwaki, H. Sarcopenia impairs prognosis of patients with liver cirrhosis. *Nutrition* **2015**, *31*, 193–199. [CrossRef] [PubMed]
51. Anastácio, L.R.; Davisson Correia, M.I.T. Nutrition therapy: Integral part of liver transplant care. *World J. Gastroenterol.* **2016**, *22*, 1513–1522. [CrossRef] [PubMed]
52. Thibault, R.; Chikhi, M.; Clerc, A.; Darmon, P.; Chopard, P.; Genton, L.; Kossovsky, M.P.; Pichard, C. Assessment of food intake in hospitalised patients: A 10-year comparative study of a prospective hospital survey. *Clin. Nutr.* **2011**, *30*, 289–296. [CrossRef] [PubMed]
53. Van Bokhorst-de van der Schueren, M.A.; Roosemalen, M.M.; Weijs, P.J.; Langius, J.A. High waste contributes to low food intake in hospitalized patients. *Nutr. Clin. Pract.* **2012**, *27*, 274–280. [CrossRef] [PubMed]
54. Navarro, D.A.; Boaz, M.; Krause, I.; Elis, A.; Chernov, K.; Giabra, M.; Levy, M.; Giboreau, A.; Kosak, S.; Mouhieddine, M.; et al. Improved meal presentation increases food intake and decreases readmission rate in hospitalized patients. *Clin. Nutr.* **2016**, *35*, 1153–1158. [CrossRef] [PubMed]
55. Sorensen, J.; Holm, L.; Frost, M.B.; Kondrup, J. Food for patients at nutritional risk: A model of food sensory quality to promote intake. *Clin. Nutr.* **2012**, *31*, 637–646. [CrossRef] [PubMed]
56. Forde, C.G.; van Kuijk, N.; Thaler, T.; de Graaf, C.; Martin, N. Texture and savoury taste influences on food intake in a realistic hot lunch time meal. *Appetite* **2013**, *60*, 180–186. [CrossRef] [PubMed]

57. Lorefalt, B.; Wissing, U.; Unosson, M. Smaller but energy and protein-enriched meals improve energy and nutrient intakes in elderly patients. *J. Nutr. Health Aging* **2005**, *9*, 243–247. [PubMed]
58. Poulsen, I.; Vendel Petersen, H.; Rahm Hallberg, I.; Schroll, M. Lack of nutritional and functional effects of nutritional supervision by nurses: A quasi-experimental study in geriatric patients. *Scand. J. Food Nutr.* **2007**, *51*, 6–12. [CrossRef]
59. Campbell, K.L.; Webb, L.; Vivanti, A.; Varghese, P.; Ferguson, M. Comparison of three interventions in the treatment of malnutrition in hospitalised older adults: A clinical trial. *Nutr. Diet.* **2013**, *70*, 325–331. [CrossRef]
60. Kozeniecki, M.; Fritzshall, R. Enteral nutrition for adults in the hospital setting. *Nutr. Clin. Pract.* **2015**, *30*, 634–651. [CrossRef] [PubMed]

6

Beneficial and Paradoxical Roles of Anti-Oxidative Nutritional Support for Non-Alcoholic Fatty Liver Disease

Daisuke Uchida, Akinobu Takaki *, Takuya Adachi and Hiroyuki Okada

Department of Gastroenterology and Hepatology, Okayama University Graduate School of Medicine, Dentistry and Pharmaceutical Sciences, 2-5-1 Shikata-cho, Kita-ku, Okayama 700-8558, Japan; d.uchida0309@gmail.com (D.U.); adataku719@yahoo.co.jp (T.A.); hiro@md.okayama-u.ac.jp (H.O.)

* Correspondence: akitaka@md.okayama-u.ac.jp

Abstract: Oxidative stress is being recognized as a key factor in the progression of chronic liver disease (CLD), especially non-alcoholic fatty liver disease (NAFLD). Many NAFLD treatment guidelines recommend the use of antioxidants, especially vitamin E. Many prospective studies have described the beneficial effects of such agents for the clinical course of NAFLD. However, as these studies are usually short-term evaluations, lasting only a few years, whether or not antioxidants continue to exert favorable long-term effects, including in cases of concomitant hepatocellular carcinoma, remains unclear. Antioxidants are generally believed to be beneficial for human health and are often commercially available as health-food products. Patients with lifestyle-related diseases often use such products to try to be healthier without practicing lifestyle intervention. However, under some experimental NAFLD conditions, antioxidants have been shown to encourage the progression of hepatocellular carcinoma, as oxidative stress is toxic for cancer cells, just as for normal cells. In this review, we will highlight the paradoxical effects of antioxidants against NAFLD and related hepatocellular carcinoma.

Keywords: non-alcoholic fatty liver disease; hepatocellular carcinoma; anti-oxidant

---

1. Introduction

Non-alcoholic fatty liver disease (NAFLD) is a common chronic liver disease associated with obesity and metabolic syndrome [1,2]. The deposition of lipids in the liver induces inflammation, insulin resistance, and hepatic steatosis [3]. Non-alcoholic steatohepatitis (NASH) is a severe form of NAFLD that causes cirrhosis and hepatocellular carcinoma (HCC) because of persistent inflammation associated with hepatic steatosis [4,5]. The mechanism underlying the development of NASH from simple steatosis, namely non-alcoholic fatty liver (NAFL), has been considered as either a two-hit theory or a multiple hit-process [6–8]. The two-hit theory comprises a first hit of hepatic steatosis and second hit of several cellular stress responses, such as oxidative stress or endoplasmic reticulum (ER) stress. Given that the second hits are multifactorial and hepatic steatosis may be induced via hepatic inflammation, the process has recently been expressed as a multiple parallel hit process or multiple hit process [8].

Oxidative stress is a cellular stress associated with NASH progression. Reactive oxygen species (ROS) are generated during free fatty acid metabolism in microsomes, peroxisomes, and mitochondria, and comprise an established source of oxidative stress [9]. Oxidative stress is increased through the generation of ROS, as well as by defects in redox defense mechanisms involving glutathione (GSH), catalase or superoxide dismutase (SOD), and it induces various events related to not only NASH progression but also carcinogenesis such as DNA damage, tissue remodeling, and alterations in gene expression [10,11]. Mitochondria play a key role in the development of oxidative stress, and the dysfunction of mitochondria may induce NASH progression. Some reports have shown that antioxidant therapies, such as vitamin E, improve NASH, but the mechanism, especially concerning malignant tumor progression, and long-term outcomes are not clear [12,13].

In the present study, we reviewed the relationship between antioxidant nutrients and NASH progression including the carcinogenic risk.

2. The Relationship between NAFLD and Oxidative Stress

Oxidative stress is strongly related to chronic hepatic inflammation, and NAFLD/NASH is no exception, being included in the "second hit" of NASH progression as well as apoptosis, ER stress, and intestinal environment. It is widely known that oxidative stress functions as an important regulator of the progression of liver steatosis [14–16]. Various cellular stresses, including oxidative stress, apoptosis, and gut-derived signals such as lipopolysaccharide (LPS), trigger an inflammatory response and progressive liver damage [17]. Chronic oxidative stress correlates with a variety of pathologies such as malignant diseases, diabetes mellitus, cardiovascular diseases, chronic inflammatory diseases, and aging acceleration. Oxidative stress is caused by the generation of ROS, which have various causes, including interactions among gut microbiota. When excess ROS are produced excessively or the endogenous antioxidant capacity is diminished, indiscriminate oxidation elicits harmful effects resulting in oxidative stress [18].

Insulin resistance and dyslipidemia are widely accepted as disease progression factors in NAFLD [7]. Insulin signals suppress gluconeogenesis and enhance lipid synthesis in the liver. A human hepatic mRNA analysis revealed that the expression of insulin receptor substrate (IRS)-2, which mediates the effects of insulin by acting as a molecular adopter, was decreased while that of gluconeogenesis enzymes was increased in both NAFL and NASH [19]. Insulin resistance is clinically evident in the advanced stage of NAFLD; however, hepatic insulin resistance at the molecular level started from the NAFL stage. Altered cholesterol homeostasis such as increased cholesterol synthesis and uptake or reduced cholesterol excretion have been shown in NAFLD [20]. The hepatic free cholesterol accumulation has been shown to damage mitochondria and ER function thereby inducing hepatic inflammation and fibrosis [21]. Lipoprotein lipase (LPL), a key regulator of fatty acid release from triglyceride-rich lipoproteins, controls the cellular uptake of fatty acid and triglyceride accumulation [22]. The inhibition of LPL may prevent the accumulation of hepatic lipid [23].

Changes in the alimentary tract environment, which is connected to the liver via the portal vein, including the oral microbiota to the intestinal and colorectal microbiota have been shown to be strongly related to various diseases. The gut microbiota, which comprise various species such as *Bifidobacterium*, *Bacteroides*, *Clostridium*, *Lactobacillales*, and *Prevotella*, produce endogenous ethanol that induces the formation of ROS by hepatic stellate cells and Kupffer cells [24]. The composition of the microbiota depends on the age, health history, food intake, and probiotics consumed [25]. The food intake strongly correlates with dyslipidemia and is a crucial factor to consider when deciding on treatments for NAFLD, as it influences the gut microbiota [26].

An imbalance in the microbiome can affect the intestine and liver via microbiota-related signaling pathways such as toll-like receptor (TLR) signaling activation. LPL can also be suppressed by a fasting-induced adipose factor, which is regulated by the gut microbiota via TLR ligands [7,27]. A TLR-4 ligand LPS is liberated from the outer membrane of Gram-negative bacteria and binds to lipopolysaccharide binding protein (LBP). These ligands stimulate TLR signals, including nuclear factor kappa (NF-kB) with cluster of differentiation (CD) 14, and induce the production of inflammatory cytokines [28]. LPS is increased by a high-fat, high-calorie diet, as well as dyslipidemia and insulin resistance, which are related to NASH progression. The involvement of TLR-2 in NASH inflammation and fibrosis has been investigated in mouse NASH models [29]. A serum multiple cytokine analysis revealed that the levels of the chemokine interferon gamma inducible protein 10 (Interferon gamma-induced protein (IP)-10; C-X-C motif chemokine (CXCL)-10 increased stepwise from healthy volunteers to NAFL and NASH patients. A TLR-2 ligand peptidoglycan in combination with an in vitro insulin resistance condition (i.e., high glucose with insulin in the culture medium) increased the expression of IP-10 mRNA, indicating the importance of insulin resistance with bacterial signals in NASH progression [30]. Therefore, the diet helps to establish a close relationship among the gut microbiota, oxidative stress and NAFLD/NASH.

3. Treatments for NAFLD/NASH

The treatment strategy of NAFLD involves intervention with diet, exercise, and drugs [13,31–34]. Lifestyle interventions, including diet and exercise, are strongly related to insulin resistance and dyslipidemia. A randomized, controlled trial testing simple weight loss gain by lifestyle intervention using a combination of diet, exercise, and behavior modification resulted in NASH pathological improvement [35]. Insulin resistance has been shown to be an independent predictor of NASH in biopsy-proven cases that were likely to be controllable by any method, including lifestyle intervention [36]. Dyslipidemia has various causes, such as hereditary predisposition, a sedentary lifestyle, and a high calorie intake. The improvement of dyslipidemia may resolve NASH progression, and nutritional support, such as low-fat and low-calorie diets, holds a prominent position in treatment approaches [37,38].

Vitamin E is the most commonly used antioxidant treatment for NASH [39]. Pioglitazone, an antihyperglycemic drug, is reported to ameliorate liver injury and fibrosis in patients with NASH with and without diabetes [33]. Sanyal et al. reported that vitamin E therapy was effective for NAFLD improvement compared with pioglitazone and placebo and recommended antioxidant treatment as well as lifestyle intervention, bariatric surgery, dyslipidemia treatment, and diabetes treatment [13]. On the basis of these data, the American Association for the Study of Liver Diseases (AASLD) recommends treating NASH with vitamin E [40]. However, the Treatment of NAFLD in Children (TONIC) randomized trial showed that neither metformin nor vitamin E improved the liver function in patients with NAFLD [41]. A meta-analysis of randomized controlled trials revealed that vitamin E and pioglitazone but not metformin improved the histological activity of NASH [42]. However, the efficacy of these drugs is still controversial, and further clinical studies including assessments of long-term outcomes should be conducted.

Probiotics are reported to be a promising treatment option for NAFLD, improving the liver function, obesity, and insulin resistance [43]. Shavakhi et al. reported that metformin in combination with probiotics improved liver inflammation to a significantly greater degree than metformin alone [44]. This effect may be caused by the association between the gut microbiota and liver, which receives blood from the intestine through the portal vein.

Surgical treatments, such as bariatric surgery and liver transplantation, are conceivable treatments for NAFLD/NASH. Bariatric surgery for obesity is effective for improving NASH, as weight loss can improve dyslipidemia and hepatic fibrosis [45,46]. It also decreases the mortality rate due to diabetes, cardiology events, and malignant tumors. Liver transplantation is another treatment option for NAFLD/NASH related end-stage cirrhosis [47]. However, NASH can occur after liver transplantations, and continuous medical approaches are needed [48].

4. Carcinogenesis and Cancer Progression in Correlation with Oxidative Stress and Antioxidant Treatment

Hepatocellular carcinoma (HCC) is the major malignant liver tumor and the main cause of death in NAFLD/NASH patients. Oxidative stress is strongly associated with hepatocarcinogenesis and cancer progression. However, the effects on cancer-free patients and patients with HCC are likely different. Oxidative stress has a driving effect on carcinogenesis while also exerting toxicity against cancer cells. This contradiction will be discussed in this section.

4.1. Oxidative Stress in NASH-Hepatocarcinogenesis

Oxidative stress is reported to induce various events related to carcinogenesis such as DNA damage, tissue remodeling, and alterations in gene expression [11,49,50]. ROS production is stimulated by inflammatory factors, and oxidative stress promotes oncogenic transformation due to DNA-damage. ROS activates various pathways, such as Wingless-type MMTV intefration site family (Wnt) / β-catenin, NF-kB, or myc proto-oncogene protein (c-Myc)/Transforming growth factor (TGF)-α. This activation also occurs in carcinogenesis in liver cancer. Inducible nitric oxide synthase (iNOS), which produces nitrogen monoxides (NO), correlates with chronic inflammation, cell proliferation, DNA repair, migration, and angiogenesis [51]. The iNOS activity is important for endothelial stress gene expression, which protects against oxidative stress, and may be the key modulator of hepatocarcinogenesis.

8-hydroxydeoxyguanosine (8-OHdG), which is produced by DNA-damage with ROS, reflects the amount of oxidative stress and generates a point mutation in DNA double strands. Kawanishi et al. reported that 8-OHdG, which is a reliable marker for oxidative stress in the liver, strongly correlates with infection-related carcinogenesis via chronic inflammation [52]. Seki et al. reported that the 8-OHdG expression in the liver tissue is related to the pathological features of NAFLD and hepatocarcinogenesis [53].

Adenosine monophosphate activated protein kinase (AMPK) is a highly conserved heterodimeric serine-threonine kinase that plays a role in cellular energy homeostasis and different fundamental cellular processes such as the cellular proliferation, survival, and metabolism. It serves as an energy sensor in eukaryotic cells and bridges metabolism to carcinogenesis [54]. Its activated form (phospho (p)-AMPK) is down-regulated in HCC tissues from patients and low levels of p-AMPK correlate with a poor prognosis, indicating the importance of AMPK signaling in HCC [55]. AMPK signaling has recently been indicated to correlate with inflammatory responses, as the energy metabolism in immune cells is related to immunoregulation [56]. Under many oxidative stress-related conditions, such as diabetes or dyslipidemia, a diminished AMPK activity has been shown to be associated with tissue oxidative stress [57,58].

As mentioned above, oxidative stress is linked to the progression from NAFLD to HCC. The correlation of AMPK and clinical conditions encourage us to control AMPK as a cancer regulator.

4.2. Antioxidant Treatment Effects on Prevention of NASH-Hepatocarcinogenesis

Given that advanced chronic liver disease is the strongest risk factor for hepatocarcinogenesis, antioxidant treatments can be an important approach to preventing HCC development from NASH. The effect of these agents concerning whether they have the properties to protect against hepatocarcinogenesis should include an improvement in liver fibrosis improvement.

Vitamin E was reported to prevent hepatocarcinogenesis via the down-regulation of iNOS and nicotinamide adenine dinucleotide phosphate (NADPH) oxidase [59]. Many clinical studies have reported that vitamin E improves NAFLD and prevents the development of HCC [13,60–62]. However, these studies were all performed over a relatively short period (i.e., within two years). Hepatocarcinogenesis progresses from NAFL/NASH to cirrhosis over a long period of time, and middle-aged men carry risks of hepatocarcinogenesis even at an early stage of NAFLD [63]. The long-term outcomes must be evaluated in order to judge the true efficacy of antioxidant therapy for NASH-hepatocarcinogenesis.

Many candidate antioxidant agents may show favorable effects on NASH and NASH-related hepatocarcinogenesis.

Anti-diabetic agents such as metformin, pioglitazone, glucagon-like peptide 1-receptor agonists (GLP-1 RAs), and dipeptidyl-peptidase-4 inhibitors (DPP-4Is) were recently found to show favorable effects on the NAFLD clinical course [7,64,65]. Metformin and pioglitazone in particular are regarded as anti-oxidant agents. Metformin is the most well-studied AMPK-activating agent. Metformin-related AMPK pathway activation is involved in many cell types including T cells, B cells, hepatocytes, and even liver fibrosis-inducing hepatic stellate cells (HSCs). In in vitro and in vivo models (mice), metformin suppressed alpha smooth muscle actin (α-SMA) expression via AMPK activation and the inhibition of the succinate-related pathway in (HSCs) [66]. HSC activation is an important step in hepatocarcinogenesis. In addition, metformin induces the production of the antioxidant enzyme, heme oxygenase-1 (HO-1) in human endothelial cells via the nuclear factor erythroid 2-related factor (Nrf2) signaling pathway [67]. Determining metformin's long-term effects on reducing the risk of hepatocarcinogenesis might require further long-term studies.

Pioglitazone is a thiazolidinedione activating peroxisome proliferator-activated receptor (PPAR) γ that improves the insulin resistance and is used to treat type 2 diabetes. A six-month randomized study of pioglitazone revealed a reduction in necroinflammation of liver histopathology with no reduction in fibrosis [68]. L-carnitine is an essential nutrient and an important molecule in regulating mitochondrial and peroxisomal metabolism [69]. A recent randomized controlled study indicated histological improvement of liver fibrosis after 18 months with pioglitazone for NASH in patients with concomitant type 2 diabetes [70]. This agent may therefore be effective for inhibiting NAFL progression to NASH and hepatocarcinogenesis.

Flavonoids are heterogeneous polyphenols found in various plants, such as fruits, vegetables, and green tea that reportedly exert antioxidative function protecting the liver tissue from damage caused by ROS [71]. A mixture of flavonolignans and minor polyphenolic compounds, derived from the milk thistle plant (*Silybum marianum*) known as silymarin, is said to be an antioxidative agent [72]. Salomone et al. reported that silibinin, the main component of silymarin, restored nicotinamide adenine dinucleotide (NAD+) levels, and played a protective role against NAFLD [73]. In a randomized, double-blind, placebo-controlled study, silymarin at 700 mg three times daily for 48 weeks significantly ameliorated liver fibrosis in NASH patients [74]. Silymarin may therefore be a promising agent for the treatment of NAFLD/NASH patients.

L-carnitine acts as an antioxidant mediator by controlling the β-oxidation cycle and adenosine triphosphate (ATP) generation [75]. L-carnitine is well known as a fat-burning supplement; however, it has recently attracted attention as an anti-cancer agent because of its effects as an antioxidant, apoptosis inducer, and inhibitor of histone deacetylase [76–79]. We previously reported that L-carnitine controls the mitochondrial function in hepatic non-cancerous tissue from a mouse NASH model by upregulating the *Lactobacillales* population related to the secondary bile acid production in the gut microbiota [76]. L-carnitine does not eliminate oxidative stress but rather controls the oxidative balance to aid the mitochondrial function. This might be a better approach to regulating oxidative stress.

High levels of plasma free fatty acids increase the levels of hepatic free fatty acids. Long-chain fatty acids taken up by mitochondria as complexes with L-carnitine are subsequently metabolized in β-oxidation pathways. Under oxidative stress, oxidative reactions convert oxidized cofactors (NAD+ and flavin adenine dinucleotide (FAD)) into reduced cofactors (nicotinamide adenine dinucleotide (NADH) and flavin adenine dinucleotide H2 (FADH2)) and deliver electrons to the respiratory chain. An imbalance between the increased delivery of electrons to the respiratory chain and the decreased outflow from the respiratory chain causes electrons and ROS products to accumulate. Antioxidant defenses, such as superoxide dismutase (SOD), glutathione peroxidase (GPx), or catalase, can metabolize $O_2\cdot$ and H_2O_2 to non-toxic H_2O. However, the Fenton and/or Haber-Weiss reactions generate highly reactive, toxic, hydroxyl radicals (OH). Vitamin E as a general cytotoxic ROS scavenger erases oxidative stress. Metformin activates AMPK and induces antioxidant gene transcription, and 5-aminoimidazole-4-carboxamide-1-β-D-ribofuranoside (AICAR) activates Nrf2 via a mechanism possibly similar to that of metformin. L-carnitine supports the mitochondrial function to increase the long-chain fatty acid uptake. In NASH patients, oxidative stress works as toxic from NASH progression to cancer development. However, in cancer patients, oxidative stress should be maintained to some degree in order to control cancer via toxic oxidative stress reactions. To control cancer progression, AMPK/mammalian target of rapamycin (mTOR) signaling has an important function that would be a target to intervene.

4.3. Antioxidant Treatment Effects on Liver Cancer

Various treatments have been proposed for HCC, such as surgical approaches (e.g., liver resection, liver transplantation), radio frequency ablation, transcatheter arterial chemoembolization, and chemotherapy [80]. However, HCC remains incurable because of the low response rate and frequent recurrence based on chronic liver inflammation and fibrosis. Many reports have described the usage of antioxidant therapies for HCC, but their efficacy still remains unclear [81–83].

Metformin inhibits the cell growth of HCC by regulating AMPK activation and inducing apoptosis [84]. The effect of metformin on NASH-related HCC in mouse models has been reported, but the clinical effect in humans is unclear [85].

The AMPK activator 5-aminoimidazole-4-carboxamide-1-β-D-ribofuranoside (AICAR) activates Nrf2 protein, which binds to Kelch-like ECH associated protein 1 (Keap1), a protein that exists in the cytoplasm in an inactive form [86]. AICAR may be a candidate for treating liver cancer.

Flavonoid and polyphenols have been shown to exert antitumor effects through the control of various molecular pathways [81,87]. Curcumin is an antioxidant polyphenol compound reported to exert antitumor activities by inhibiting the vascular endothelial growth factor (VEGF) expression and phosphoinositide 3-kinase (PI3K)/v-Akt murine thymoma viral oncogene (Akt) signaling [82]. The newly confirmed antioxidant silymarin has also been analyzed for its utility in preventing hepaticarcinogenesis [73].

L-carnitine is a mitochondria supporting agent that may be useful for controlling oxidative stress in HCC patients. Our previous report showed that the tumor number and maximum tumor size were decreased in NASH-HCC mouse models than control diet [76]. In that experiment, L-carnitine was administered from the early onset of NASH, and the liver tumor outcomes were assessed afterwards. Under such conditions, L-carnitine improved the NASH pathogenesis resulting in decreased NASH related hepatocarcinogenesis and so is difficult to conclude whether its use is beneficial for HCC. To answer this point, we next examined the effect of L-carnitine administration after hepatocarcinogenesis in NASH-related cholangiocarcinoma-like tumors [88]. L-carnitine resulted in a good outcome for this model, suggesting it might be an effective antioxidant even after cancer development.

As above, many candidate antioxidant treatments have been proposed for HCC; however, the clinical investigations on this point are inadequate at present. To administer antioxidants for cancer stages, we must consider the oxidative stress-related environment adequately (Figure 1).

Recently, oral chemotherapeutic multi-kinase inhibitors such as sorafenib have been widely used to control advanced-stage HCC. Sorafenib inhibits tumor cell proliferation and angiogenesis through the inactivation of vascular endothelial growth factor receptor (VEGFR), platelet-derived growth factor receptor (PDGFR), and the serine-threonine kinase Raf-1, which participates in the Rat sarcoma (Ras)/rapidly accelerated fibrosarcoma (Raf)/mitogen-activated protein kinase kinase (MEK)/mitogen-activated protein kinase (MAPK) signal cascade [89]. Recently, other multi-kinase inhibitors such as lenvatinib, regorafenib, cabozantinib, and ramucirumab have also been developed [90–92]. Recent clinical experience with sorafenib has indicated that acquired drug resistance can occur over a long period of drug administration. Thus, in these stages of HCC, the effects of accompanying agents such as antioxidants on the drug resistance should be investigated. Accumulating data indicate that autophagy and phosphoinositide 3-kinase (PI3K)/Akt signaling are associated with acquired resistance to sorafenib in HCC. The AMPK/mTOR signaling pathway had been demonstrated to be important in autophagy. A high sustained glucose condition produces advanced glycation products (AGEs) which damage many organs including the liver. The receptor for AGE (RAGE) has been shown to be overexpressed in HCC promoting proliferation. In addition, RAGE induced sorafenib resistance in in vitro and in vivo xenograft models [93]. A reduction in RAGE was also found to be able to increase autophagy and eliminate sorafenib resistance in vitro via the AMPK pathway activation. Metformin was able to reduce RAGE expression and helped rescue cells from sorafenib resistance. Metformin might therefore be useful for eliminating sorafenib resistance in

HCC; however, one clinical study reported a bad outcome for patients administered metformin with sorafenib [94].

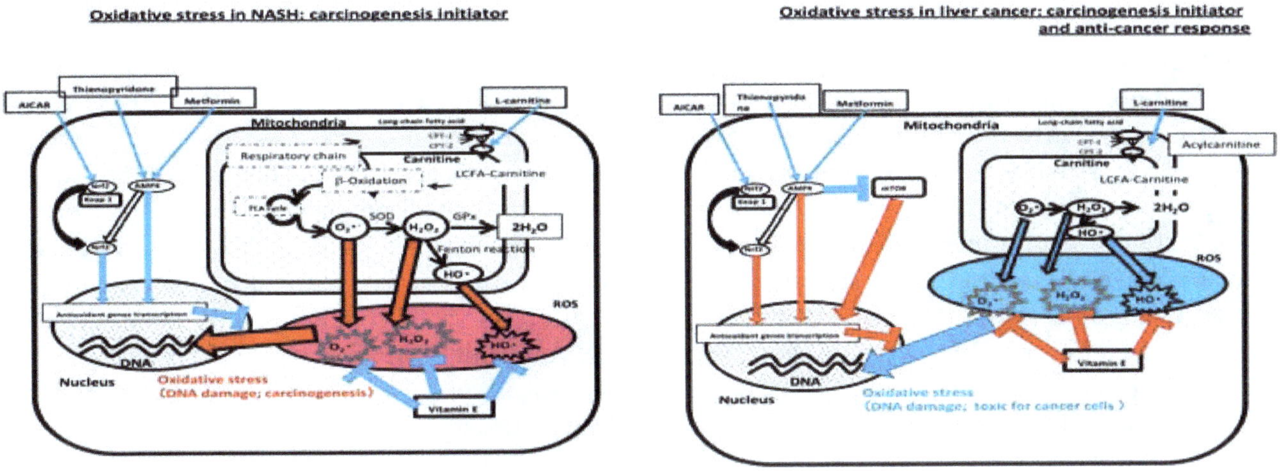

Figure 1. Oxidative stress and anti-oxidant in non-alcoholic steatohepatitis (NASH) and liver cancer. Red lines; unfavorable effects, Blue lines; favorable effects, AICAR, 5-aminoimidazole-4-carboxamide-1-β-D-ribofuranoside; Nrf2, nuclear factor erythroid 2-related factor; AMPK, AMP-activated protein kinase; Keap1, Kelch-like enoyl-CoA hydratase (ECH) associated protein; Nrf2, nuclear factor erythroid 2-related factor; CPT, carnitine palmitoyltransferase; SOD, superoxide dismutase; GPx, glutathione peroxidase; LCFA-carnitine, long-chain acylcarnitine; TCA-cycle, tricarboxylic acid cycle.

Administering sorafenib efficacy-supporting agents is an approach to resolving drug resistance as mentioned above with metformin. The oxidative stress-inducing agent tetrandrine, a bisbenzylisoquinoline alkaloid, has been shown to exert synergistic anti-tumor activity with sorafenib by increasing ROS [95]. More data on such combination therapy with sorafenib will be required to draw more solid conclusions.

Immune checkpoint molecules including programmed cell death-1 (PD-1) and programmed cell death-1 ligand (PD-L1), are promising new therapeutic agents for the treatment of various cancers including HCC [96]. Nivolumab, an anti-PD-1 antibody, was approved by the Food and Drug Administration (FDA) and is a key drug for the treatment of HCC dramatically improving the survival of many cancers, including solid-tumors; however, 30 to 50% of patients are unresponsive [97]. To overcome this unresponsiveness, several combination treatments have been attempted. An in vivo analysis of CD8+ T cells treated with PD-1 antibody revealed that a highly proliferative fraction could be found in the draining lymph node indicating that tumor priming was necessary for CD8+ T cell activation [98]. These highly proliferative CD8+ T cells contained more cellular ROS, a larger mitochondrial mass, higher mitochondrial potential, and more mitochondrial superoxide than CD8+ T cells without PD-1 antibody treatment, indicating the activation of mitochondria in T cells. Several mitochondrial function activators have been tested for their additive effects of PD-1 blockade with successful results. Of them, the PPAR-α agonist bezafibrate showed a particularly promising response. Given that bezafibrate is a standard agent for treating high triglyceride levels, this combination might be useful for combination therapy. The relationship between oxidative stress, antioxidants, and PD-1/PD-L1 needs further study and clinical trials to resolve the issue of a lack of responsiveness to anti-PD-1 antibody therapy.

4.4. Cautions of Antioxidants on Liver Cancer Initiation and Maintenance

Whether or not antioxidant agents prevent cancer risks remains controversial. The U.S. Preventive Services Task Force (USPSTF) stated that the current evidence is insufficient to assess the balance of benefits and harms of vitamins [99]. In particular, excessive doses of vitamins may induce negative effects. Four randomized controlled trials (RCTs) of vitamin E included in the USPSTF comments showed no significant effect on the incidence of all types of cancer or cancer mortality rates. However, one RCT assessing the risk of prostate cancer with vitamin E administration found a 17% increase in the prostate cancer incidence with this supplement [100]. Since a large prospective study to confirm the HCC risks for NASH is difficult to perform and requires a long observation time (although there are some ongoing studies), we should attempt to determine the optimum treatment approach based on short-term data from small populations and experimental data.

Oxidative stress is a crucial event for cancer initiation; however, it also has important roles in cancer prevention. Stem cell-like cancer cells have powerful antioxidative properties that protect them from oxidative stress and thus prevent self-apoptosis [101]. The expression of CD44 variant 9 (CD44v9) has recently been investigated as a functional marker of stem-like cells in many types of cancers [102]. The interaction of CD44v9 with xc- Substrate-specific Subunit (xCT), also called the glutamate/cysteine antiporter solute carrier family 7 member 11 (SLC7A11), a subunit of the glutamate-cystine transporter system xc-, stabilizes the latter and thereby potentiates cancer cells to promote glutathione synthesis and reduce the activity of cellular redox system, resulting in resistance to toxic oxidative stresses [103]. Inducing oxidative stress in cancer patients is an approach that is being investigated as a cancer treatment in several clinical trials [104]. However, this approach is likely to also be toxic to normal cells and may lead to the induction of further carcinogenesis. Furthermore, given that treatment-resistant cancer stem cells can still escape toxic oxidative stress, maintaining moderate oxidative stress is a critical point of anti-oxidative stress treatment for cancer patients.

Mitochondrial function-supporting agents, such as metformin or L-carnitine, might be good therapies to investigate in large-scale prospective studies in humans. In cancer patients, the drug effects should be analyzed according to the stages of the cancer. When tumors have been completely resected or ablated, a standard anti-oxidant approach may be effective for preventing new hepatocarcinogenesis. When tumors have not been ablated completely but can be managed with local treatment, such as transcatheter arterial chemo-embolization (TACE), mitochondrial function-supporting agents, such as metformin or L-carnitine, might be useful approaches for controlling the oxidative-antioxidative stress balance. When tumors are not being treated with local therapies but instead managed with anti-cancer agents, presently multi-kinase inhibitors such as sorafenib, regorafenib and lenvatinib, oxidative stress may be an important cellular stress to cancer cells not to be eliminated. As mentioned in previous section, oxidative stress-inducing agents may compound the effects of sorafenib [95]. However, even the favorably reported antioxidant metformin might adversely affect the clinical outcome in patients with HCC receiving the multi-kinase inhibitor sorafenib [94].

L-carnitine is a candidate drug that has shown good efficacy even after cancer has already developed. We previously investigated the effects of the standard anti-oxidant agents vitamin E and L-carnitine and found that only L-carnitine reduced the number of liver tumors [88]. Vitamin E administration induced HO-1 protein expression in cancer tissue, resulting in an increase in the number of stem-like cancer cells. Furthermore, L-carnitine administration improved the *Lactobacillales* population and the balance of bile acid (primary to secondary bile acid), while vitamin E did not affect the intestinal environment. These findings show that vitamin E strongly ameliorates the oxidative stress in both cancer cells and normal cells, while L-carnitine works as an "oxidative stress balancer". An "oxidative stress eraser" such as vitamin E might therefore be unsuitable for the treatment of cancer patients. However, even L-carnitine carries the possibility of an increased risk of experimental HCC [105]. A mouse HCC model of diethylnitrosamine (DEN)-injected mice fed a high-fat diet showed the predominance of acylcarnitine species in the tumors according to a metabolomic profiling analysis. Intracellular long-chain fatty acids are esterified to acyl-coenzyme A and conjugated with carnitine resulting in acylcarnitine by carnitine palmitoyltransferase 1 (CPT 1). The acylcarnitine is then converted back to acyl-coenzyme A by CPT2 and enters the β-oxidation pathway. Of note, the CPT2 expression was diminished in the HCC tumors inducing acylcarnitine deposition. In this mouse model, L-carnitine supplementation resulted in an increased amount of acylcarnitines and enhanced HCC tumorigenesis. These conflicting results suggest that the HCC-preventive effects of L-carnitine might require a preserved CPT2 function in order to avoid inducing the accumulation of acylcarnitines.

It should be noted that almost all antioxidants can elicit unfavorable effects on carcinogenesis under certain conditions. We must bear these facts in mind and thus perform antioxidant supplementation judiciously. We can use antioxidant for NASH, while should decide whether to stop after HCC development (Figure 2).

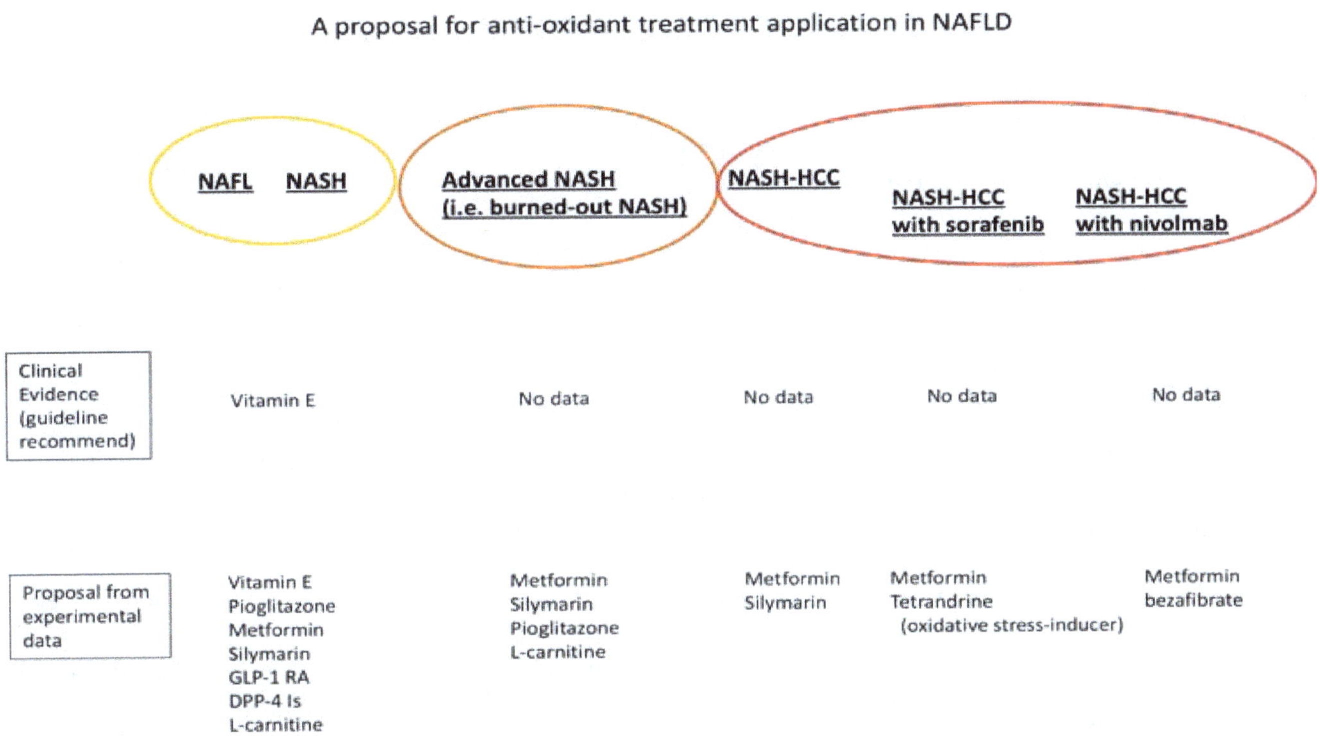

Figure 2. A proposal for the antioxidant treatment application in non-alcoholic fatty liver disease (NAFLD). NAFL, non-alcoholic fatty liver; NASH, Non-alcoholic steatohepatitis; HCC, hepatocellular carcinoma; GLP-1 RA, glucagon-like peptide 1-receptor agonist; DPP-4 Is, dipeptidyl-peptidase-4 inhibitors.

Several guidelines recommend vitamin E be administered for NASH, as some prospective studies proved to be beneficial for laboratory data and histological activity. However, there are no prospective data on NASH with diminished activity and steatosis with advanced fibrosis, such as burned-out NASH. There are also no data on NASH-HCC. Many experimental studies recommend antioxidant agents be administered for patients with NAFL and NASH. Given that advanced NASH often shows no steatosis, some antioxidants may be more suitable for these patients than others. For NASH-HCC, given that oxidative stress is an important stress response for regulating cancer cells, strong antioxidants may actually be harmful. When we administer oxidative stress-related agents together with sorafenib and other multi-kinase inhibitors, combination effects may be exerted by oxidative stress-inducing agents. The AMPK activator metformin has been shown to be beneficial for HCC, although clinical evidence is still being discussed. Nivolmab is a next-step HCC treatment approach for activating the cancer immune response. Bezafibrate has been shown to exert additive effects to activate the T cell response.

5. Conclusions

NAFLD is a major lifestyle-related disease, and nutritional support is an important approach to its treatment. Antioxidant therapy, such as vitamin E administration, is effective for preventing NASH progression; however, the long-term outcomes of this therapy are unclear, especially in precancerous and cancer patients. Antioxidant therapy should be prescribed according to the clinical condition of the patients, such as those with NAFL, NASH, advanced NASH, cancer with successful ablation, cancer with relative ablation, and advanced cancer requiring anti-cancer agents. In HCC patients, antioxidant treatment should be carefully managed, as these agents can also act against tumor resolution.

Author Contributions: Conceptualization, A.T. and D.U.; Methodology, A.T. and D.U.; Writing-Original Draft Preparation, D.U.; Writing-Review & Editing, A.T., T.A.; Supervision, H.O.

References

1. Pacifico, L.; Anania, C.; Martino, F.; Poggiogalle, E.; Chiarelli, F.; Arca, M.; Chiesa, C. Management of metabolic syndrome in children and adolescents. *Nutr. Metab. Cardiovasc. Dis.* **2011**, *21*, 455–466. [CrossRef] [PubMed]
2. Doycheva, I.; Watt, K.D.; Alkhouri, N. Nonalcoholic fatty liver disease in adolescents and young adults: The next frontier in the epidemic. *Hepatology* **2017**, *65*, 2100–2109. [CrossRef] [PubMed]
3. Smith, B.W.; Adams, L.A. Non-alcoholic fatty liver disease. *Crit. Rev. Clin. Lab. Sci.* **2011**, *48*, 97–113. [CrossRef] [PubMed]
4. Matteoni, C.A.; Younossi, Z.M.; Gramlich, T.; Boparai, N.; Liu, Y.C.; McCullough, A.J. Nonalcoholic fatty liver disease: A spectrum of clinical and pathological severity. *Gastroenterology* **1999**, *116*, 1413–1419. [CrossRef]
5. Ono, M.; Saibara, T. Clinical features of nonalcoholic steatohepatitis in Japan: Evidence from the literature. *J. Gastroenterol.* **2006**, *41*, 725–732. [CrossRef] [PubMed]
6. Gentile, C.L.; Pagliassotti, M.J. The role of fatty acids in the development and progression of nonalcoholic fatty liver disease. *J. Nutr. Biochem.* **2008**, *19*, 567–576. [CrossRef] [PubMed]
7. Takaki, A.; Kawai, D.; Yamamoto, K. Molecular mechanisms and new treatment strategies for non-alcoholic steatohepatitis (NASH). *Int. J. Mol. Sci.* **2014**, *15*, 7352–7379. [CrossRef] [PubMed]
8. Tilg, H.; Moschen, A.R. Evolution of inflammation in nonalcoholic fatty liver disease: The multiple parallel hits hypothesis. *Hepatology* **2010**, *52*, 1836–1846. [CrossRef] [PubMed]
9. Pessayre, D. Role of mitochondria in non-alcoholic fatty liver disease. *J. Gastroenterol. Hepatol.* **2007**, *22* (Suppl. S1), 20–27. [CrossRef] [PubMed]
10. Muriel, P. Role of free radicals in liver diseases. *Hepatol. Int.* **2009**, *3*, 526–536. [CrossRef] [PubMed]
11. Yongvanit, P.; Pinlaor, S.; Bartsch, H. Oxidative and nitrative DNA damage: Key events in opisthorchiasis-induced carcinogenesis. *Parasitol. Int.* **2012**, *61*, 130–135. [CrossRef] [PubMed]
12. Al-Busafi, S.A.; Bhat, M.; Wong, P.; Ghali, P.; Deschenes, M. Antioxidant therapy in nonalcoholic steatohepatitis. *Hepat. Res. Treat.* **2012**, *2012*, 947575. [CrossRef] [PubMed]
13. Sanyal, A.J.; Chalasani, N.; Kowdley, K.V.; McCullough, A.; Diehl, A.M.; Bass, N.M.; Neuschwander-Tetri, B.A.; Lavine, J.E.; Tonascia, J.; Unalp, A.; et al. Pioglitazone, vitamin E, or placebo for nonalcoholic steatohepatitis. *N. Engl. J. Med.* **2010**, *362*, 1675–1685. [CrossRef] [PubMed]
14. Albano, E.; Mottaran, E.; Occhino, G.; Reale, E.; Vidali, M. Review article: Role of oxidative stress in the progression of non-alcoholic steatosis. *Aliment. Pharmacol. Ther.* **2005**, *22* (Suppl. S2), 71–73. [CrossRef] [PubMed]
15. Seki, S.; Kitada, T.; Yamada, T.; Sakaguchi, H.; Nakatani, K.; Wakasa, K. In situ detection of lipid peroxidation and oxidative DNA damage in non-alcoholic fatty liver diseases. *J. Hepatol.* **2002**, *37*, 56–62. [CrossRef]
16. Begriche, K.; Igoudjil, A.; Pessayre, D.; Fromenty, B. Mitochondrial dysfunction in NASH: Causes, consequences and possible means to prevent it. *Mitochondrion* **2006**, *6*, 1–28. [CrossRef] [PubMed]
17. Csak, T.; Ganz, M.; Pespisa, J.; Kodys, K.; Dolganiuc, A.; Szabo, G. Fatty acid and endotoxin activate inflammasomes in mouse hepatocytes that release danger signals to stimulate immune cells. *Hepatology* **2011**, *54*, 133–144. [CrossRef] [PubMed]
18. Ohta, S. Molecular hydrogen as a preventive and therapeutic medical gas: Initiation, development and potential of hydrogen medicine. *Pharmacol. Ther.* **2014**, *144*, 1–11. [CrossRef] [PubMed]
19. Honma, M.; Sawada, S.; Ueno, Y.; Murakami, K.; Yamada, T.; Gao, J.; Kodama, S.; Izumi, T.; Takahashi, K.; Tsukita, S.; et al. Selective insulin resistance with differential expressions of IRS-1 and IRS-2 in human NAFLD livers. *Int. J. Obes.* **2018**. [CrossRef] [PubMed]

20. Musso, G.; Gambino, R.; Cassader, M. Cholesterol metabolism and the pathogenesis of non-alcoholic steatohepatitis. *Prog. Lipid Res.* **2013**, *52*, 175–191. [CrossRef] [PubMed]
21. Van Rooyen, D.M.; Larter, C.Z.; Haigh, W.G.; Yeh, M.M.; Ioannou, G.; Kuver, R.; Lee, S.P.; Teoh, N.C.; Farrell, G.C. Hepatic free cholesterol accumulates in obese, diabetic mice and causes nonalcoholic steatohepatitis. *Gastroenterology* **2011**, *141*, 1393–1403. [CrossRef] [PubMed]
22. Preiss-Landl, K.; Zimmermann, R.; Hammerle, G.; Zechner, R. Lipoprotein lipase: The regulation of tissue specific expression and its role in lipid and energy metabolism. *Curr. Opin. Lipidol.* **2002**, *13*, 471–481. [CrossRef] [PubMed]
23. Zhang, L.; Zhang, Z.; Li, Y.; Liao, S.; Wu, X.; Chang, Q.; Liang, B. Cholesterol induces lipoprotein lipase expression in a tree shrew (Tupaia belangeri chinensis) model of non-alcoholic fatty liver disease. *Sci. Rep.* **2015**, *5*, 15970. [CrossRef] [PubMed]
24. Su, G.L. Lipopolysaccharides in liver injury: Molecular mechanisms of Kupffer cell activation. *Am. J. Physiol.-Gastrointest. Liver Physiol.* **2002**, *283*, G256–G265. [CrossRef] [PubMed]
25. Gratz, S.W.; Mykkanen, H.; El-Nezami, H.S. Probiotics and gut health: A special focus on liver diseases. *World J. Gastroenterol.* **2010**, *16*, 403–410. [CrossRef] [PubMed]
26. Backhed, F.; Ding, H.; Wang, T.; Hooper, L.V.; Koh, G.Y.; Nagy, A.; Semenkovich, C.F.; Gordon, J.I. The gut microbiota as an environmental factor that regulates fat storage. *Proc. Natl. Acad. Sci. USA* **2004**, *101*, 15718–15723. [CrossRef] [PubMed]
27. Zak-Golab, A.; Olszanecka-Glinianowicz, M.; Kocelak, P.; Chudek, J. The role of gut microbiota in the pathogenesis of obesity. *Postepy Hig. Med. Dosw. (Online)* **2014**, *68*, 84–90. [CrossRef] [PubMed]
28. Miller, Y.I.; Choi, S.H.; Wiesner, P.; Bae, Y.S. The SYK side of TLR4: Signalling mechanisms in response to LPS and minimally oxidized LDL. *Br. J. Pharmacol.* **2012**, *167*, 990–999. [CrossRef] [PubMed]
29. Miura, K.; Yang, L.; van Rooijen, N.; Brenner, D.A.; Ohnishi, H.; Seki, E. Toll-like receptor 2 and palmitic acid cooperatively contribute to the development of nonalcoholic steatohepatitis through inflammasome activation in mice. *Hepatology* **2013**, *57*, 577–589. [CrossRef] [PubMed]
30. Wada, N.; Takaki, A.; Ikeda, F.; Yasunaka, T.; Onji, M.; Nouso, K.; Nakatsuka, A.; Wada, J.; Koike, K.; Miyahara, K.; et al. Serum-inducible protein (IP)-10 is a disease progression-related marker for non-alcoholic fatty liver disease. *Hepatol. Int.* **2017**, *11*, 115–124. [CrossRef] [PubMed]
31. Ekstedt, M.; Franzen, L.E.; Mathiesen, U.L.; Thorelius, L.; Holmqvist, M.; Bodemar, G.; Kechagias, S. Long-term follow-up of patients with NAFLD and elevated liver enzymes. *Hepatology* **2006**, *44*, 865–873. [CrossRef] [PubMed]
32. Bradford, V.; Dillon, J.; Miller, M. Lifestyle interventions for the treatment of non-alcoholic fatty liver disease. *Hepat. Med.* **2014**, *6*, 1–10. [PubMed]
33. Aithal, G.P.; Thomas, J.A.; Kaye, P.V.; Lawson, A.; Ryder, S.D.; Spendlove, I.; Austin, A.S.; Freeman, J.G.; Morgan, L.; Webber, J. Randomized, placebo-controlled trial of pioglitazone in nondiabetic subjects with nonalcoholic steatohepatitis. *Gastroenterology* **2008**, *135*, 1176–1184. [CrossRef] [PubMed]
34. Nelson, J.E.; Roth, C.L.; Wilson, L.A.; Yates, K.P.; Aouizerat, B.; Morgan-Stevenson, V.; Whalen, E.; Hoofnagle, A.; Mason, M.; Gersuk, V.; et al. Vitamin D Deficiency Is Associated with Increased Risk of Non-alcoholic Steatohepatitis in Adults with Non-alcoholic Fatty Liver Disease: Possible Role for MAPK and NF-kappaB? *Am. J. Gastroenterol.* **2016**, *111*, 852–863. [CrossRef] [PubMed]
35. Promrat, K.; Kleiner, D.E.; Niemeier, H.M.; Jackvony, E.; Kearns, M.; Wands, J.R.; Fava, J.L.; Wing, R.R. Randomized controlled trial testing the effects of weight loss on nonalcoholic steatohepatitis. *Hepatology* **2010**, *51*, 121–129. [CrossRef] [PubMed]
36. Ballestri, S.; Nascimbeni, F.; Romagnoli, D.; Lonardo, A. The independent predictors of non-alcoholic steatohepatitis and its individual histological features. Insulin resistance, serum uric acid, metabolic syndrome, alanine aminotransferase and serum total cholesterol are a clue to pathogenesis and candidate targets for treatment. *Hepatol. Res.* **2016**, *46*, 1074–1087. [PubMed]
37. Targher, G.; Bertolini, L.; Rodella, S.; Tessari, R.; Zenari, L.; Lippi, G.; Arcaro, G. Nonalcoholic fatty liver disease is independently associated with an increased incidence of cardiovascular events in type 2 diabetic patients. *Diabetes Care* **2007**, *30*, 2119–2121. [CrossRef] [PubMed]
38. Corey, K.E.; Vuppalanchi, R.; Wilson, L.A.; Cummings, O.W.; Chalasani, N.; Nash, C.R.N. NASH resolution

is associated with improvements in HDL and triglyceride levels but not improvement in LDL or non-HDL-C levels. *Aliment. Pharmacol. Ther.* **2015**, *41*, 301–309. [CrossRef] [PubMed]
39. Watanabe, S.; Hashimoto, E.; Ikejima, K.; Uto, H.; Ono, M.; Sumida, Y.; Seike, M.; Takei, Y.; Takehara, T.; Tokushige, K.; et al. Evidence-based clinical practice guidelines for nonalcoholic fatty liver disease/nonalcoholic steatohepatitis. *J. Gastroenterol.* **2015**, *50*, 364–377. [CrossRef] [PubMed]
40. Chalasani, N.; Younossi, Z.; Lavine, J.E.; Diehl, A.M.; Brunt, E.M.; Cusi, K.; Charlton, M.; Sanyal, A.J. The diagnosis and management of non-alcoholic fatty liver disease: Practice Guideline by the American Association for the Study of Liver Diseases, American College of Gastroenterology, and the American Gastroenterological Association. *Hepatology* **2012**, *55*, 2005–2023. [CrossRef] [PubMed]
41. Lavine, J.E.; Schwimmer, J.B.; Van Natta, M.L.; Molleston, J.P.; Murray, K.F.; Rosenthal, P.; Abrams, S.H.; Scheimann, A.O.; Sanyal, A.J.; Chalasani, N.; et al. Effect of vitamin E or metformin for treatment of nonalcoholic fatty liver disease in children and adolescents: The TONIC randomized controlled trial. *JAMA* **2011**, *305*, 1659–1668. [CrossRef] [PubMed]
42. Said, A.; Akhter, A. Meta-Analysis of Randomized Controlled Trials of Pharmacologic Agents in Non-alcoholic Steatohepatitis. *Ann. Hepatol.* **2017**, *16*, 538–547. [CrossRef] [PubMed]
43. Lavekar, A.S.; Raje, D.V.; Manohar, T.; Lavekar, A.A. Role of Probiotics in the Treatment of Nonalcoholic Fatty Liver Disease: A Meta-analysis. *Euroasian J. Hepatogastroenterol.* **2017**, *7*, 130–137. [CrossRef] [PubMed]
44. Shavakhi, A.; Minakari, M.; Firouzian, H.; Assali, R.; Hekmatdoost, A.; Ferns, G. Effect of a Probiotic and Metformin on Liver Aminotransferases in Non-alcoholic Steatohepatitis: A Double Blind Randomized Clinical Trial. *Int. J. Prev. Med.* **2013**, *4*, 531–537. [PubMed]
45. Adams, T.D.; Gress, R.E.; Smith, S.C.; Halverson, R.C.; Simper, S.C.; Rosamond, W.D.; Lamonte, M.J.; Stroup, A.M.; Hunt, S.C. Long-term mortality after gastric bypass surgery. *N. Engl. J. Med.* **2007**, *357*, 753–761. [CrossRef] [PubMed]
46. Lassailly, G.; Caiazzo, R.; Buob, D.; Pigeyre, M.; Verkindt, H.; Labreuche, J.; Raverdy, V.; Leteurtre, E.; Dharancy, S.; Louvet, A.; et al. Bariatric Surgery Reduces Features of Nonalcoholic Steatohepatitis in Morbidly Obese Patients. *Gastroenterology* **2015**, *149*, 379–388. [CrossRef] [PubMed]
47. Wang, X.; Li, J.; Riaz, D.R.; Shi, G.; Liu, C.; Dai, Y. Outcomes of liver transplantation for nonalcoholic steatohepatitis: A systematic review and meta-analysis. *Clin. Gastroenterol. Hepatol.* **2014**, *12*, 394–402. [CrossRef] [PubMed]
48. Dare, A.J.; Plank, L.D.; Phillips, A.R.; Gane, E.J.; Harrison, B.; Orr, D.; Jiang, Y.; Bartlett, A.S. Additive effect of pretransplant obesity, diabetes, and cardiovascular risk factors on outcomes after liver transplantation. *Liver Transpl.* **2014**, *20*, 281–290. [CrossRef] [PubMed]
49. Georgakilas, A.G. Oxidative stress, DNA damage and repair in carcinogenesis: Have we established a connection? *Cancer Lett.* **2012**, *327*, 3–4. [CrossRef] [PubMed]
50. Vallee, A.; Lecarpentier, Y. Crosstalk between peroxisome proliferator-activated receptor gamma and the canonical wnt/beta-catenin pathway in chronic inflammation and oxidative stress during carcinogenesis. *Front. Immunol.* **2018**, *9*, 745. [CrossRef] [PubMed]
51. Sawa, T.; Ohshima, H. Nitrative DNA damage in inflammation and its possible role in carcinogenesis. *Nitric Oxide* **2006**, *14*, 91–100. [CrossRef] [PubMed]
52. Kawanishi, S.; Ohnishi, S.; Ma, N.; Hiraku, Y.; Oikawa, S.; Murata, M. Nitrative and oxidative DNA damage in infection-related carcinogenesis in relation to cancer stem cells. *Genes Environ.* **2016**, *38*, 26. [CrossRef] [PubMed]
53. Seki, S.; Kitada, T.; Sakaguchi, H. Clinicopathological significance of oxidative cellular damage in non-alcoholic fatty liver diseases. *Hepatol. Res.* **2005**, *33*, 132–134. [CrossRef] [PubMed]
54. Hardie, D.G.; Carling, D.; Carlson, M. The AMP-activated/SNF1 protein kinase subfamily: Metabolic sensors of the eukaryotic cell? *Annu. Rev. Biochem.* **1998**, *67*, 821–855. [CrossRef] [PubMed]
55. Zheng, L.; Yang, W.; Wu, F.; Wang, C.; Yu, L.; Tang, L.; Qiu, B.; Li, Y.; Guo, L.; Wu, M.; et al. Prognostic significance of AMPK activation and therapeutic effects of metformin in hepatocellular carcinoma. *Clin. Cancer Res.* **2013**, *19*, 5372–5380. [CrossRef] [PubMed]
56. Gubser, P.M.; Bantug, G.R.; Razik, L.; Fischer, M.; Dimeloe, S.; Hoenger, G.; Durovic, B.; Jauch, A.; Hess, C. Rapid effector function of memory CD8+ T cells requires an immediate-early glycolytic switch. *Nat. Immunol.* **2013**, *14*, 1064–1072. [CrossRef] [PubMed]

57. Cheng, X.; Siow, R.C.; Mann, G.E. Impaired redox signaling and antioxidant gene expression in endothelial cells in diabetes: A role for mitochondria and the nuclear factor-E2-related factor 2-Kelch-like ECH-associated protein 1 defense pathway. *Antioxid. Redox Signal.* **2011**, *14*, 469–487. [CrossRef] [PubMed]
58. Yamauchi, T.; Kamon, J.; Minokoshi, Y.; Ito, Y.; Waki, H.; Uchida, S.; Yamashita, S.; Noda, M.; Kita, S.; Ueki, K.; et al. Adiponectin stimulates glucose utilization and fatty-acid oxidation by activating AMP-activated protein kinase. *Nat. Med.* **2002**, *8*, 1288–1295. [CrossRef] [PubMed]
59. Calvisi, D.F.; Ladu, S.; Hironaka, K.; Factor, V.M.; Thorgeirsson, S.S. Vitamin E down-modulates iNOS and NADPH oxidase in c-Myc/TGF-alpha transgenic mouse model of liver cancer. *J. Hepatol.* **2004**, *41*, 815–822. [CrossRef] [PubMed]
60. Foster, T.; Budoff, M.J.; Saab, S.; Ahmadi, N.; Gordon, C.; Guerci, A.D. Atorvastatin and antioxidants for the treatment of nonalcoholic fatty liver disease: The St Francis Heart Study randomized clinical trial. *Am. J. Gastroenterol.* **2011**, *106*, 71–77. [CrossRef] [PubMed]
61. Dufour, J.F.; Oneta, C.M.; Gonvers, J.J.; Bihl, F.; Cerny, A.; Cereda, J.M.; Zala, J.F.; Helbling, B.; Steuerwald, M.; Zimmermann, A.; et al. Randomized placebo-controlled trial of ursodeoxycholic acid with vitamin e in nonalcoholic steatohepatitis. *Clin. Gastroenterol. Hepatol.* **2006**, *4*, 1537–1543. [CrossRef] [PubMed]
62. Kawanaka, M.; Mahmood, S.; Niiyama, G.; Izumi, A.; Kamei, A.; Ikeda, H.; Suehiro, M.; Togawa, K.; Sasagawa, T.; Okita, M.; et al. Control of oxidative stress and reduction in biochemical markers by Vitamin E treatment in patients with nonalcoholic steatohepatitis: A pilot study. *Hepatol. Res.* **2004**, *29*, 39–41. [CrossRef] [PubMed]
63. Tokushige, K.; Hyogo, H.; Nakajima, T.; Ono, M.; Kawaguchi, T.; Honda, K.; Eguchi, Y.; Nozaki, Y.; Kawanaka, M.; Tanaka, S.; et al. Hepatocellular carcinoma in Japanese patients with nonalcoholic fatty liver disease and alcoholic liver disease: Multicenter survey. *J. Gastroenterol.* **2016**, *51*, 586–596. [CrossRef] [PubMed]
64. Carbone, L.J.; Angus, P.W.; Yeomans, N.D. Incretin-based therapies for the treatment of non-alcoholic fatty liver disease: A systematic review and meta-analysis. *J. Gastroenterol. Hepatol.* **2016**, *31*, 23–31. [CrossRef] [PubMed]
65. Takaki, A.; Kawai, D.; Yamamoto, K. Multiple hits, including oxidative stress, as pathogenesis and treatment target in non-alcoholic steatohepatitis (NASH). *Int. J. Mol. Sci.* **2013**, *14*, 20704–20728. [CrossRef] [PubMed]
66. Nguyen, G.; Park, S.Y.; Le, C.T.; Park, W.S.; Choi, D.H.; Cho, E.H. Metformin ameliorates activation of hepatic stellate cells and hepatic fibrosis by succinate and GPR91 inhibition. *Biochem. Biophys. Res. Commun.* **2018**, *495*, 2649–2656. [CrossRef] [PubMed]
67. Liu, X.M.; Peyton, K.J.; Shebib, A.R.; Wang, H.; Korthuis, R.J.; Durante, W. Activation of AMPK stimulates heme oxygenase-1 gene expression and human endothelial cell survival. *Am. J. Physiol. Heart Circ. Physiol.* **2011**, *300*, H84–H93. [CrossRef] [PubMed]
68. Belfort, R.; Harrison, S.A.; Brown, K.; Darland, C.; Finch, J.; Hardies, J.; Balas, B.; Gastaldelli, A.; Tio, F.; Pulcini, J.; et al. A placebo-controlled trial of pioglitazone in subjects with nonalcoholic steatohepatitis. *N. Engl. J. Med.* **2006**, *355*, 2297–2307. [CrossRef] [PubMed]
69. Walter, P.; Schaffhauser, A.O. L-Carnitine, a Vitamin-like Substance for functional food. *Ann Nutr. Metabol.* **2000**, *44*, 75–96. [CrossRef] [PubMed]
70. Bril, F.; Kalavalapalli, S.; Clark, V.C.; Lomonaco, R.; Soldevila-Pico, C.; Liu, I.C.; Orsak, B.; Tio, F.; Cusi, K. Response to Pioglitazone in Patients With Nonalcoholic Steatohepatitis with vs. without Type 2 Diabetes. *Clin. Gastroenterol. Hepatol.* **2018**, *16*, 558–566. [CrossRef] [PubMed]
71. Bubols, G.B.; Vianna Dda, R.; Medina-Remon, A.; von Poser, G.; Lamuela-Raventos, R.M.; Eifler-Lima, V.L.; Garcia, S.C. The antioxidant activity of coumarins and flavonoids. *Mini. Rev. Med. Chem.* **2013**, *13*, 318–334. [PubMed]
72. Loguercio, C.; Festi, D. Silybin and the liver: From basic research to clinical practice. *World J. Gastroenterol.* **2011**, *17*, 2288–2301. [CrossRef] [PubMed]
73. Salomone, F.; Barbagallo, I.; Godos, J.; Lembo, V.; Currenti, W.; Cina, D.; Avola, R.; D'Orazio, N.; Morisco, F.; Galvano, F.; et al. Silibinin Restores NAD (+) Levels and Induces the SIRT1/AMPK Pathway in Non-Alcoholic Fatty Liver. *Nutrients* **2017**, *9*, 1086. [CrossRef] [PubMed]
74. Wah Kheong, C.; Nik Mustapha, N.R.; Mahadeva, S. A Randomized Trial of Silymarin for the Treatment of Nonalcoholic Steatohepatitis. *Clin. Gastroenterol. Hepatol.* **2017**, *15*, 1940–1949. [CrossRef] [PubMed]

75. Sharma, S.; Black, S.M. Carnitine Homeostasis, Mitochondrial Function, and Cardiovascular Disease. *Drug Discov. Today Dis. Mech.* **2009**, *6*, e31–e39. [CrossRef] [PubMed]
76. Ishikawa, H.; Takaki, A.; Tsuzaki, R.; Yasunaka, T.; Koike, K.; Shimomura, Y.; Seki, H.; Matsushita, H.; Miyake, Y.; Ikeda, F.; et al. L-carnitine prevents progression of non-alcoholic steatohepatitis in a mouse model with upregulation of mitochondrial pathway. *PLoS ONE* **2014**, *9*, e100627. [CrossRef] [PubMed]
77. Park, S.J.; Park, S.H.; Kim, J.O.; Kim, J.H.; Park, S.J.; Hwang, J.J.; Jin, D.H.; Jeong, S.Y.; Lee, S.J.; Kim, J.C.; et al. Carnitine sensitizes TRAIL-resistant cancer cells to TRAIL-induced apoptotic cell death through the up-regulation of Bax. *Biochem. Biophys. Res. Commun.* **2012**, *428*, 185–190. [CrossRef] [PubMed]
78. Huang, H.; Liu, N.; Guo, H.; Liao, S.; Li, X.; Yang, C.; Liu, S.; Song, W.; Liu, C.; Guan, L.; et al. L-carnitine is an endogenous HDAC inhibitor selectively inhibiting cancer cell growth in vivo and in vitro. *PLoS ONE* **2012**, *7*, e49062. [CrossRef] [PubMed]
79. Huang, H.; Liu, N.; Yang, C.; Liao, S.; Guo, H.; Zhao, K.; Li, X.; Liu, S.; Guan, L.; Liu, C.; et al. HDAC inhibitor L-carnitine and proteasome inhibitor bortezomib synergistically exert anti-tumor activity in vitro and in vivo. *PLoS ONE* **2012**, *7*, e52576. [CrossRef] [PubMed]
80. Li, M.; Zhang, W.; Wang, B.; Gao, Y.; Song, Z.; Zheng, Q.C. Ligand-based targeted therapy: A novel strategy for hepatocellular carcinoma. *Int. J. Nanomed.* **2016**, *11*, 5645–5669. [CrossRef] [PubMed]
81. Garcia, E.R.; Gutierrez, E.A.; de Melo, F.; Novaes, R.D.; Goncalves, R.V. Flavonoids Effects on Hepatocellular Carcinoma in Murine Models: A Systematic Review. *Evid. Based Complement. Alternat. Med.* **2018**, *2018*, 6328970. [CrossRef] [PubMed]
82. Pan, Z.; Zhuang, J.; Ji, C.; Cai, Z.; Liao, W.; Huang, Z. Curcumin inhibits hepatocellular carcinoma growth by targeting VEGF expression. *Oncol. Lett.* **2018**, *15*, 4821–4826. [CrossRef] [PubMed]
83. Liu, H.T.; Huang, Y.C.; Cheng, S.B.; Huang, Y.T.; Lin, P.T. Effects of coenzyme Q10 supplementation on antioxidant capacity and inflammation in hepatocellular carcinoma patients after surgery: A randomized, placebo-controlled trial. *Nutr. J.* **2016**, *15*, 85. [CrossRef] [PubMed]
84. Cai, X.; Hu, X.; Cai, B.; Wang, Q.; Li, Y.; Tan, X.; Hu, H.; Chen, X.; Huang, J.; Cheng, J.; et al. Metformin suppresses hepatocellular carcinoma cell growth through induction of cell cycle G1/G0 phase arrest and p21CIP and p27KIP expression and downregulation of cyclin D1 in vitro and in vivo. *Oncol. Rep.* **2013**, *30*, 2449–2457. [CrossRef] [PubMed]
85. Tajima, K.; Nakamura, A.; Shirakawa, J.; Togashi, Y.; Orime, K.; Sato, K.; Inoue, H.; Kaji, M.; Sakamoto, E.; Ito, Y.; et al. Metformin prevents liver tumorigenesis induced by high-fat diet in C57Bl/6 mice. *Am. J. Physiol. Endocrinol. Metab.* **2013**, *305*, E987–E998. [CrossRef] [PubMed]
86. Sid, B.; Glorieux, C.; Valenzuela, M.; Rommelaere, G.; Najimi, M.; Dejeans, N.; Renard, P.; Verrax, J.; Calderon, P.B. AICAR induces Nrf2 activation by an AMPK-independent mechanism in hepatocarcinoma cells. *Biochem. Pharmacol.* **2014**, *91*, 168–180. [CrossRef] [PubMed]
87. Kim, H.; Lee, H.J.; Kim, D.J.; Kim, T.M.; Moon, H.S.; Choi, H. Panax ginseng exerts antiproliferative effects on rat hepatocarcinogenesis. *Nutr. Res.* **2013**, *33*, 753–760. [CrossRef] [PubMed]
88. Uchida, D.; Takaki, A.; Ishikawa, H.; Tomono, Y.; Kato, H.; Tsutsumi, K.; Tamaki, N.; Maruyama, T.; Tomofuji, T.; Tsuzaki, R.; et al. Oxidative stress balance is dysregulated and represents an additional target for treating cholangiocarcinoma. *Free Radic. Res.* **2016**, *50*, 732–743. [CrossRef] [PubMed]
89. Liu, L.; Cao, Y.; Chen, C.; Zhang, X.; McNabola, A.; Wilkie, D.; Wilhelm, S.; Lynch, M.; Carter, C. Sorafenib blocks the RAF/MEK/ERK pathway, inhibits tumor angiogenesis, and induces tumor cell apoptosis in hepatocellular carcinoma model PLC/PRF/5. *Cancer Res.* **2006**, *66*, 11851–11858. [CrossRef] [PubMed]
90. Eso, Y.; Marusawa, H. Novel approaches for molecular targeted therapy against hepatocellular carcinoma. *Hepatol. Res.* **2018**, *48*, 597–607. [CrossRef] [PubMed]
91. Abou-Alfa, G.K.; Meyer, T.; Cheng, A.L.; El-Khoueiry, A.B.; Rimassa, L.; Ryoo, B.Y.; Cicin, I.; Merle, P.; Chen, Y.; Park, J.W.; et al. Cabozantinib in Patients with Advanced and Progressing Hepatocellular Carcinoma. *N. Eng. J. Med.* **2018**, *379*, 54–63. [CrossRef] [PubMed]
92. Chau, I.; Peck-Radosavljevic, M.; Borg, C.; Malfertheiner, P.; Seitz, J.F.; Park, J.O.; Ryoo, B.Y.; Yen, C.J.; Kudo, M.; Poon, R.; et al. Ramucirumab as second-line treatment in patients with advanced hepatocellular carcinoma following first-line therapy with sorafenib: Patient-focused outcome results from the randomised phase III REACH study. *Eur. J. Cancer* **2017**, *81*, 17–25. [PubMed]

93. Li, J.; Wu, P.W.; Zhou, Y.; Dai, B.; Zhang, P.F.; Zhang, Y.H.; Liu, Y.; Shi, X.L. Rage induces hepatocellular carcinoma proliferation and sorafenib resistance by modulating autophagy. *Cell Death Dis.* **2018**, *9*, 225. [CrossRef] [PubMed]
94. Casadei Gardini, A.; Faloppi, L.; De Matteis, S.; Foschi, F.G.; Silvestris, N.; Tovoli, F.; Palmieri, V.; Marisi, G.; Brunetti, O.; Vespasiani-Gentilucci, U.; et al. Metformin and insulin impact on clinical outcome in patients with advanced hepatocellular carcinoma receiving sorafenib: Validation study and biological rationale. *Eur. J. Cancer* **2017**, *86*, 106–114. [CrossRef] [PubMed]
95. Wan, J.; Liu, T.; Mei, L.; Li, J.; Gong, K.; Yu, C.; Li, W. Synergistic antitumour activity of sorafenib in combination with tetrandrine is mediated by reactive oxygen species (ROS)/Akt signaling. *Br. J. Cancer* **2013**, *109*, 342–350. [CrossRef] [PubMed]
96. El-Khoueiry, A.B.; Sangro, B.; Yau, T.; Crocenzi, T.S.; Kudo, M.; Hsu, C.; Kim, T.Y.; Choo, S.P.; Trojan, J.; Welling, T.H.R.; et al. Nivolumab in patients with advanced hepatocellular carcinoma (CheckMate 040): An open-label, non-comparative, phase 1/2 dose escalation and expansion trial. *Lancet* **2017**, *389*, 2492–2502. [CrossRef]
97. Zou, W.; Wolchok, J.D.; Chen, L. PD-L1 (B7-H1) and PD-1 pathway blockade for cancer therapy: Mechanisms, response biomarkers, and combinations. *Sci. Transl. Med.* **2016**, *8*, 328rv4. [CrossRef] [PubMed]
98. Chamoto, K.; Chowdhury, P.S.; Kumar, A.; Sonomura, K.; Matsuda, F.; Fagarasan, S.; Honjo, T. Mitochondrial activation chemicals synergize with surface receptor PD-1 blockade for T cell-dependent antitumor activity. *Proc. Natl. Acad. Sci. USA* **2017**, *114*, E761–E770. [CrossRef] [PubMed]
99. Moyer, V.A.; Force, U.S.P.S.T. Vitamin, mineral, and multivitamin supplements for the primary prevention of cardiovascular disease and cancer: U.S. Preventive services Task Force recommendation statement. *Ann. Int. Med.* **2014**, *160*, 558–564. [CrossRef] [PubMed]
100. Klein, E.A.; Thompson, I.M., Jr.; Tangen, C.M.; Crowley, J.J.; Lucia, M.S.; Goodman, P.J.; Minasian, L.M.; Ford, L.G.; Parnes, H.L.; Gaziano, J.M.; et al. Vitamin E and the risk of prostate cancer: The Selenium and Vitamin E Cancer Prevention Trial (SELECT). *JAMA* **2011**, *306*, 1549–1556. [CrossRef] [PubMed]
101. Yae, T.; Tsuchihashi, K.; Ishimoto, T.; Motohara, T.; Yoshikawa, M.; Yoshida, G.J.; Wada, T.; Masuko, T.; Mogushi, K.; Tanaka, H.; et al. Alternative splicing of CD44 mRNA by ESRP1 enhances lung colonization of metastatic cancer cell. *Nat. Commun.* **2012**, *3*, 883. [CrossRef] [PubMed]
102. Wada, T.; Ishimoto, T.; Seishima, R.; Tsuchihashi, K.; Yoshikawa, M.; Oshima, H.; Oshima, M.; Masuko, T.; Wright, N.A.; Furuhashi, S.; et al. Functional role of CD44v-xCT system in the development of spasmolytic polypeptide-expressing metaplasia. *Cancer Sci.* **2013**, *104*, 1323–1329. [CrossRef] [PubMed]
103. Yoshikawa, M.; Tsuchihashi, K.; Ishimoto, T.; Yae, T.; Motohara, T.; Sugihara, E.; Onishi, N.; Masuko, T.; Yoshizawa, K.; Kawashiri, S.; et al. xCT inhibition depletes CD44v-expressing tumor cells that are resistant to EGFR-targeted therapy in head and neck squamous cell carcinoma. *Cancer Res.* **2013**, *73*, 1855–1866. [CrossRef] [PubMed]
104. Trachootham, D.; Alexandre, J.; Huang, P. Targeting cancer cells by ROS-mediated mechanisms: A radical therapeutic approach? *Nat. Rev. Drug Discov.* **2009**, *8*, 579–591. [CrossRef] [PubMed]
105. Fujiwara, N.; Nakagawa, H.; Enooku, K.; Kudo, Y.; Hayata, Y.; Nakatsuka, T.; Tanaka, Y.; Tateishi, R.; Hikiba, Y.; Misumi, K.; et al. CPT2 downregulation adapts HCC to lipid-rich environment and promotes carcinogenesis via acylcarnitine accumulation in obesity. *Gut* **2018**, *67*, 1493–1504. [CrossRef] [PubMed]

7

Nutrition and Liver Disease

Claudia Mandato [1], Antonella Di Nuzzi [2] and Pietro Vajro [2,*]

[1] Pediatrics, Santobono - Pausilipon Pediatric Hospital, 80100 Naples, Italy; cla.mandato@gmail.com
[2] Department of Medicine, Surgery and Dentistry "Scuola Medica Salernitana", Pediatrics Section, University of Salerno, 84081 Baronissi (Salerno), Italy; antonelladinuzzi@gmail.com
* Correspondence: pvajro@unisa.it

Abstract: Malnutrition in children and adults with advanced liver disease represents a tremendous challenge as the nutritional problems are multifactorial. This Editorial comments the articles appearing in this special issue of *Nutrients*, "Nutrition and Liver disease" dealing with multiple diagnostic and therapeutic features that relate the outcomes of liver disease to nutrition. To improve quality of life and prevent nutrition-related medical complications, patients diagnosed with advanced liver disease should have their nutritional status promptly assessed and be supported by appropriate dietary interventions. Furthermore specific food supplements and/or restriction diets are often necessary for those with hepatic conditions associated with an underlying metabolic or nutritional or intestinal disease.

Keywords: nutrition; liver disease; cholestasis; liver transplantation; assessment; support

---

Despite advances in both the assessment and management of patients with liver disease, the provision of appropriate nutritional support for these patients is frequently lacking, an omission that has a large impact on clinical outcomes and quality of life. Except for elimination diets indicated for some hereditary or metabolic diseases that affect the liver, the general nutritional recommendations for most cases of compensated liver disease are analogous to the customary recommendations for a balanced diet. Malnutrition in children and adults with advanced liver disease, however, remains a tremendous challenge. The nutritional problems of these patients are multifactorial, and commonly include decreased intake due to anorexia, hypermetabolism, increased energy loss, and increased energy needs (Figure 1). The complicated underlying metabolic scenario is characterized by reduced glycogen stores, reduced protein synthesis, decreased branched-chain amino acid (BCAA)/aromatic amino acid (AAA) or BCCA/tyrosine (BT) ratios (3.5:1→1:1), and disturbances in fat metabolism during fasting.

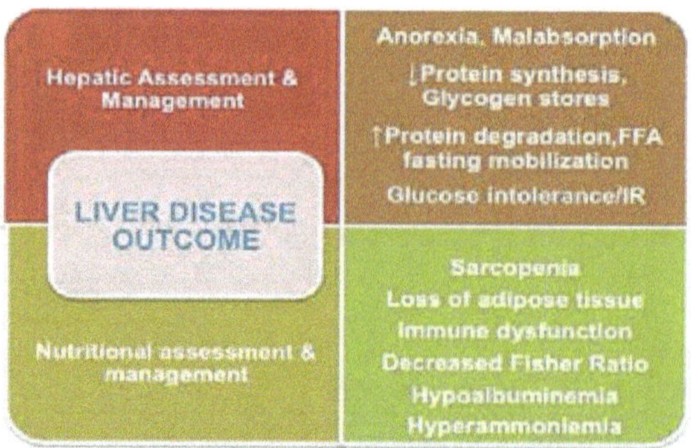

Figure 1. Diagnostic and therapeutic issues that link outcomes of liver diseases to nutrition.

In this special issue of *Nutrients*, which focuses on "Nutrition and Liver Disease," a number of contributors have presented novel information and additional perspectives on multiple diagnostic and therapeutic features that relate the outcomes of patients with liver disease to nutrition.

1. Skeletal Muscle Mass

Skeletal muscle mass (SMM) is determined by the balance between protein synthesis and breakdown. Skeletal muscle loss (SML) is a major complication of liver cirrhosis (LC). In clinical settings, the assessment of skeletal muscle mass (SMM) to identifysevere SML (or sarcopenia) has long represented a very simple and objective bedside clinical measure of liver disease severity, because SML is associated with liver disease prognosis. It has now recently enhanced thanks to the support of various new imaging methods for assessing core SMM.

In this issue of *Nutrients*, the prognostic value of SMM was reported by studies in various categories of hepatic conditions, and the information has furthered our knowledge on the following issues:

- Strict interdependence exists between (1) the prevention of depletion of SMM,(2) the early diagnosis of and curative therapy for hepatocellular carcinoma (HCC),(3) the preservation of liver functional reserve, and (4) improved liver disease outcomes [1]. Age of male patients, female gender, a Child–Pugh score, and increased tumor size were significantly related to the SMM index, as measured at the third lumbar vertebra by transverse computed tomography (CT) imaging, which is a commonly used tool for HCC in the clinical setting. The results of the study by Imai et al. overall confirmed that sarcopenia negatively impacts the survival of patients with HCC, and is a valuable prognostic factor that might be impacted by liver functional reserve and the clinical stage of HCC.
- Therelationship between the loss of SMM, as assessed by bioelectric impedance analysis (BIA), and liver fibrosis, as measured by virtual-touch-quantification (VTQ) and acoustic-radiation-force-impulse elastography in patients with chronic liver disease (CLD), was reported by Nishikawa et al. [2]. Interestingly, BCAAs-to-tyrosine ratio (BTR) showed the second strongest correlation with the VTQ level, and was an independent predictor for decreased SMM index.
- BothBTR and SMM, as evaluated by BIA, were also confirmed to be reliable predictors of outcome in patients with liver diseases in another study, which found that increased values of BTR and SMM were associated with the resolution of chronic hepatitis C in patients treated with interferon-free direct-acting-antiviral therapy [3].
- However, all that glitters is not gold, and these studies have both strengths and limitations. The study by Imai et al. [1] was based on imaging techniques, and, although these assessments are objective and not affected by defects in hepatic synthesis or retention of NaCl and water, they are either expensive or involve radiation and cannot easily be repeated to monitor progress. The other twostudies [2,3] that used BIA, which is based on a two-component model of body composition (fat and fat-free mass), may have drawbacks. As recently emphasized by Amodio et al. [4] the validity of this technique is in fact critically dependent on assumptions relating to tissue density and hydration.

In future clinical and research settings, hand-grip dynamometry, which can provide measures for risk stratification for all-cause death, cardiovascular death, and cardiovascular disease in the general population [5], should be also implemented for the assessment of muscle strength. Indeed, for patients with cirrhosis, muscle strength, as assessed by hand-grip dynamometry, appears to be an easy-to-measure, sensitive, and specific marker for depletion of SMM [6] and ispositively correlated with total body protein [5,7].

2. Nutritional Assessment and Support

Another major issue concerns the fine line between the need for a hypercaloric diet rich in proteins and the risk of hepatic encephalopathy and hyperammonemia in sarcopenic, chronically malnourished patients with end-stage liver disease. The appropriate nutritional support of adult cirrhosis before and after liver transplantation was the focus of three articles in this issue.

- The first article [8] recommends the performance of an accurate multidisciplinary assessment of malnutrition in order to optimize nutritional support, especially for those patients with elevated risk for malnutrition because of the severity of their native liver disease. The recommended daily requirements for nutrients and energy intake should be achieved through oral intake, oral supplementation, and enteral nutrition. Parenteral nutrition (PN) should be used for moderately or severely malnourished patients with cirrhosis who cannot be fed orally or enterally, or if they have fasted longer than 72 h [9].
- The important and difficult issues concerned with the careful assessment of nutritional status of patients who are candidates for liver transplantation were also emphasized in the articles by Ahmed Hammad et al. [10] and Yang et al. [11]. The perioperative nutritional interventions, including the use of synbiotics, micronutrients, branched-chain amino acid (BCAA) supplements, and immunonutrients; fluid and electrolyte balance, the partial substitution of conventional fats with medium-chain triglycerides, and carefully monitored supplementation using fat soluble vitamins for cholestasis were reviewed for both adult and pediatric patients. Children with chronic liver disease are particularly vulnerable to malnutrition, which can compromise growth and brain development. They should benefit from early intervention provided by a multidisciplinary team. Yang et al. in particular have focused on the nutritional needs and support of children with chronic liver disease [11]; they revised the issues by providing conclusions that are consistent with the most recent guidelines of the European Society of Paediatric Gastroenterology Hepatology and Nutrition (ESPGHAN) [12].

3. Hepatopathies due to Inherited Metabolic/Genetic Defects

A number of inherited metabolic/genetic defects, including those that require (a) specific well established dietary restrictions (galactosemia, hereditary fructose intolerance, inborn errors of the urea cycle such as citrin deficiency and related metabolic pathways),(b) the addition of specific drugs (e.g., tyrosinemia; Wilson disease), or (c) special food supplements such as uncooked starch (e.g., glycogen storage diseases), represent a further challenge not only for pediatricians but also for adult hepatologists at the time of transition of care [13]. A dietician familiar with metabolic disorders is often needed on the team caring for these patients [14].

Dietary intervention is an evolving and increasingly used therapy also for the novel group of Congenital Disorders of Glycosylation (CDG). Glycosylation consists in the covalent binding ofan oligosaccharide chain to the polypeptide side chains of a glycoprotein. The carbohydrate consists of a simple sugar (e.g., glucose, galactose, mannose, and xylose), an amino sugar (e.g., *N*-acetylglucosamine or *N*-acetylgalactosamine), or an acidic sugar (e.g., sialic acid or *N*-acetylneuraminic acid). Monosaccharide supplements are being evaluated in trials for more and more subtypes of CDG, because monosaccharides have relatively high safety, especially compared to experimental drugs, and are easy to administer. The mechanism is still poorly understood, although in CDG-Ib, alimentary addition of mannose appear to bypass the defective step (conversion of fructose-6-phosphate to mannose-6-phosphate) by allowing for the formation of mannose-6-phosphate via the action of hexokinase [15]. In their article, Morava and her group presented an accurate overview of very recent data on the contributions of nutritional therapy by evaluating many of the different options for nutritional therapy that have somehow been associated with a positive effect on liver function in CDG [16]. The questions these authors, however, pose include whether or not these dietary interventions are sufficient and whether these dietary interventions are the most efficient therapies for CDG. They remind the reader that mannose therapy for patients with mannose phosphate isomerase (MPI)-CDG has not only been found to be possibly hazardous at higher doses, but unfortunately also cannot prevent progressive fibrotic liver disease in about one third of affected patients. In addition, recent experience with galactose therapy has been found beneficial for several CDGs [17–19] without, however, completely alleviating all clinical symptoms. While recognizing the progress this approach represents, they also suggest that future therapy for CDG therapy will most likely include administration of activated monosaccharides instead of single dietary sugars. The efficacy and toxicity of these novel drugs, however, remain to be investigated in human trials as well after careful preliminary evaluations in animal models are made.

4. Hepatopathies Driven by Primary Nutritional/Intestinal Tract Diseases

A number of liver diseases that are driven by primary nutritional/intestinal tract diseases (e.g., inflammatory bowel disease (IBD), celiac disease, cystic fibrosis (CF), alcoholic steatohepatitis (ASH), and non-alcoholic steatohepatitis (NASH) parenteral nutrition-associated liver disease(PNALD)), which are included under the umbrella term *gut-liver axisdysfunction* [20,21], also represent specific challenges. Investigations of the associations between the liver and diseased intestine are still preliminary, and further studies are essential for the clinical management of these complicated conditions (Figure 2).

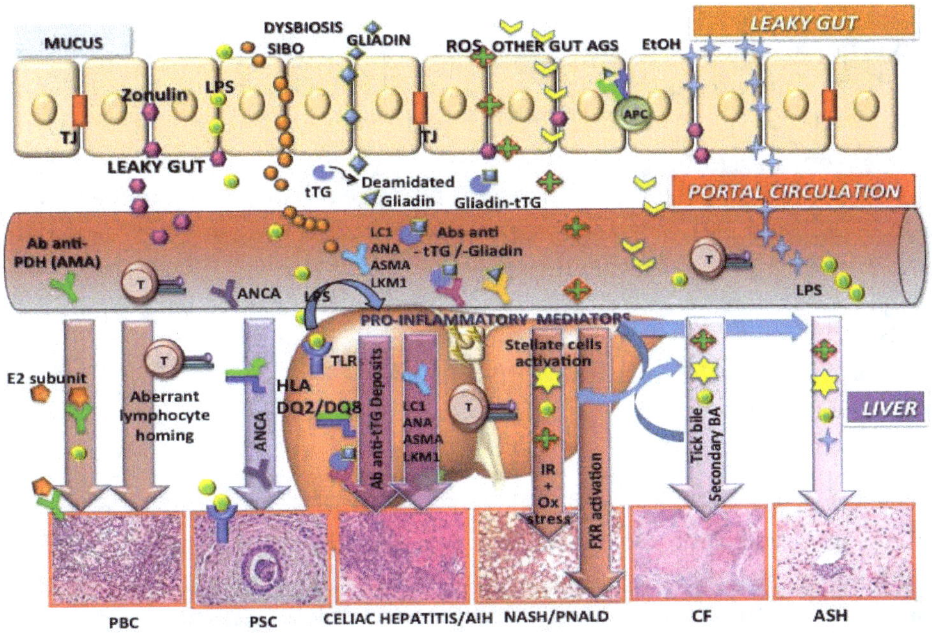

Figure 2. Gut-liver axis and liver diseases. Increased intestinal permeability and dysbiosis are common features linking the liver to a number of nutritional/gastrointestinal (GI) diseases depicted in the figure. The toll-like receptor (TLR)–bacterial lipopolysaccharide (LPS) interaction is one of the mechanisms involved in the release of proinflammatory mediators (cytokines), leading to liver inflammation and stellate-cell-activation-dependent fibrosis. Emerging therapeutic approaches that target the gut-liver axis therefore represent promising therapies to prevent or halt liver disease progression.

Genetic predisposition and environmental stimulation determine the loss of tolerance in primary biliary cholangitis (PBC) where antimitochondrial antibodies (AMAs) cross-react with proteins from intestinal bacteria (E2 subunit), possibly because of molecular mimicry. Aberrant homing of intestinal lymphocytes also occurs. The association between celiac disease and PBC is also well established.

Closely associated with inflammatory bowel disease, primary sclerosing cholangitis (PSC) is also a heterogeneous disease that involves marked interactions between altered immune status (human leucocyte antigen (HLA)), altered bile composition, and host microbiome. Some subgroups of antineutrophil cytoplasmic antibodies (ANCAs) in the blood and bile are associated with increased liver enzyme levels and are biomarkers of liver disease with a possible role in the pathogenesis of the disease as well.

In celiac disease, immunoactive molecules generated from cross-linking between tissue transglutaminase and food/bacterial antigens reach the liver through the portal circulation and are responsible for transglutaminase antigen (tTG)–antibody complex hepatic deposits. The liver may respond to gluten either as a reactive "celiac hepatitis" or a true autoimmune hepatitis (with anti-liver cytosol (LC1), anti-nuclear antibodies (ANA), anti-smoot muscle antibodies (ASMA), anti-liver kidney microsomes (LKM1)) based on the DQ2 strong linkage disequilibrium with the DR3 and DR4, the latter being the major HLA risk factor for autoimmune liver disease.

Increased levels of bacterial endotoxin in the portal circulation suggest a role for gut-derived toxins also in the alcoholic liver diseasesteatohepatitis (ASH), non-alcoholic fatty liver disease (NAFLD/NASH), and parenteral nutrition liver disease (PNALD). Alcohol (EtOH) consumption and endogenous alcohol production by gut bacteria in obese individuals can disrupt the tight junctions (TJ) of the intestinal epithelial barrier, resulting in increased gut permeability. The bacterial endotoxin (lypopolisaccharides, LPS) contributes to inflammation through activation of toll-like receptor 4 (TLR4). Oxidative stress with reactive oxygen species (ROS), insulin resistance (IR), secondary bile acids (BAs), and farnesoid X receptor activation (FXR) represent major mechanisms of pathogenesis.

Animals with cystic fibrosis transmembrane conductance regulator defects and patients with cystic fibrosis have microbiomes that are different from individuals without CF, which might be accounted for by altered bile properties, prolonged small bowel transit, frequent antibiotic exposure, and small intestinal bacterial overgrowth (SIBO) (adapted and modified from [20]).

For celiac disease [22] and NASH [23,24], nutritional correction of the underlying gastrointestinal/nutritional disease may be effective in preventing the progression of liver disease. Readers are also referredto the 2017 *Nutrients* issue (ISSN 2072-6643) edited by Nobili and Alisi, where specific measures for the treatment of obesity-related NAFLD are specifically discussed.

Unfortunately, for some nutritional/intestinal conditions such as IBD and CF, the liver disease does not seem to be affected by decreases in the inflammatory activity in the intestinal tract [25] or improved function of the pancreas/respiratory tract [26].

Impaired intestinal function, directly or indirectly associated with gut dysbiosis, may also be one of the main pathogenic mechanisms of PNALD [27] (Figure 2).

- In this issue of *Nutrients*, Cahova et al. [28] reviewed studies of animal models and humans that suggested that chronic parenteral nutrition-related liver damage depends on intestinal failure and associated complications rather than PN administration per se. The prominent factors appear to be increased permeability of the intestinal barrier, which facilitates translocation of bacterial toxins and microorganisms into the portal circulation, mesenteric lymph nodes, and liver, and the overall proinflammatory status of the compromised intestine. The gut microbiota play a weighty role in the maintenance of the functional intestinal barrier and the establishment of either an immunotolerant or inflammatory intestinal setting [23,27]. Therapeutic strategies that focus on improving the composition of the microbiota through the targeted delivery of beneficial microbiota or by supplementation with immunomodulators are attractive areas of investigation.
- Alcoholic liver disease (ALD) is a strong predictor of malnutrition because of the numerous risk factors for malnutrition that are associated with both acute and chronic alcohol abuse. Due to complicated pathogenetic mechanisms, therapies for ALD and especially for severe alcoholic hepatitis (AH) are thorny problems in clinical practice. For severe acute AH, specific drug treatments, including glucorticoids and pentoxifylline, have been identified and currently are recommended by international guidelines. However, further elucidation of the mechanisms of pathogenesis is still needed [29]. In this context, the article by Xuchong Tang et al. [30] in this issue of *Nutrients* is particularly welcome. The study revealed that an artichoke extract exhibited

significant preventive hepatoprotective effects not only for the carbon-tetrachloride-induced hepatoxicity [31,32] and NAFLD/NASH [33] as previously demonstrated but also against acute alcohol-induced liver injury (ASH). The effects probably depend on the ability of components of the extract not only to attenuate oxidative stress but also to suppress the toll-like receptor 4/nuclear factor kappa-light-chain-enhancer of activated Bcells (TLR4/NFkB) inflammatory pathway, a signaling pathway suggested to be one of the mechanisms of pathogenesis also of NAFLD through the overexpression of hepcidin [34].

5. Conclusions

In conclusion, to improve quality of life and prevent nutrition-related medical complications, patients diagnosed with advanced liver disease should have their nutritional status promptly assessed and be supported by appropriate dietary interventions. Furthermore, a dietary approach that uses specific food supplements and/or restriction diets is often necessary for patients with hepatic conditions associated with an underlying metabolic or nutritional or intestinal disease, due to the hepatoprotective and/or anti-oxidant and/or anti-inflammatory effects of these measures.

Author Contributions: The authors contributed equally.

References

1. Imai, K.; Takai, K.; Watanabe, S.; Hanai, T.; Suetsugu, A.; Shiraki, M.; Shimizu, M. Sarcopenia Impairs Prognosis of Patients with Hepatocellular Carcinoma: The Role of Liver Functional Reserve and Tumor-Related Factors in Loss of Skeletal Muscle. *Nutrients* **2017**, *9*, 1054. [CrossRef] [PubMed]
2. Nishikawa, H.; Nishimura, T.; Enomoto, H.; Iwata, Y.; Ishii, A.; Miyamoto, Y.; Ishii, N.; Yuri, Y.; Takata, R.; Hasegawa, K.; et al. Impact of Virtual Touch Quantification in Acoustic Radiation Force Impulse for Skeletal Muscle Mass Loss in Chronic Liver Diseases. *Nutrients* **2017**, *9*, 620. [CrossRef] [PubMed]
3. Yoh, K.; Nishikawa, H.; Enomoto, H.; Ishii, A.; Iwata, Y.; Miyamoto, Y.; Ishii, N.; Yuri, Y.; Hasegawa, K.; Nakano, C.; et al. Predictors Associated with Increase in Skeletal Muscle Mass after Sustained Virological Response in Chronic Hepatitis C Treated with Direct Acting Antivirals. *Nutrients* **2017**, *9*, 1135. [CrossRef] [PubMed]
4. Amodio, P.; Bemeur, C.; Butterworth, R.; Cordoba, J.; Kato, A.; Montagnese, S.; Uribe, M.; Vilstrup, H.; Morgan, M.Y. The nutritional management of hepatic encephalopathy in patients with cirrhosis: International Society for Hepatic Encephalopathy and Nitrogen Metabolism Consensus. *Hepatology* **2013**, *58*, 325–336. [CrossRef] [PubMed]
5. Leong, D.P.; Teo, K.K.; Rangarajan, S.; Lopez-Jaramillo, P.; Avezum, A., Jr.; Orlandini, A.; Seron, P.; Ahmed, S.H.; Rosengren, A.; Kelishadi, R.; et al. Prognostic value of grip strength: Findings from the Prospective Urban Rural Epidemiology (PURE) study. *Lancet* **2015**, *386*, 266–273. [CrossRef]
6. Huisman, E.J.; Trip, E.J.; Siersema, P.D.; van Hoek, B.; van Erpecum, K.J. Protein energy malnutrition predicts complications in liver cirrhosis. *Eur. J. Gastroenterol. Hepatol.* **2011**, *23*, 982–989. [CrossRef] [PubMed]
7. Dasarathy, S. Consilience in sarcopenia of cirrhosis. *J. Cachexia Sarcopenia Muscle* **2012**, *3*, 225–237. [CrossRef] [PubMed]
8. Perumpail, B.J.; Li, A.A.; Cholankeril, G.; Kumari, R.; Ahmed, A. Optimizing the Nutritional Support of Adult Patients in the Setting of Cirrhosis. *Nutrients* **2017**, *9*, 1114. [CrossRef] [PubMed]
9. Plauth, M.; Cabré, E.; Campillo, B.; Kondrup, J.; Marchesini, G.; Schütz, T.; Shenkin, A.; Wendon, J.; ESPEN. ESPEN Guidelines on Parenteral Nutrition: Hepatology. *Clin. Nutr.* **2009**, *28*, 436–444. [CrossRef] [PubMed]
10. Hammad, A.; Kaido, T.; Aliyev, V.; Mandato, C.; Uemoto, S. Nutritional Therapy in Liver Transplantation. *Nutrients* **2017**, *9*, 1126. [CrossRef] [PubMed]
11. Yang, C.H.; Perumpail, B.J.; Yoo, E.R.; Ahmed, A.; Kerner, J.A., Jr. Nutritional Needs and Support for Children with Chronic Liver Disease. *Nutrients* **2017**, *9*, 1127. [CrossRef] [PubMed]
12. McLin, V.A.; Allen, U.; Boyer, O.; Bucuvalas, J.; Colledan, M.; Cuturi, M.C.; d'Antiga, L.; Debray, D.; Dezsofi, A.; Goyet, J.V.; et al. Early and Late Factors Impacting Patient and Graft Outcome in Pediatric Liver

Transplantation: Summary of an ESPGHAN Monothematic Conference. *J. Pediatr. Gastroenterol. Nutr.* **2017**, *65*, 53–59. [CrossRef] [PubMed]

13. Guercio Nuzio, S.; Ann Tizzard, S.; Vajro, P. Tips and hints for the transition: What adult hepatologists should know when accept teens with a pediatric hepatobiliary disease. *Clin. Res. Hepatol. Gastroenterol.* **2014**, *38*, 277–283. [CrossRef] [PubMed]
14. Thompson, R.J.; Azevedo, R.A.; Galoppo, C.; Lewindon, P.; McKiernan, P. Cholestatic and metabolic liver diseases: Working Group report of the second World Congress of Pediatric Gastroenterology, Hepatology, and Nutrition. *J. Pediatr. Gastroenterol. Nutr.* **2004**, *39*, 611–615. [CrossRef]
15. Péanne, R.; de Lonlay, P.; Foulquier, F.; Kornak, U.; Lefeber, D.J.; Morava, E.; Pérez, B.; Seta, N.; Thiel, C.; Van Schaftingen, E.; et al. Congenital disorders of glycosylation (CDG): Quo vadis? *Eur. J. Med. Genet.* **2017**. [CrossRef]
16. Witters, P.; Cassiman, D.; Morava, E. Nutritional Therapies in Congenital Disorders of Glycosylation (CDG). *Nutrients* **2017**, *9*, 1222. [CrossRef] [PubMed]
17. Morelle, W.; Potelle, S.; Witters, P.; Wong, S.; Climer, L.; Lupashin, V.; Matthijs, G.; Gadomski, T.; Jaeken, J.; Cassiman, D.; et al. Galactose supplementation in patients with tmem165-CDG rescues the glycosylation defects. *J. Clin. Endocrinol. Metab.* **2017**, *102*, 1375–1386. [CrossRef] [PubMed]
18. Morava, E. Galactose supplementation in phosphoglucomutase-1 deficiency; review and outlook for a novel treatable CDG. *Mol. Genet. Metab.* **2014**, *112*, 275–279. [CrossRef] [PubMed]
19. Wong, S.Y.; Gadomski, T.; van Scherpenzeel, M.; Honzik, T.; Hansikova, H.; Holmefjord, K.S.B.; Mork, M.; Bowling, F.; Sykut-Cegielska, J.; Koch, D.; et al. Oral D-galactose supplementation in PGM1-CDG. *Genet. Med.* **2017**, *19*, 1226–1235. [CrossRef] [PubMed]
20. Poeta, M.; Pierri, L.; Vajro, P. Gut-Liver Axis Derangement in Non-Alcoholic Fatty Liver Disease. *Children* **2017**, *4*, 66. [CrossRef] [PubMed]
21. Troisi, J.; Pierri, L.; Landolfi, A.; Marciano, F.; Bisogno, A.; Belmonte, F.; Palladino, C.; Guercio Nuzio, S.; Campiglia, P.; Vajro, P. Urinary Metabolomics in Pediatric Obesity and NAFLD Identifies Metabolic Pathways/Metabolites Related to Dietary Habits and Gut-Liver Axis Perturbations. *Nutrients* **2017**, *9*, 485. [CrossRef] [PubMed]
22. Marciano, F.; Savoia, M.; Vajro, P. Celiac disease-related hepatic injury: Insights into associated conditions and underlying pathomechanisms. *Dig. Liver Dis.* **2016**, *48*, 112–119. [CrossRef] [PubMed]
23. Vajro, P.; Paolella, G.; Fasano, A. Microbiota and gut-liver axis: Their influences on obesity and obesity-related liver disease. *J. Pediatr. Gastroenterol. Nutr.* **2013**, *56*, 461–468. [CrossRef] [PubMed]
24. Ma, J.; Zhou, Q.; Li, H. Gut Microbiota and Nonalcoholic Fatty Liver Disease: Insights on Mechanisms and Therapy. *Nutrients* **2017**, *9*, 1124. [CrossRef] [PubMed]
25. Vavricka, S.R.; Schoepfer, A.; Scharl, M.; Lakatos, P.L.; Navarini, A.; Rogler, G. Extraintestinal Manifestations of Inflammatory Bowel Disease. *Inflamm. Bowel Dis.* **2015**, *21*, 1982–1992. [CrossRef] [PubMed]
26. Debray, D.; Narkewicz, M.R.; Bodewes, F.A.J.A.; Colombo, C.; Housset, C.; de Jonge, H.R.; Jonker, J.W.; Kelly, D.A.; Ling, S.C.; Poynard, T.; et al. Cystic Fibrosis–related Liver Disease: Research Challenges and Future Perspectives. *J. Pediatr. Gastroenterol. Nutr.* **2017**, *65*, 443–448. [CrossRef] [PubMed]
27. Orso, G.; Mandato, C.; Veropalumbo, C.; Cecchi, N.; Garzi, A.; Vajro, P. Pediatric parenteral nutrition-associated liver disease and cholestasis: Novel advances in pathomechanisms-based prevention and treatment. *Dig. Liver Dis.* **2016**, *48*, 215–222. [CrossRef] [PubMed]
28. Cahova, M.; Bratova, M.; Wohl, P. Parenteral Nutrition-Associated Liver Disease: The Role of the Gut Microbiota. *Nutrients* **2017**, *9*, 987. [CrossRef] [PubMed]
29. Abenavoli, L.; Masarone, M.; Federico, A.; Rosato, V.; Dallio, M.; Loguercio, C.; Persico, M. Alcoholic Hepatitis: Pathogenesis, Diagnosis and Treatment. *Rev. Recent. Clin. Trials.* **2016**, *11*, 159–166. [CrossRef] [PubMed]
30. Tang, X.; Wei, R.; Deng, A.; Lei, T. Protective Effects of Ethanolic Extracts from Artichoke, an Edible Herbal Medicine, against Acute Alcohol-Induced Liver Injury in Mice. *Nutrients* **2017**, *9*, 1000. [CrossRef] [PubMed]
31. Colak, E.; Ustuner, M.C.; Tekin, N.; Colak, E.; Burukoglu, D.; Degirmenci, I.; Gunes, H.V. The hepatocurative effects of *Cynara scolymus* L. leaf extract on carbon tetrachloride-induced oxidative stress and hepatic injury in rats. *Springerplus* **2016**, *5*, 216. [CrossRef] [PubMed]

32. Mehmetçik, G.; Ozdemirler, G.; Koçak-Toker, N.; Cevikbaş, U.; Uysal, M. Effect of pretreatment with artichoke extract on carbon tetrachloride-induced liver injury and oxidative stress. *Exp. Toxicol. Pathol.* **2008**, *60*, 475–480. [CrossRef] [PubMed]
33. Rangboo, V.; Noroozi, M.; Zavoshy, R.; Rezadoost, S.A.; Mohammadpoorasl, A. The Effect of Artichoke Leaf Extract on Alanine Aminotransferase and Aspartate Aminotransferase in the Patients with Nonalcoholic Steatohepatitis. *Int. J. Hepatol.* **2016**. [CrossRef] [PubMed]
34. Chen, W.; Wang, X.; Huang, L.; Liu, B. Hepcidin in non-alcoholic fatty liver disease regulated by the TLR4/NF-κB signaling pathway. *Exp. Ther. Med.* **2016**, *11*, 73–76. [CrossRef] [PubMed]

8

Circulating Phospholipid Patterns in NAFLD Patients Associated with a Combination of Metabolic Risk Factors

Shilpa Tiwari-Heckler, Hongying Gan-Schreier, Wolfgang Stremmel, Walee Chamulitrat and Anita Pathil *

Department of Internal Medicine IV, Gastroenterology and Hepatology, University of Heidelberg, Im Neuenheimer Feld 410, 69120 Heidelberg, Germany; Shilpa.Tiwari-Heckler@med.uni-heidelberg.de (S.T.-H.); Hongying.Gan-Schreier@med.uni-heidelberg.de (H.G.-S.); Wolfgang.Stremmel@med.uni-heidelberg.de (W.S.); Walee.Chamulitrat@med.uni-heidelberg.de (W.C.)

* Correspondence: Anita.Pathil-Warth@med.uni-heidelberg.de

Abstract: Background: Non-alcoholic fatty liver disease (NAFLD) is associated with inefficient macro- and micronutrient metabolism, and alteration of circulating phospholipid compositions defines the signature of NAFLD. This current study aimed to assess the pattern of serum phospholipids in the spectrum of NAFLD, and its related comorbidities and genetic modifications. Methods: 97 patients with diagnosed NAFLD were recruited at a single center during 2013–2016. Based on histological and transient elastography assessment, 69 patients were divided into non-alcoholic steatohepatitis (NASH) and non-alcoholic fatty liver (NAFL) subgroups. 28 patients served as healthy controls. Serum phospholipids were determined by liquid-chromatography mass spectrometry (LC-MS/MS). Results: The total content of phosphatidylcholine (PC) and sphingomyelin in the serum was significantly increased in NAFL and NASH patients, compared to healthy controls. In addition, serum lysophospatidylethanolamine levels were significantly decreased in NAFL and NASH individuals. Circulating PC species, containing linoleic and α-linolenic acids, were markedly increased in NAFLD patients with hypertension, compared to NAFLD patients without hypertension. The pattern of phospholipids did not differ between NAFLD patients with diabetes and those without diabetes. However, NAFLD patients with hyperglycemia (blood glucose level (BGL) >100 mg/dL) exhibited significantly a higher amount of monounsaturated phosphatidylethanolamine than those with low blood glucose levels. In addition, NAFLD patients with proven GG-genotype of PNPLA3, who were at higher risk for the development of progressive disease with fibrosis, showed lower levels of circulating plasmalogens, especially 16:0, compared to those with CC- and CG-allele. Conclusions: Our extended lipidomic study presents a unique metabolic profile of circulating phospholipids associated with the presence of metabolic risk factors or the genetic background of NAFLD patients.

Keywords: non-alcoholic fatty liver disease; NAFLD; phospholipids; metabolic disease

1. Introduction

Non-alcoholic fatty liver disease (NAFLD) is one of the most common causes of chronic liver disease in the western world, and is linked to increasing prevalence of obesity and diabetes [1,2]. One of the major contributors to this issue is overconsumption with an inefficient metabolism of macro- and micronutrients, affecting immune response and consequently leading to chronic liver disease [3]. NAFLD extends from lipid accumulation in the liver (non-alcoholic fatty liver (NAFL)) to non-alcoholic steatohepatitis (NASH), which may progress to liver cirrhosis and end-stage liver disease [4,5]. Disturbed hepatic lipid metabolism is a hallmark of NAFLD. Certain lipids, such as diacylglycerol, free fatty acids and ceramides, seem to mediate inflammatory pathways leading to lipotoxicity and oxidative stress, which finally may contribute to disease progression [6]. Previous metabolic studies have provided new insights into altered phospholipid metabolism in NAFLD, implicating an important pathophysiological role for this lipid class [7–9]. Puri et al. showed a significant decrease of hepatic phosphatidiylcholine (PC) levels and hepatic lipid subclasses containing arachidonic acid (AA) in NAFLD patients [7]. The progression of NAFL to NASH is characterized by an altered monounsaturated (MUFA) and n3- and n6-polyunsaturated (PUFA) metabolism, probably due to deranged activities of δ-5, -6, and -9 desaturases, as well as by an impaired PUFA oxidation process, leading to an increase in the total plasma content of non-enzymatic autoxidation products of PUFA lipids, e.g. 11-Hydroxyeicosatetraenoic acid (11-HETE) [7,10], 9-Hydroxyoctadecadienoic acid (9-HODE) and 13-Hydroxyoctadecadienoic acid (13-HODE) [11] or 20-carboxy arachidonic acid (20-COOH AA) [12]. NAFLD is associated with different clinical manifestations of the metabolic syndrome, including obesity, diabetes and hypertension [2,5]. Development of hepatic steatosis and progression to NASH is also linked to genetic background. Genetic association studies recently suggested that the G-allele in patatin-like phospholipase-3 (PNPLA3), which encodes adiponutrin, is strongly associated with hepatic fat content, and more importantly, promotes the susceptibility to develop advanced disease stages with fibrosis [13,14]. Thus, the aim of the present study was to extend lipidomic analysis data on the spectrum of NAFLD, and its associated comorbidities as well as its genetic modifications. Therefore, we performed lipidomic profiling in the serum of healthy controls and patients with NAFLD in order to (1) quantify and compare different circulating phospholipid metabolites; (2) to analyze phospholipids in NAFLD-associated metabolic diseases; and finally to (3) study the association between specific circulating lipids and PNPLA3 polymorphism.

2. Materials and Methods

2.1. Study Cohort

97 patients were recruited from the Department of Internal Medicine at the University Hospital of Heidelberg from 2013–2016. 28 patients served as healthy controls. These control patients had normal liver enzyme levels and did not have any record of liver disease, and therefore showed no indication for liver biopsy. All individuals had routine clinical and hematological examinations. NAFLD was suspected by the presence of elevated liver enzymes and after exclusion of other causes of liver disease (e.g., viral or autoimmune hepatitis, M. Wilson, hemochromatosis, significant alcohol use). In addition, ultrasound examinations and transient elastography with FibroScan® 502 Touch (Echosens™) were conducted. Liver biopsy was performed in 41 patients. The diagnosis of NASH was based on the following criteria: (1) Elevated liver enzymes (AST > 46 U/L, ALT > 50 U/L); (2) hepatic steatosis on ultrasound; and (3) histological examination or (4) elevated Fibroscan results (>7 kPa). 42 patients were assigned to the NASH cohort according to these criteria. 25 patients were included in the NAFL group: 5 patients because of liver histology results and 20 patients who exhibited only one or two of the above mentioned criteria. Blood samples of the 97 patients were taken and immediately prepared, and stored at −80 °C for further analysis, as shown below. Genotype of the PNPLA3 rs738409 gene of 52 patients was investigated after patient informed consent. The institutional review board approved the study.

2.2. Profiling of Phospholipids and Sphingolipids

The patterns of phospholipids and sphingolipids were determined by using XBridge C18 Column from Waters, Milford, MA, USA and HPLC-ESI/MSMS (triple-quadrupole Micro Mass Quattro 81 Premier, Waters, Milford, MA, USA, coupled with HTC Pal auto sampler, CTC Analytics, Zwingen, Switzerland), as described in Jiao et al. [15]. In brief, a constant amount of internal standards, containing 17:0 lysophosphatidylcholine (lysoPC), 14:0/14:0 phosphatidylcholine (PC), 12:0/12:0 phosphatidylethanolamine (PE), and 17:0 Ceramide (Cer), were added to each serum sample.

A classical Folch method, which uses chloroform/methanol (3:2, *v/v*), was applied to the glass tubes [16]. After evaporation, lipid extracts were resolved in methanol and were analyzed using HPLC-ESI/MSMS. For the purpose of data acquisition and processing, Masslynx version 4.1 software (Waters, Milford, MA, USA) was used.

2.3. Data Analysis

Data are presented as mean ± SEM and were analyzed with GraphPad Prism 5.0 (GraphPad Software, La Jolla, CA, USA). Groups were compared using unpaired two-tailed students' *t*-test. One-way ANOVA, including Bonferroni post-hoc test, was used for comparing three or more groups. A *p*-value less than 0.05 was considered statistically significant.

3. Results

3.1. Baseline Characteristics

The study population included 69 patients, who presented at the Department of Internal Medicine at the University Hospital of Heidelberg with the suspected diagnosis of NAFLD. 28 patients served as healthy controls. All patients underwent clinical examination, laboratory data were collected and additionally, ultrasound examinations and transient elastography were performed. Forty-one patients underwent liver biopsy. According to the histological assessment, 5 patients were diagnosed with NAFL and 34 patients were grouped as NASH patients. Two patients were excluded from the study, as they had no pathological findings indicating NAFLD. Based on Fibroscan values (F2–F4), further 8 patients were added to the NASH group. 20 patients were included in the NAFL cohort, as they presented with Fibroscan values under F2. NASH (n = 42) and NAFL (n = 25) patients had significantly higher levels of liver enzymes, triglycerides and total cholesterol in comparison to healthy controls (n = 28) (Table 1).

Table 1. Baseline characteristics and laboratory results from healthy controls, NAFL and NASH patients.

	Control (n = 28)	NAFL (n = 25)	NASH (n = 42)
Age (years)	39.4 ± 2.6	46.4 ± 2.9	43.7 ± 2.2
Sex (M/F)	13/15	14/11	29/13
AST (U/L)	20.7 ± 1.3	43.6 ± 5.8 ***	55.3 ± 6.0 ***
ALT (U/L)	22.0 ± 1.7	68.9 ± 7.9 ***	86.3 ± 9.5 ***
GGT (U/L)	21.8 ± 2.4	144.4 ± 24.6 ***	218.1 ± 49.6 **
Bilirubin (mg/dL)	0.6 ± 0.04	0.9 ± 0.2	1.4 ± 0.6
Triglycerides (mg/dL)	83.4 ± 5.9	152.2 ± 12.6 ***	187.3 ± 14.6 ***
Total cholesterol (mg/dL)	182.2 ± 9.0	213.2 ± 7.8 *	169.3 ± 12.2
HDL cholesterol (mg/dL)	54.7 ± 3.9	53.1 ± 3.7	46.7 ± 2.2
LDL cholesterol (mg/dL)	110.8 ± 6.4	128.2 ± 6.6	113.3 ± 6.2

M = Male, F = Female, AST = Aspartate aminotransaminase, ALT = Alanine aminotransaminase, GGT = Gamma-glutamyl transpeptidase, HDL = High-density lipoproteins, LDL = Low-density lipoprotein. Values are represented in mean ± SEM. *p*-values vs. control. * p-value < 0.05, ** p-value < 0.01, *** p-value < 0.001.

3.2. Increase of Circulating PC and Sphingomyelin and Decrease of Phosphatidylethanolamine in NAFL and NASH

By using LC-MS/MS, we identified and quantified 140 species of phospholipids and sphingomyelin (SM) in the serum. The total content of PC and SM in the serum was significantly increased in NAFL and NASH patients, compared to healthy controls (Figure 1A,C). Contrary to PC, the level of lysophosphatidylcholine (LPC) showed a trend to be decreased in both the NAFL and NASH groups, without reaching significance (Figure 1D). Circulating phosphatidylethanolamine (PE) was elevated in patients with NASH, compared to those with NAFL (Figure 1B). The amount of lysophosphatidylethanolamine (LPE) was significantly decreased in NAFL and NASH patients in comparison to controls (Figure 1E). The level of phosphatidylinositol (PI) and plasmalogens did not differ between all groups (Figure 1F,G).

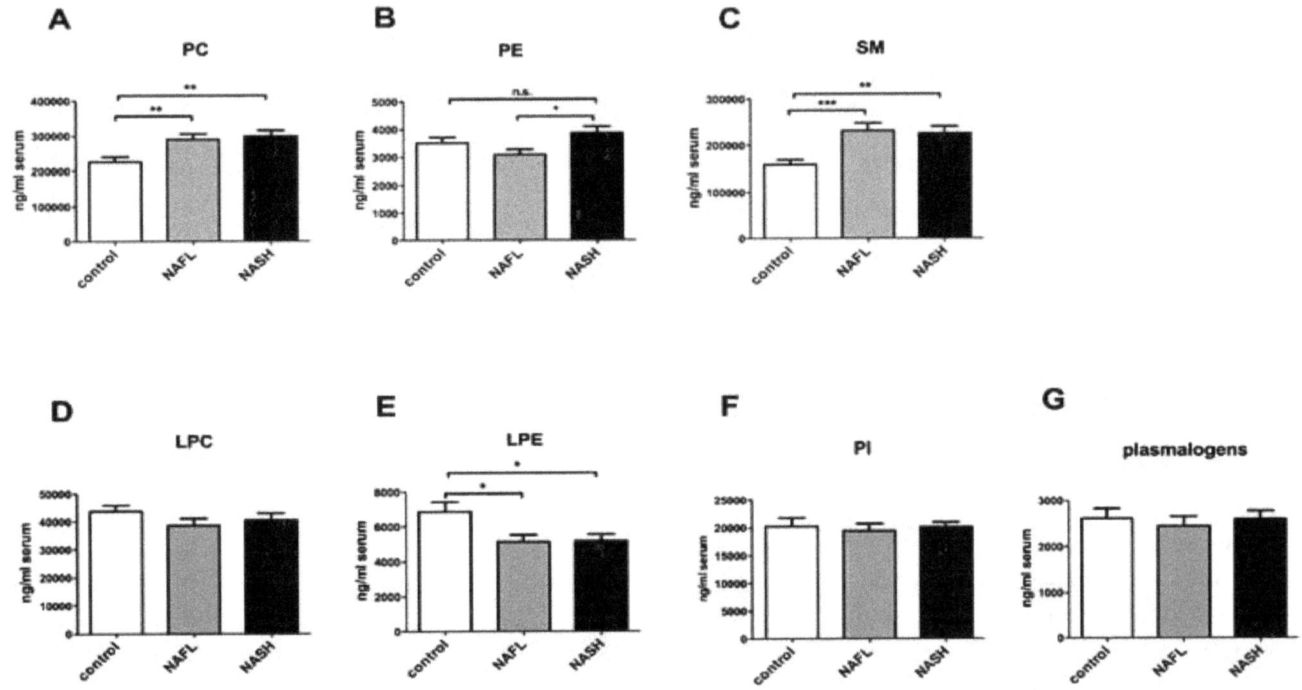

Figure 1. Circulating phospholipids in control (n = 28), NAFL (n = 25) and NASH (n = 42) cohorts. Results of lipid profiling of 95 patients by using LC-MS/MS method. Patients were divided in NAFL and NASH cohorts. 28 patients served as healthy control. Quantification of (**A**) PC; (**B**) PE; (**C**) SM; (**D**) LPC; (**E**) LPE; (**F**) PI; and (**G**) plasmalogens in the serum of healthy, NAFL and NASH patients in ng/mL serum. All the values are presented in mean ± SEM. * $p < 0.05$, ** $p < 0.01$, *** $p < 0.001$, n.s. = not significant ($p > 0.05$).

3.3. Altered Phospholipid Composition in NASH Patients with Metabolic Risk Factors

We investigated the contribution of phospholipid species in NAFLD-associated comorbidities. NAFL and NASH patients were enrolled in groups regarding the presence of diabetes, hypertension and obesity. Interestingly, NAFLD patients with hypertension exhibited significantly higher levels of PC and SM (Figure 2A,B) in the serum than NAFLD patients without hypertension. Circulating PC species, containing linoleic acids (PC 34:2, PC 36:2, PC 38:2) and α-linolenic acids (PC 34:3, PC 36:3, PC 38:3), were markedly increased in these patients, whereas those containing arachidonic acid remained unaffected (Figure 2D–G). The sum of phospholipids, including PC, PE and SM, did not differ between diabetes (n = 18) and non-diabetes NAFLD patients (n = 49) (Figure 3A). However, further analysis revealed a correlation between MUFA-PE and hyperglycemia within the NAFLD cohort. 16 patients with a blood glucose level (BGL) over 100 mg/dL showed higher levels of serum PE, which was due to a significant elevation of MUFA-PE, whereas PUFA-PE remained unchanged (Figure 3B). Obese NAFLD patients (body mass index (BMI) > 30 kg/m^2) showed no significant differences, compared to healthy (BMI < 25 kg/m^2) and overweight (BMI 25–30 kg/m^2) NAFLD patients (Supplementary Materials Figure S1).

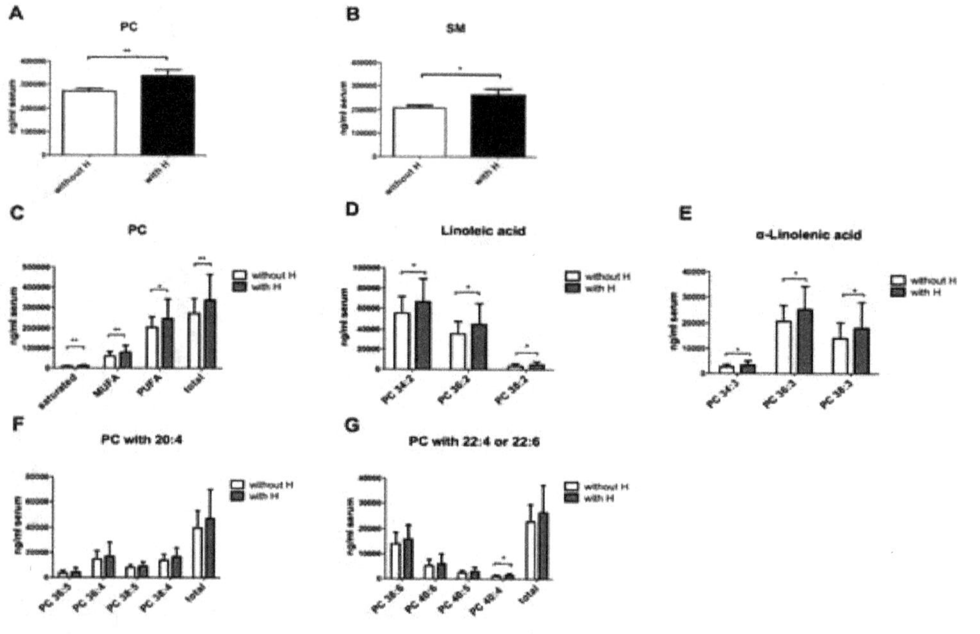

Figure 2. Overview of circulating phospholipids in NAFLD patients with and without hypertension. NAFLD patients were divided into patients with hypertension (with H; n = 24) and without hypertension (without H; n = 43). (**A**) Quantification of circulating PC and SM is represented in ng/mL serum. (**B**) Distribution of PC subtypes, namely saturated, mono- and poly-unsaturated PC levels, are displayed in these two groups in ng/mL serum. The total content of PC is evaluated as a sum of saturated and unsaturated PC. (**C–E**) Circulating PC, containing linoleic acids (PC 34:2, PC 36:2, PC 38:2) and α-linolenic acids (PC 34:3, PC 36:3, PC 38:3), are compared between hypertensive and normotensive NAFLD patients. (**F,G**) The amount of arachidonic acid (PC 20:4, 22:4 and 22:6) in PC is demonstrated in this graphic. All the values are presented in mean ± SEM. * $p < 0.05$, ** $p < 0.01$.

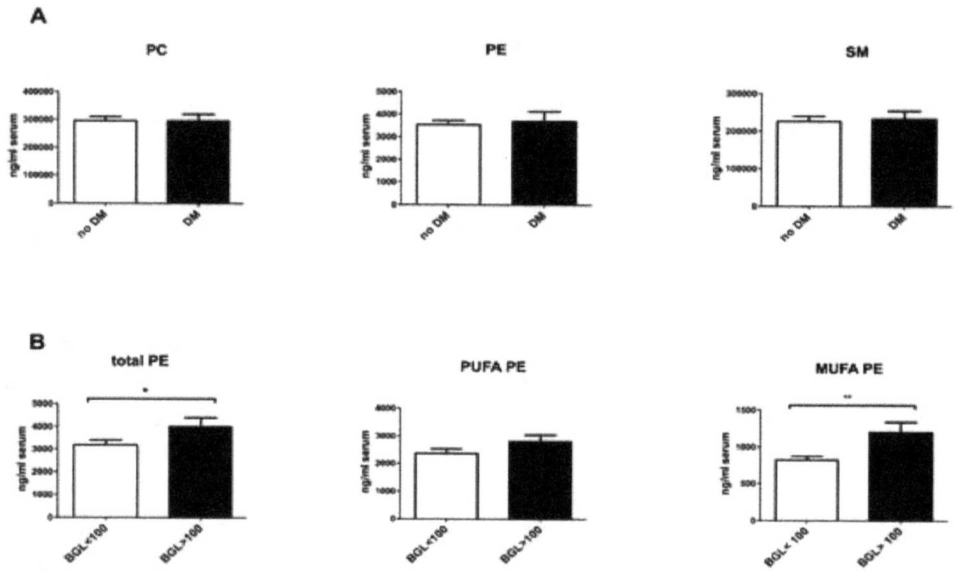

Figure 3. MUFA-PE is increased in NAFLD patients with hyperglycemia. (**A**) Quantification of circulating PC, PE and SM in ng/mL serum in NAFLD patients who were divided into patients with diabetes mellitus (DM; n = 18) and without diabetes mellitus (no DM; n = 49). (**B**) Quantification of total PE, PUFA-PE and MUFA-PE in ng/mL serum in NAFLD patients with a BGL over 100 mg/dL (BGL > 100; n = 16) or under 100 mg/dL (BGL < 100; n = 22). All the values are presented in mean ± SEM. * $p < 0.05$, ** $p < 0.01$.

3.4. *Reduction of Circulating Plasmalogens in Patients with PNPLA3 GG-Genotype*

Genetic analysis regarding the determination of the PNPLA3 rs738409 genotype was performed in 52 NAFLD patients. Lipid profiling of these patients showed lower levels of total plasmalogens, especially 16:0 and 18:1, in patients with PNPLA3 GG-genotype (n = 14), compared to those with CC- (n = 20) or CG- (n = 18) allele (Figure 4).

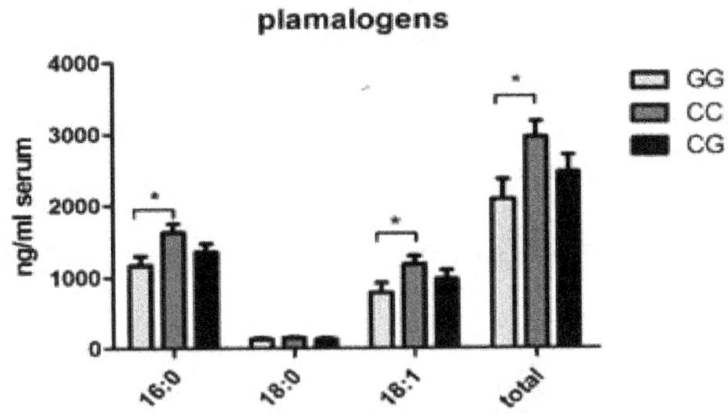

Figure 4. Association between plasmalogens and PNPLA3 gene polymorphism. The PNPLA3 rs738409 genotype was determined in 52 NAFLD patients. The total level of plasmalogen was the sum of plasmalogen 16:0, 18:0 and 18:1. The amount of these plasmalogen subtypes was quantified in NAFLD patients with GG- (n = 14), CC- (n = 20) and CG-allele (n = 18) of PNPLA3. Circulating plasmalogen subclasses are displayed in ng/mL serum. All the values are presented in mean ± SEM. * $p < 0.05$.

4. Discussion

It is well known that NAFLD is the hepatic manifestation of the metabolic syndrome [1]. Our extended lipidomic analysis provides an insight into the complex changes in circulating lipid patterns and lipid levels related to NAFLD-associated metabolic risk factors, as well as to the individual genetic background, potentially provoking metabolic and immunomodulatory responses in liver.

It has been recently discovered that altered PC metabolism is involved in the progression of human NAFL to NASH [7]. We also confirm hereby that the content of circulating PC is increased in NAFL and NASH patients, compared to healthy controls. We could not measure a significant change in the PC product, i.e., LPC in our cohorts. One possible explanation is the further utilization of LPC, e.g., by autotaxin. It has been recently reported that plasma autotaxin levels are increased in different chronic liver diseases, including NASH [17]. Total PE content was elevated in NASH patients, compared to NAFL in our study. However, data on PE analysis were inconsistent. Puri et al. and Wattacheril et al. showed that PE levels seemed to be unchanged in NASH compared to healthy liver [7,9], but as recently presented by Ma et al., accumulation of PE could be associated with disease progression [18].

However, we discovered that LPE might serve as a novel biomarker for NAFL and NASH, as this phospholipid subgroup was significantly reduced in the NAFLD cohort. We suggest that the lack of LPE and consequently the inability to further metabolize LPE to PC, can lead to disease progression. To compensate the decrease of hepatocellular PC, therapeutic approaches, including PC supplementation by food intake, were conducted [19]. Stremmel et al. showed a protective and anti-inflammatory role of topical PC in chronic ulcerative colitis [20]. However, the treatment of liver diseases with PC was not as successful in humans as in mouse models, because a replenishment of high PC levels in hepatocytes was not easily achievable [21,22]. As direct application of PC is of no therapeutic benefit, pro-drugs, serving as PC precursors, have been developed [23,24]. For instance, our group synthetized a drug candidate, which consists of the bile acid (UDCA) and the PC precursor LPE [25], and which owns hepatoprotective and anti-inflammatory functions in a high fat diet mouse model of NAFLD by changing hepatic fatty acid composition [24,26].

Our LC-MS/MS analyses revealed that circulating PC, containing linoleic (LA) and α-linolenic acids (ALA), was increased in NAFLD patients with hypertension. With changing nutritional behavior over the last few decades, western diet is now characterized by high fat diet and suboptimal micronutrient intake [3]. In particular, intake and metabolism of essential fatty acids are relevant to the pathogenesis of different chronic diseases [27,28]. Essential PUFAs, which are not produced by the human body, include LA and ALA [19,29]. Few epidemiological studies suggest a positive impact of dietary intake of essential PUFAs on cholesterol profiling or blood pressure [19,30]. However, these associations seem to be inconsistent in the literature, as other investigations imply the opposite effect or do not recognize any difference [27,31]. Additionally, an excess of LA can lead to adverse effects because of an increase of oxidized LA metabolites [29]. For instance, oxidized LDL compounds derive from LA and contribute to atherosclerosis [32]. In vitro studies demonstrate pro-inflammatory properties of LA, during liver injury by stimulating endoplasmatic reticulum stress and hepatocyte apoptosis and by increasing pro-inflammatory cytokines, such as TNFα, which leads to Kupffer cell activation [33,34]. Accordingly, in clinical settings, oxidized derivates of LA, such as 9- and 13-HODE, are correlated with NASH [11]. LA and ALA can also be converted to arachidonic acids [29], which remained unaltered in our cohorts. Our data indicate a positive association between circulating essential fatty acids and NAFLD-associated hypertension.

Although we did not discover lipid alterations by comparing diabetes and non-diabetes NAFLD patients, further analysis regarding BGLs revealed an increase of PE, especially MUFA-PE, in NAFLD patients with a BGL over 100 mg/dL. Glycation of PE could lead to an Amadori-linked product, which could induce lipid peroxidation. The level of Amadori-PE was increased in diabetic patients and was considered as a possible marker of a hyperglycemic condition, particularly in the early stage of diabetes [35,36].

In our next step, our lipid profiling in the NAFLD group identified a decrease of plasmalogens in patients with the GG-genotype of PNPLA3, compared to those with the CC- and CG-genotypes.

Recent studies highlighted a strong association between a variant (rs738409 C>G p. I148M) in the *PNPLA3* gene and steatosis, fibrosis and the development of hepatocellular carcinoma in multiple chronic liver diseases, including metabolic disorders, alcoholic liver disease and chronic viral hepatitis. The I148M substitution represents a loss of function mutant that contributes to triglyceride accumulation in hepatocytes, which may lead to increased lipid peroxidation and oxidative stress (lipotoxicity) [37,38]. A recent study by Carpino et al. analyzed serum from NAFLD patients with I148M variant, showing high levels of serum systemic oxidative stress markers, such as F2-isoprostanes and Nox2 activity [37].

Plasmalogens are synthesized in peroxisomes and prevent cellular damage induced by oxidative stress, and thus, seem to have anti-inflammatory functions [39,40]. As recently published by Jang and colleagues, endogenous hepatic plasmalogens appear to be involved in fatty acid metabolism and inhibit steatosis and NASH progression through PPARα-dependent signaling [41]. It is known that oxidative stress-induced peroxisome dysfunction limits plasmalogen biosynthesis, and thus, attenuates the release of plasmalogens to the blood [39]. Puri et al. reported low circulating serum plasmalogen levels in patients presenting with NASH in their lipidomics study [10].

Interestingly, we discovered a positive association of PNPLA3 I148M carriers and low levels of circulating plasmalogens, compared to patients with CC- or CG-genotype. This observation suggests a possible pathogenetic link on the cellular level, underlining the association between triglyceride accumulation, oxidative stress, peroxisome dysfunction and accordingly, defects of plasmologens biosynthesis. Moreover, their loss of function may aggravate NASH progression. This molecular mechanism between PNPLA3 I148M mutant and plasmologens still remains unclear and needs to be elucidated in further experimental and clinical studies.

In recent publications, the most frequently used categorization of NAFLD patients in NASH and NAFL was due to histological assessment. In our cohort study, 28 patients denied liver biopsy in spite of medical recommendation. Ultrasound examination and transient elastography with Fibroscan were performed in all sessions. Therefore, 39 patients could be divided in NAFL and NASH subgroups based on histological analyses. Eight patients exhibited liver stiffness >F2 by transient elastography and were included to the NASH group. This kind of categorization may lead to sample selection bias. However, lipid profiling in 39 patients with only histological assessment revealed a significant increase of high levels of PC and SM and a marked decrease of LPE in the NASH cohort (34 patients), compared to healthy controls, consistent with the lipid analysis in our groups with results of histology and transient elastography. No significant deviation could be detected between NAFL and control patients. It should be noted that only 5 individuals from 39 patients with histological analyses could be assigned to the NAFL group (Supplementary Materials Figure S2).

5. Conclusions

In summary, this lipidomic profiling investigated circulating phospholipid metabolites in NAFLD patients. This current study confirmed that PC is significantly increased in the serum of NASH patients and is identified as a possible novel biomarker in the pathogenesis of NAFLD, namely LPE. Our analysis elucidated lipidomic alterations in NAFLD patients with hypertension, demonstrating a key role for PC species containing essential fatty acids in NAFLD-associated hypertension. Furthermore, metabolic profiling in this NAFLD cohort determined a correlation between high levels of MUFA-PE and hyperglycemia. Finally, we discovered a link between low levels of circulating plasmalogens and NAFLD patients with the unfavorable GG genotype of PNPLA3.

Author Contributions: S.T.-H. and A.P. conceived and designed the experiments; S.T.-H. and H.G.-S. performed the experiments; S.T.-H. and W.C. analyzed the data; A.P. contributed reagents/materials/analysis tools; S.T.-H. and A.P. wrote the paper.

References

1. Williams, C.D.; Stengel, J.; Asike, M.I.; Torres, D.M.; Shaw, J.; Contreras, M.; Landt, C.L.; Harrison, S.A. Prevalence of Nonalcoholic Fatty Liver Disease and Nonalcoholic Steatohepatitis among a Largely Middle-Aged Population Utilizing Ultrasound and Liver Biopsy: A Prospective Study. *Gastroenterology* **2011**, *140*, 124–131. [CrossRef] [PubMed]
2. Bellentani, S.; Scaglioni, F.; Marino, M.; Bedogni, G. Epidemiology of non-alcoholic fatty liver disease. *Dig. Dis.* **2010**, *28*, 155–161. [CrossRef] [PubMed]
3. Myles, I.A. Fast food fever: Reviewing the impacts of the Western diet on immunity. *Nutr. J.* **2014**, *13*, 61. [CrossRef] [PubMed]
4. Contos, M.J.; Sanyal, A.J. The clinicopathologic spectrum and management of nonalcoholic fatty liver disease. *Adv. Anat. Pathol.* **2002**, *9*, 37–51. [CrossRef] [PubMed]
5. Bedossa, P.; Poitou, C.; Veyrie, N.; Bouillot, J.L.; Basdevant, A.; Paradis, V.; Tordjman, J.; Clement, K. Histopathological algorithm and scoring system for evaluation of liver lesions in morbidly obese patients. *Hepatology* **2012**, *56*, 1751–1759. [CrossRef] [PubMed]
6. Malhi, H.; Gores, G. Molecular Mechanisms of Lipotoxicity in Nonalcoholic Fatty Liver Disease. *Semin. Liver Dis.* **2008**, *28*, 360–369. [CrossRef] [PubMed]
7. Puri, P.; Baillie, R.A.; Wiest, M.M.; Mirshahi, F.; Choudhury, J.; Cheung, O.; Sargeant, C.; Contos, M.J.; Sanyal, A.J. A lipidomic analysis of nonalcoholic fatty liver disease. *Hepatology* **2007**, *46*, 1081–1090. [CrossRef] [PubMed]
8. Anjani, K.; Lhomme, M.; Sokolovska, N.; Poitou, C.; Aron-Wisnewsky, J.; Bouillot, J.-L.; Lesnik, P.; Bedossa, P.; Kontush, A.; Clement, K.; et al. Circulating phospholipid profiling identifies portal contribution to NASH signature in obesity. *J. Hepatol.* **2015**, *62*, 905–912. [CrossRef] [PubMed]
9. Wattacheril, J.; Seeley, E.H.; Angel, P.; Chen, H.; Bowen, B.P.; Lanciault, C.; Caprioli, R.M.; Abumrad, N.; Flynn, C.R. Differential Intrahepatic Phospholipid Zonation in Simple Steatosis and Nonalcoholic Steatohepatitis. *PLoS ONE* **2013**, *8*, e57165. [CrossRef] [PubMed]

10. Puri, P.; Wiest, M.M.; Cheung, O.; Mirshahi, F.; Sargeant, C.; Min, H.-K.; Contos, M.J.; Sterling, R.K.; Fuchs, M.; Zhou, H.; et al. The plasma lipidomic signature of nonalcoholic steatohepatitis. *Hepatology* **2009**, *50*, 1827–1838. [CrossRef] [PubMed]
11. Feldstein, A.E.; Lopez, R.; Tamimi, T.A.-R.; Yerian, L.; Chung, Y.-M.; Berk, M.; Zhang, R.; McIntyre, T.M.; Hazen, S.L. Mass spectrometric profiling of oxidized lipid products in human nonalcoholic fatty liver disease and nonalcoholic steatohepatitis. *J. Lipid Res.* **2010**, *51*, 3046–3054. [CrossRef] [PubMed]
12. Loomba, R.; Quehenberger, O.; Armando, A.; Dennis, E.A. Polyunsaturated fatty acid metabolites as novel lipidomic biomarkers for noninvasive diagnosis of nonalcoholic steatohepatitis. *J. Lipid Res.* **2015**, *56*, 185–192. [CrossRef] [PubMed]
13. Romeo, S.; Kozlitina, J.; Xing, C.; Pertsemlidis, A.; Cox, D.; Pennacchio, L.A.; Boerwinkle, E.; Cohen, J.C.; Hobbs, H.H. Genetic variation in PNPLA3 confers susceptibility to nonalcoholic fatty liver disease. *Nat. Genet.* **2008**, *40*, 1461–1465. [CrossRef] [PubMed]
14. Krawczyk, M.; Grünhage, F.; Zimmer, V.; Lammert, F. Variant adiponutrin (PNPLA3) represents a common fibrosis risk gene: Non-invasive elastography-based study in chronic liver disease. *J. Hepatol.* **2011**, *55*, 299–306. [CrossRef] [PubMed]
15. Jiao, L.; Gan-Schreier, H.; Zhu, X.; Wei, W.; Tuma-Kellner, S.; Liebisch, G.; Stremmel, W.; Chamulitrat, W. Ageing sensitized by iPLA2β deficiency induces liver fibrosis and intestinal atrophy involving suppression of homeostatic genes and alteration of intestinal lipids and bile acids. *Biochim. Biophys. Acta Mol. Cell Biol. Lipids* **2017**, *1862*, 1520–1533. [CrossRef] [PubMed]
16. Folch, J.; Lees, M.; Sloane Stanley, G.H. A simple method for the isolation and purification of total lipides from animal tissues. *J. Biol. Chem.* **1957**, *226*, 497–509. [PubMed]
17. Kaffe, E.; Katsifa, A.; Xylourgidis, N.; Ninou, I.; Zannikou, M.; Harokopos, V.; Foka, P.; Dimitriadis, A.; Evangelou, K.; Moulas, A.N.; et al. Hepatocyte autotaxin expression promotes liver fibrosis and cancer. *Hepatology* **2017**, *65*, 1369–1383. [CrossRef] [PubMed]
18. Ma, D.W.L.; Arendt, B.M.; Hillyer, L.M.; Fung, S.K.; McGilvray, I.; Guindi, M.; Allard, J.P. Plasma phospholipids and fatty acid composition differ between liver biopsy-proven nonalcoholic fatty liver disease and healthy subjects. *Nutr. Diabetes* **2016**, *6*, e220. [CrossRef] [PubMed]
19. Küllenberg, D.; Taylor, L.A.; Schneider, M.; Massing, U. Health effects of dietary phospholipids. *Lipids Health Dis.* **2012**, *11*, 3. [CrossRef] [PubMed]
20. Stremmel, W.; Merle, U.; Zahn, A.; Autschbach, F.; Hinz, U.; Ehehalt, R. Retarded release phosphatidylcholine benefits patients with chronic active ulcerative colitis. *Gut* **2005**, *54*, 966–971. [CrossRef] [PubMed]
21. Lieber, C.S. Alcoholic fatty liver: Its pathogenesis and mechanism of progression to inflammation and fibrosis. *Alcohol* **2004**, *34*, 9–19. [CrossRef] [PubMed]
22. Lieber, C.S.; Weiss, D.G.; Groszmann, R.; Paronetto, F.; Schenker, S.; Veterans Affairs Cooperative Study 391 Group II. Veterans Affairs Cooperative Study of Polyenylphosphatidylcholine in Alcoholic Liver Disease. *Alcohol. Clin. Exp. Res.* **2003**, *27*, 1765–1772. [CrossRef] [PubMed]
23. Abdelmalek, M.F.; Angulo, P.; Jorgensen, R.A.; Sylvestre, P.B.; Lindor, K.D. Betaine, a promising new agent for patients with nonalcoholic steatohepatitis: Results of a pilot study. *Am. J. Gastroenterol.* **2001**, *96*, 2711–2717. [CrossRef] [PubMed]
24. Chamulitrat, W.; Liebisch, G.; Xu, W.; Gan-Schreier, H.; Pathil, A.; Schmitz, G.; Stremmel, W. Ursodeoxycholyl Lysophosphatidylethanolamide Inhibits Lipoapoptosis by Shifting Fatty Acid Pools toward Monosaturated and Polyunsaturated Fatty Acids in Mouse Hepatocytes. *Mol. Pharmacol.* **2013**, *84*, 696–709. [CrossRef] [PubMed]
25. Chamulitrat, W.; Burhenne, J.; Rehlen, T.; Pathil, A.; Stremmel, W. Bile salt-phospholipid conjugate ursodeoxycholyl lysophosphatidylethanolamide as a hepatoprotective agent. *Hepatology* **2009**, *50*, 143–154. [CrossRef] [PubMed]
26. Pathil, A.; Mueller, J.; Warth, A.; Chamulitrat, W.; Stremmel, W. Ursodeoxycholyl lysophosphatidylethanolamide improves steatosis and inflammation in murine models of nonalcoholic fatty liver disease. *Hepatology* **2012**, *55*, 1369–1378. [CrossRef] [PubMed]
27. Bemelmans, W.J.E.; Lefrandt, J.D.; Feskens, E.J.M.; van Haelst, P.L.; Broer, J.; Meyboom-de Jong, B.; May, J.F.; Tervaert, J.W.C.; Smit, A.J. Increased α-linolenic acid intake lowers C-reactive protein, but has no effect on markers of atherosclerosis. *Eur. J. Clin. Nutr.* **2004**, *58*, 1083–1089. [CrossRef] [PubMed]

28. Berry, E. Are diets high in omega-6 polyunsaturated fatty acids unhealthy? *Eur. Heart J. Suppl.* **2001**, *3*, D37–D41. [CrossRef]
29. Santoro, N.; Caprio, S.; Feldstein, A.E. Oxidized metabolites of linoleic acid as biomarkers of liver injury in nonalcoholic steatohepatitis. *Clin. Lipidol.* **2013**, *8*, 411–418. [CrossRef] [PubMed]
30. Stamler, J.; Rose, G.; Stamler, R.; Elliott, P.; Dyer, A.; Marmot, M.; Brown, I.J.; Tzoulaki, I.; Saitoh, S.; Dyer, A.R.; et al. INTERSALT study findings. Public health and medical care implications. *Hypertension* **1989**, *14*, 570–577. [CrossRef] [PubMed]
31. Scherhag, R.; Kramer, H.J.; Düsing, R. Dietary administration of eicosapentaenoic and linolenic acid increases arterial blood pressure and suppresses vascular prostacyclin synthesis in the rat. *Prostaglandins* **1982**, *23*, 369–382. [CrossRef]
32. Spiteller, D.; Spiteller, G. Oxidation of Linoleic Acid in Low-Density Lipoprotein: An Important Event in Atherogenesis. *Angew. Chem. Int. Ed.* **2000**, *39*, 585–589. [CrossRef]
33. Böhm, T.; Berger, H.; Nejabat, M.; Riegler, T.; Kellner, F.; Kuttke, M.; Sagmeister, S.; Bazanella, M.; Stolze, K.; Daryabeigi, A.; et al. Food-derived peroxidized fatty acids may trigger hepatic inflammation: A novel hypothesis to explain steatohepatitis. *J. Hepatol.* **2013**, *59*, 563–570. [CrossRef] [PubMed]
34. Zhang, Y.; Xue, R.; Zhang, Z.; Yang, X.; Shi, H. Palmitic and linoleic acids induce ER stress and apoptosis in hepatoma cells. *Lipids Health Dis.* **2012**, *11*, 1. [CrossRef] [PubMed]
35. Sookwong, P.; Nakagawa, K.; Fujita, I.; Shoji, N.; Miyazawa, T. Amadori-Glycated Phosphatidylethanolamine, a Potential Marker for Hyperglycemia, in Streptozotocin-Induced Diabetic Rats. *Lipids* **2011**, *46*, 943–952. [CrossRef] [PubMed]
36. Miyazawa, T.; Oak, J.-H.; Nakagawa, K. Tandem Mass Spectrometry Analysis of Amadori-Glycated Phosphatidylethanolamine in Human Plasma. *Ann. N. Y. Acad. Sci.* **2005**, *1043*, 280–283. [CrossRef] [PubMed]
37. Carpino, G.; Pastori, D.; Baratta, F.; Overi, D.; Labbadia, G.; Polimeni, L.; Di Costanzo, A.; Pannitteri, G.; Carnevale, R.; Del Ben, M.; et al. PNPLA3 variant and portal/periportal histological pattern in patients with biopsy-proven non-alcoholic fatty liver disease: A possible role for oxidative stress. *Sci. Rep.* **2017**, *7*, 15756. [CrossRef] [PubMed]
38. Trépo, E.; Romeo, S.; Zucman-Rossi, J.; Nahon, P. PNPLA3 gene in liver diseases. *J. Hepatol.* **2016**, *65*, 399–412. [CrossRef] [PubMed]
39. Wallner, S.; Schmitz, G. Plasmalogens the neglected regulatory and scavenging lipid species. *Chem. Phys. Lipids* **2011**, *164*, 573–589. [CrossRef] [PubMed]
40. Brites, P.; Waterham, H.R.; Wanders, R.J. Functions and biosynthesis of plasmalogens in health and disease. *Biochim. Biophys. Acta Mol. Cell Biol. Lipids* **2004**, *1636*, 219–231. [CrossRef] [PubMed]
41. Jang, J.E.; Park, H.-S.; Yoo, H.J.; Baek, I.-J.; Yoon, J.E.; Ko, M.S.; Kim, A.-R.; Kim, H.S.; Park, H.-S.; Lee, S.E.; et al. Protective role of endogenous plasmalogens against hepatic steatosis and steatohepatitis in mice. *Hepatology* **2017**, *66*, 416–431. [CrossRef] [PubMed]

9

Impact of Virtual Touch Quantification in Acoustic Radiation Force Impulse for Skeletal Muscle Mass Loss in Chronic Liver Diseases

Hiroki Nishikawa, Takashi Nishimura, Hirayuki Enomoto *, Yoshinori Iwata, Akio Ishii, Yuho Miyamoto, Noriko Ishii, Yukihisa Yuri, Ryo Takata, Kunihiro Hasegawa, Chikage Nakano, Kazunori Yoh, Nobuhiro Aizawa, Yoshiyuki Sakai, Naoto Ikeda, Tomoyuki Takashima, Shuhei Nishiguchi and Hiroko Iijima

Division of Hepatobiliary and Pancreatic disease, Department of Internal Medicine, Hyogo College of Medicine, Hyogo 6638501, Japan; nishikawa_6392@yahoo.co.jp (H.N.); tk-nishimura@hyo-med.ac.jp (T.N.); yo-iwata@hyo-med.ac.jp (Y.I.); akio0010@yahoo.co.jp (A.I.); yuho.0818.1989@gmail.com (Y.M.); ishinori1985@yahoo.co.jp (N.I.); gyma27ijo04td@gmail.com (Y.Y.); chano_chano_rt@yahoo.co.jp (R.T.); hiro.red1230@gmail.com (K.H.); chikage@hyo-med.ac.jp (C.N.); mm2wintwin@ybb.ne.jp (K.Y.); nobu23hiro@yahoo.co.jp (N.A.); sakai429@hyo-med.ac.jp (Y.S.); nikeneko@hyo-med.ac.jp (N.I.); tomo0204@yahoo.co.jp (T.T.); nishiguc@hyo-med.ac.jp (S.N.); hiroko-i@hyo-med.ac.jp (H.I.)

* Correspondence: enomoto@hyo-med.ac.jp

Abstract: Background and aims: We sought to clarify the relationship between virtual touch quantification (VTQ) in acoustic radiation force impulse and skeletal muscle mass as assessed by bio-electronic impedance analysis in patients with chronic liver diseases (CLDs, n = 468, 222 males and 246 females, median age = 62 years). Patients and methods: Decreased skeletal muscle index (D-SMI) was defined as skeletal muscle index (SMI) <7.0 kg/m^2 for males and as SMI <5.7 kg/m^2 for females, according to the recommendations in current Japanese guidelines. We examined the correlation between SMI and VTQ levels and investigated factors linked to D-SMI in the univariate and multivariate analyses. The area under the receiver operating curve (AUROC) for the presence of D-SMI was also calculated. Results: In patients with D-SMI, the median VTQ level was 1.64 meters/second (m/s) (range, 0.93–4.32 m/s), while in patients without D-SMI, the median VTQ level was 1.11 m/s (range, 0.67–4.09 m/s) (p < 0.0001). In the multivariate analysis, higher VTQ was found to be an independent predictor linked to the presence of D-SMI (p < 0.0001). In receiver operating characteristic analysis, body mass index had the highest AUROC (0.805), followed by age (0.721) and VTQ (0.706). Conclusion: VTQ levels can be useful for predicting D-SMI in patients with CLDs.

Keywords: virtual touch quantification; skeletal muscle mass; bio-electronic impedance analysis; liver fibrosis marker; predictive ability

1. Introduction

The severity of liver fibrosis in patients with chronic liver diseases (CLDs) is the major determinant of long-term clinical outcomes, driving both the development of liver-related complications and mortality [1–4]. Thus, evaluating the degree of liver fibrosis correctly plays a pivotal role for the control of disease progression and for creating treatment strategies and evaluating the prognosis for CLD patients [5,6]. High diagnostic accuracy, easy accessibility, and the possibility for follow-up examinations can lead to the implementation of non-invasive diagnostic methods into daily clinical practice.

Acoustic radiation force impulse (ARFI), which is a technology designed to measure shear wave-front at multiple sites to estimate tissue stiffness, is a novel ultrasound-based radiological technique for non-invasively assessing the degree of tissue stiffness [7–10]. This modality can evaluate the degree of liver fibrosis easily and accurately in the clinical settings [10,11]. ARFI elastography has two modes which involve qualitative response and quantitative response for virtual touch quantification (VTQ), and it measures transverse shear wave velocity values in meters/second (m/s). The shear wave velocity reflects tissue stiffness through a simple method: the stiffer the tissue, the higher shear wave velocity [7–11]. A recent meta-analysis demonstrated that ARFI elastography was a good method for evaluating the degree of liver fibrosis and had similar predictive value to transient elastography for significant fibrosis and liver cirrhosis (LC) [12]. Another recent study reported that spleen stiffness measured by ARFI imaging can predict clinical outcomes for LC patients with high accuracy [13]. On the other hand, several serum liver fibrosis markers for predicting the degree of liver fibrosis have been proposed and validated as well as radiological modalities for assessing liver fibrosis [12,14–16]. Of these, FIB-4 index and aspartate aminotransferase (AST) to platelet ratio index (APRI) have been the most widely utilized liver fibrosis markers in CLD patients [16–21].

On the other hand, skeletal muscle is regarded as having a role in maintaining energy metabolism and nutritional status, and the depletion of skeletal muscle mass may be a considerable impairment circumstance [22–25]. Skeletal muscle mass loss can be affected by aging, while LC is occasionally associated with this muscular disorder [22,23]. In our previous investigation, the percentage of skeletal muscle mass loss as determined by bio-electronic impedance analysis (BIA) in LC subjects was significantly higher than that in subjects with chronic hepatitis without LC [26]. Other studies have claimed the significant role of muscle mass assessment in LC patients as a helpful marker for reflecting malnutrition and liver function and for predicting clinical outcomes [26–30]. Recently, sarcopenic obesity, which is the coexistence of sarcopenia as defined by low muscle mass and muscle strength and obesity, has been treated with much caution due to its close linkage to clinical outcomes in CLD patients [31,32].

Considering these reports, the speculation that liver fibrosis marker level is associated with the development of skeletal muscle loss in patients with CLDs may be true. Several reports showing that the proportion of decreased skeletal muscle mass (D-SMI) demonstrated a linear increment with liver fibrosis progression in non-alcoholic fatty liver disease (NAFLD) or non-alcoholic steatohepatitis (NASH) patients support our hypothesis [33–35]. However, an extensive literature search has not shown the relationship between skeletal muscle mass and the liver fibrosis markers in CLD patients, and these clinical questions should be fully addressed. In this study, we sought to clarify the relationship between radiological or serum liver fibrosis markers (VTQ, FIB-4 index, APRI, and platelet count) and skeletal muscle mass, as well as to investigate factors linked to the decrease in skeletal muscle mass in CLD patients.

2. Patients and Methods

2.1. Patients

In this retrospective study, we analyzed 549 patients with CLD who were admitted to the Division of Hepatobiliary and Pancreatic disease, Department of Internal Medicine, Hyogo College of Medicine, Hyogo, Japan between October 2008 and May 2014, and were assessed using BIA to diagnose decreased skeletal muscle mass. All CLD patients who agreed to nutritional evaluation were included. Next, patients without data for VTQ (n = 48), those with advanced malignancies which potentially affect the development of muscle mass loss (n = 16), and those with severe ascites (n = 17) were excluded. Patients with severe ascites were excluded because body weight and body mass index (BMI) may be overestimated in these patients, and skeletal muscle index (SMI) may also be overestimated by BIA [26]. Several edematous patients with advanced cirrhosis (Child-Pugh B or C), hypoalbuminemia, and severe ascites were thus excluded from the current analysis. A total of 468 CLD patients were therefore analyzed. In this study, 447 patients underwent liver biopsy. For patients without liver biopsy data (n = 21), LC was determined by radiological findings such as deformity of the liver surface and presence of varices. We assessed skeletal muscle mass by employing SMI using BIA at baseline. SMI indicates appendicular skeletal muscle mass divided by height squared (cm^2/m^2). D-SMI was defined as SMI <7.0 kg/m^2 for males and as SMI <5.7 kg/m^2 for females, according to the recommendations in current Japanese guidelines [26]. We examined the correlation between SMI and liver fibrosis markers (VTQ, FIB-4 index, APRI, and platelet count) and investigated factors linked to D-SMI in the univariate and multivariate analyses.

APRI score was calculated as reported elsewhere: AST level/upper limit of normal level for AST/platelet count ($\times 10^9$/L) $\times$ 100 [17–20]. The FIB-4 index was calculated as reported elsewhere: age (years) $\times$ AST (IU/L) /platelet count ($\times 10^9$/L) $\times \sqrt{}$alanine aminotransferase (ALT) (IU/L) [19–21]. Our protocols for liver biopsy were detailed in our previous study, and the degrees of liver fibrosis and inflammation were determined as reported elsewhere [36]. The ethics committee meeting of Hyogo college of medicine acknowledged this study protocol (approval number: 2117, approval date: 1 March 2016). And our study protocol conformed to all of the regulations of the Declaration of Helsinki.

2.2. *Measurement for VTQ*

We have routinely used a Siemens ACUSON S2000/3000 (Mochida Siemens Medical Systems, Tokyo, Japan) for VTQ measurement. The method for VTQ measurement by ARFI was conducted as reported elsewhere [10]. Briefly, using intercostal approach by one experienced sonologist, the examination for VTQ measurement was performed on the right lobe of the liver with a measurement depth of 2–3 cm below the liver surface. When successful acquisitions for VTQ data six times at different sites in the liver were obtained on each subject, the median value of these was calculated and data were presented in m/s [10].

2.3. *Statistical Analysis*

For quantitative parameters, the statistical analysis between groups was performed using Student's t test, Mann-Whitney U-test, Kruskal-Wallis test, Fisher's exact test, or Spearman's rank correlation coefficient r_s as appropriate. Parameters with p value < 0.05 in the univariate analysis were entered into the multivariate analysis utilizing the logistic regression analysis. In the multivariate analyses, significant variables in the univariate analyses were changed to dichotomous covariates using each median value. Receiver operating characteristic curve (ROC) analysis for the presence of D-SMI was performed for calculating the area under the ROC (AUROC) in baseline quantitative variables. p values of less than 0.05 were considered to suggest significance. Data are presented as median values (range) unless otherwise mentioned. Statistical analysis was performed with the JMP 11 (SAS Institute Inc., Cary, NC, USA).

3. Results

3.1. *Baseline Characteristics*

The baseline characteristics of the analyzed subjects (n = 468) are shown in Table 1. There are 222 males and 246 females with the median (range) age of 62 (18–90) years. In terms of liver fibrosis stages, F4 was observed in 178 patients, F3 in 73, F2 in 73, F1 in 114, F0 in 9, and not tested in 21. Patients predominantly presented with hepatitis C virus (HCV) infection (57.1%, 267/468). The median (range) SMI for males and females were 7.35 (4.66–11.05) cm^2/m^2 and 5.86 (3.50–8.10) cm^2/m^2, respectively. In this analysis, there were 76 male patients with D-SMI (33.3%) and 99 female patients with D-SMI (40.2%) (p = 0.1823). VTQ ranged from 0.67 m/s to 4.32 m/s (median, 1.34 m/s). FIB-4 index ranged from 0.12 to 2.61 (median, 1.03). APRI ranged from 0.09 to 7.58 (median, 0.83). In males, a significant inverse correlation between VTQ and SMI was found ($r_s = -0.4276$, $p < 0.0001$). Similarly, in females, a significant inverse correlation between VTQ and SMI was found ($r_s = -0.2384$, $p = 0.0002$) (Figure 1A,B).

Table 1. Baseline characteristics ($n = 468$).

Variables	Number or Median (Range)
Age (years)	62 (18–90)
Gender, male/female	222/246
SMI (cm^2/m^2), male	7.35 (4.66–11.05)
SMI (cm^2/m^2), female	5.86 (3.50–8.10)
BMI (kg/m^2)	22.26 (13.05–41.94)
Cause of liver disease, B/C/B and C/alcoholic/others	47/267/4/17/133
AST (IU/L)	36 (12–182)
ALT (IU/L)	35 (7–268)
Serum albumin (g/dL)	3.9 (2.6–5.1)
Total bilirubin (mg/dL)	0.9 (0.2–5.1)
Prothrombin time (%)	89.8 (43.3–133.6)
Platelet count ($\times 10^4/mm^3$)	14.9 (2.1–50.4)
Total cholesterol (mg/dL)	167 (82–448)
Triglyceride (mg/dL)	91 (27–572)
Fasting blood glucose (mg/dL)	99 (70–298)
Serum creatinine (mg/dL)	0.67 (0.32–7.69)
BTR	5.58 (1.63–11.86)
Serum ammonia (μg/dL)	31 (5–137)
C reactive protein (mg/dL)	0.1 (0–2.4)
VTQ (m/s)	1.34 (0.67–4.32)
FIB-4 index	1.03 (0.12–2.61)
APRI	0.83 (0.09–7.58)
F stage, 0/1/2/3/4/NT	9/114/73/73/178/21

SMI: skeletal muscle index; BMI: body mass index; AST: aspartate aminotransferase; ALT: alanine aminotransferase; BTR: branched-chain amino acid to tyrosine ratio; VTQ: virtual touch quantification; APRI: AST to platelet ratio index; NT: not tested.

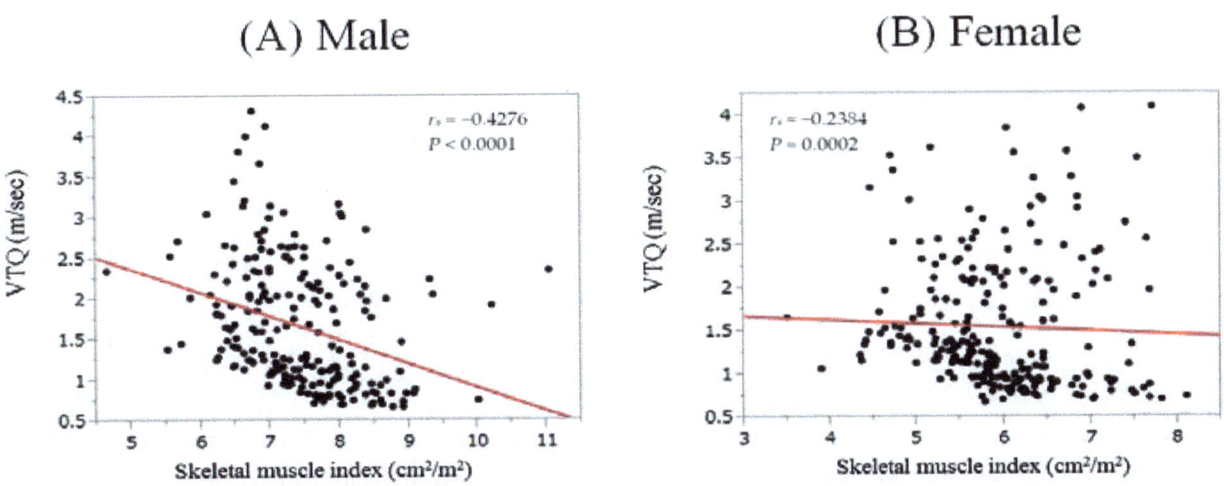

Figure 1. (**A**) Correlation between virtual touch quantification (VTQ) and skeletal muscle index (SMI) in males. Significant inverse correlation between VTQ and SMI was found ($r_s = -0.4276$, $p < 0.0001$); (**B**) Correlation between VTQ and SMI in females. Significant inverse correlation between VTQ and SMI was found ($r_s = -0.2384$, $p = 0.0002$).

3.2. VTQ Level according to The Degree of Liver Fibrosis

For the entire cohort (excluding 21 patients with missing data for liver histology, $n = 447$), the stepwise increase of VTQ level was found according to the severity of liver fibrosis (overall significance, $p < 0.0001$). (Figure 2A) Similarly, for patients with HCV (excluding patients with missing data for liver histology, $n = 246$), the stepwise increase of VTQ level was also found according to the severity of liver fibrosis (overall significance, $p < 0.0001$) (Figure 2B).

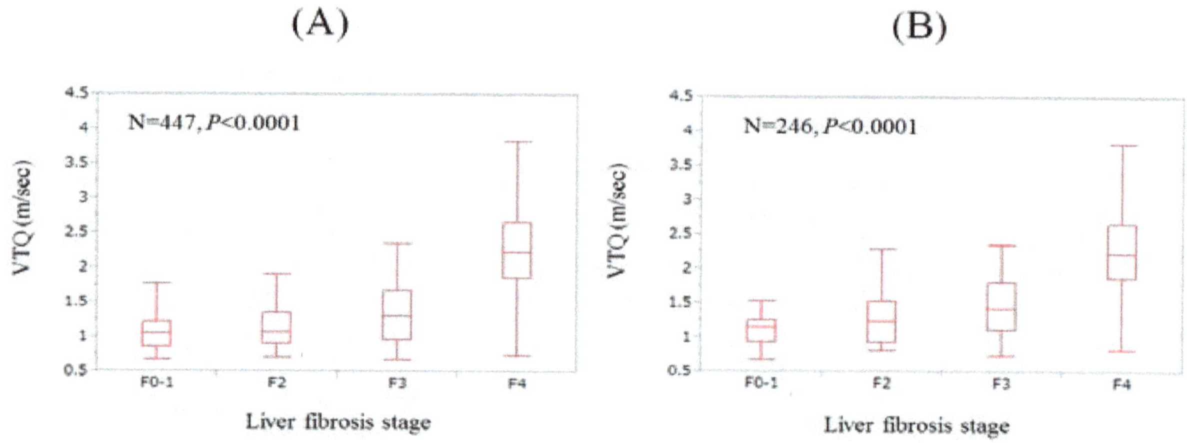

Figure 2. (**A**) VTQ level according to liver fibrosis stage for the entire cohort (excluding 21 patients with missing data for liver histology, $n = 447$). The stepwise increase of VTQ level was found according to the severity of liver fibrosis (overall significance, $p < 0.0001$); (**B**) VTQ level according to liver fibrosis stage for patients with hepatitis C virus (HCV) (excluding patients with missing data for liver histology, $n = 246$). The stepwise increase of VTQ level was found according to the severity of liver fibrosis (overall significance, $p < 0.0001$).

3.3. VTQ Level in Patients with and without D-SMI

In patients with D-SMI, the median VTQ level was 1.64 m/s (range, 0.93–4.32 m/s), while in patients without D-SMI, the median VTQ level was 1.11 m/s (range, 0.67–4.09 m/s) ($p < 0.0001$) (Figure 3A).

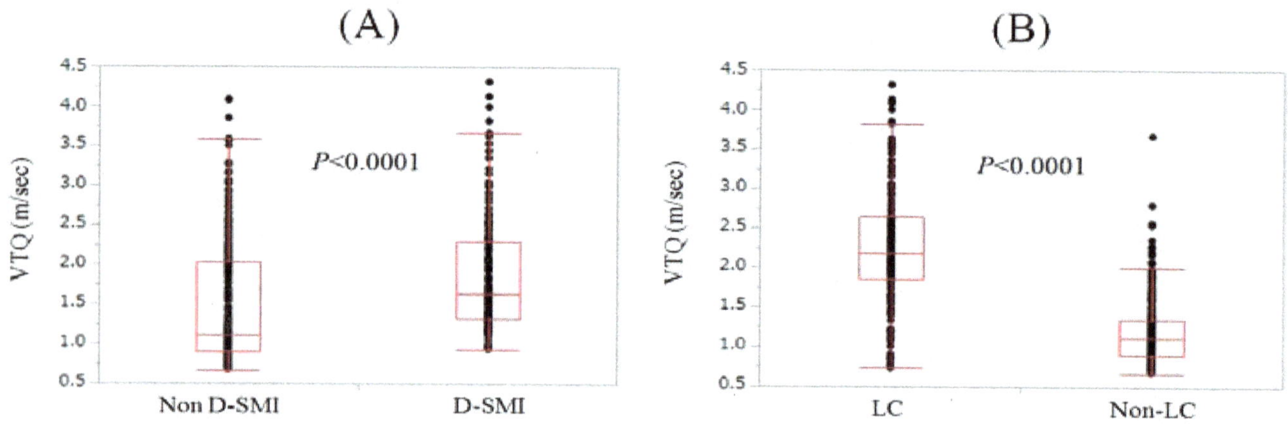

Figure 3. (**A**) VTQ level in patients with and without decreased skeletal muscle mass (D-SMI). In patients with D-SMI, the median VTQ level was 1.64 m/s (range, 0.93–4.32 m/s), while in patients without D-SMI, the median VTQ level was 1.11 m/s (range, 0.67–4.09 m/s) ($p < 0.0001$); (**B**) VTQ level according to liver cirrhosis (LC) status. In patients with LC, the median VTQ level was 2.18 m/s (range, 0.73–4.32 m/s), while in patients without LC, the median VTQ level was 1.11 m/s (range, 0.67–3.67 m/s) ($p < 0.0001$).

3.4. VTQ Level according to LC Status

In patients with LC, the median VTQ level was 2.18 m/s (range, 0.73–4.32 m/s), while in patients without LC, the median VTQ level was 1.11 m/s (range, 0.67–3.67 m/s) ($p < 0.0001$) (Figure 3B).

3.5. ROC Analysis for the Presence of D-SMI

Results for ROC analyses (AUROC, optimal cutoff point, sensitivity, and specificity) for the presence of D-SMI are presented in Table 2. BMI had the highest AUROC (0.805), followed by age (AUROC = 0.721), VTQ (AUROC = 0.706), and serum albumin (AUROC = 0.698).

Table 2. ROC analysis for decreased skeletal muscle index.

	AUROC	Cutoff Value	Sensitivity (%)	Specificity (%)
Age	0.721	62	72.57	62.80
Body mass index	0.805	22.78	85.14	61.77
AST	0.469	57.0	78.87	24.91
ALT	0.532	72.0	89.14	18.77
Serum albumin	0.698	4.0	85.14	54.27
Total bilirubin	0.535	0.80	53.4	54.95
Prothrombin time	0.504	85.7	68.57	38.91
Platelet count	0.579	17.8	76.00	41.64
Total cholesterol	0.521	192	76.57	31.06
Triglyceride	0.576	102	72.57	46.42
Fasting blood glucose	0.466	127	12.0	91.13
Serum creatinine	0.476	0.89	18.29	88.05
BTR	0.563	5.93	68.57	47.78
Serum ammonia	0.478	64	94.51	12.0
C reactive protein	0.548	0	53.71	57.68
VTQ	0.706	1.12	94.86	50.51
FIB-4 index	0.635	0.772	84.57	37.2
APRI	0.564	0.716	64.57	51.54

AUROC: area under the receiver operating curve; AST: aspartate aminotransferase; ALT: alanine aminotransferase; BTR: branched-chain amino acid to tyrosine ratio; VTQ: virtual touch quantification; APRI: AST to platelet ratio index.

3.6. Relationship between VTQ and Baseline Variables

Age ($r_s = 0.4418, p < 0.0001$), AST ($r_s = 0.3315, p < 0.0001$), total bilirubin ($r_s = 0.1994, p < 0.0001$), serum ammonia ($r_s = 0.3191, P < 0.0001$), FIB-4 index ($r_s = 0.2122, p = 0.0001$), and APRI ($r_s = 0.6011$, $p < 0.0001$) had significantly positive correlations with VTQ level. SMI in males ($r_s = -0.4276, p < 0.0001$), SMI in females ($r_s = -0.2384, p = 0.0002$), serum albumin ($r_s = -0.5538, p < 0.0001$), prothrombin time ($r_s = -0.5504$, $p < 0.0001$), platelet count ($r_s = -0.6152$, $p < 0.0001$), total cholesterol ($r_s = -0.3941$, $p < 0.0001$), triglyceride ($r_s = -0.2075, p < 0.0001$), and branched-chain amino acid to tyrosine ratio (BTR) ($r_s = -0.6061, p < 0.0001$) had significant inverse correlations with VTQ level (Table 3).

3.7. Univariate and Multivariate Analyses of Factors Contributing to The Presence of D-SMI

Significant variables linked to the presence of D-SMI in the univariate analyses are: age ($p < 0.0001$); BMI ($p < 0.0001$); serum albumin ($p < 0.0001$); platelet count ($p = 0.0044$); BTR ($p = 0.0219$); VTQ ($p < 0.0001$); FIB-4 index ($p < 0.0001$); and APRI ($p = 0.0204$) (Table 4). The odds ratios (ORs) and 95% confidence intervals calculated by using multivariate analysis for the eight significant parameters ($p < 0.05$) in the univariate analysis are presented in Table 5. BMI ($p < 0.0001$), age ($p < 0.0001$), serum albumin ($p < 0.0001$), BTR ($p = 0.0031$), VTQ ($p < 0.0001$), and FIB-4 index ($p = 0.0425$) were found to be independent predictors associated with the presence of D-SMI (Table 5).

Table 3. Relationship between VTQ level and baseline data.

	r_s	*p* Value
Age	0.4418	<0.0001
SMI, male	−0.4276	<0.0001
SMI, female	−0.2384	0.0002
Body mass index	−0.0746	0.1071
AST	0.3315	<0.0001
ALT	0.0121	0.7947
Serum albumin	−0.5538	<0.0001
Total bilirubin	0.1994	<0.0001
Prothrombin time	−0.5504	<0.0001
Platelet count	−0.6152	<0.0001
Total cholesterol	−0.3941	<0.0001
Triglyceride	−0.2075	<0.0001
Fasting blood glucose	0.0731	0.1140
Serum creatinine	0.0679	0.1427
BTR	−0.6061	<0.0001
Serum ammonia	0.3191	<0.0001
C reactive protein	0.0559	0.2277
FIB-4 index	0.2122	<0.0001
APRI	0.6011	<0.0001

VTQ: virtual touch quantification; SMI: skeletal muscle index; AST: aspartate aminotransferase; ALT: alanine aminotransferase; BTR: branched-chain amino acid to tyrosine ratio; APRI: AST to platelet ratio index.

Table 4. Comparison of baseline characteristics between patients with D-SMI (n = 185) and those without D-SMI (n = 304).

	Decreased Skeletal Muscle Mass (D-SMI) (n = 175)	**Non D-SMI (n = 293)**	*p* **Value**
Age (years)	67 (25–90)	58 (18–81)	<0.0001
Gender, male/female	76/99	146/147	0.1823
Cause of liver disease B/C/B and C/Alcohol/Others	15/113/2/6/39	32/154/2/11/94	0.0988
BMI (kg/m^2)	20.28 (13.05–31.14)	23.78 (17.21–41.94)	<0.0001
Serum albumin (g/dL)	3.7 (2.6–4.9)	4.1 (2.7–5.1)	<0.0001
Total bilirubin (mg/dL)	0.8 (0.3–5.1)	0.9 (0.2–4.7)	0.2045
Prothrombin time (%)	89.4 (55.5–123)	90.0 (43.3–133.6)	0.8143
Platelet count ($\times 10^4$/mm^3)	13.7 (3.3–40.8)	15.7 (2.1–50.4)	0.0044
AST (IU/L)	38 (13–125)	35 (12–182)	0.2571
ALT (IU/L)	34 (7–268)	36 (8–247)	0.2449
Total cholesterol (mg/dL)	166 (85–292)	167 (82–448)	0.3264
Triglyceride	85 (27–554)	97 (29–572)	0.1026
Fasting blood glucose	96 (70–298)	101 (73–249)	0.2169
BTR	5.33 (1.63–11.86)	5.83 (1.79–10.46)	0.0219
Serum creatinine (mg/dL)	0.65 (0.32–7.67)	0.68 (0.35–6.5)	0.3808
Serum ammonia	31 (10–105)	30 (5–137)	0.4519
C reactive protein	0 (0–2.3)	0.1 (0–2.4)	0.5844
VTQ	1.64 (0.93–4.32)	1.11 (0.67–4.09)	<0.0001
FIB-4 index	1.15 (0.36–2.61)	0.96 (0.12–2.60)	<0.0001
APRI	0.97 (0.20–4.23)	0.70 (0.09–7.58)	0.0204

SMI: skeletal muscle index; BMI: body mass index; AST: aspartate aminotransferase; ALT: alanine aminotransferase; BTR: branched-chain amino acid to tyrosine ratio; VTQ: virtual touch quantification; APRI: AST to platelet ratio index.

Table 5. Multivariate analyses of factors linked to the presence of D-SMI.

Variables	Multivariate Analysis		
	OR	95% CI	*p* Value
BMI (per one kg/m^2)	1.712	1.523–1.925	<0.0001
Age (per one year)	0.922	0.895–0.953	<0.0001
Platelet count (per one $\times 10^4$/mm^3)	1.017	0.969–1.068	0.5003
Serum albumin (per one g/dL)	4.832	2.148–10.872	<0.0001
BTR (per one)	1.374	1.107–1.704	0.0031
VTQ (per one m/s)	0.278	0.167–0.462	<0.0001
FIB-4 index (per one)	0.625	0.384–0.955	0.0425
APRI (per one)	0.455	0.189–1.095	0.0735

OR: Odds ratio; CI: confidence interval; BMI: body mass index; BTR: branched-chain amino acid to tyrosine ratio; VTQ: virtual touch quantification; APRI: AST to platelet ratio index.

4. Discussion and Conclusions

Radiological and serum liver fibrosis markers are useful markers and have been preferably used in the clinical settings for their non-invasiveness and easy availability [7–11,13]. Indeed, the stepwise increase of VTQ level according to the severity of liver fibrosis was found in our data. However, there have been no available data for the relationship between skeletal muscle mass and VTQ level in CLD patients. Because skeletal muscle mass in CLDs has been drawing much caution due to its prognostic significance, addressing this problem may be clinically essential [23,26,28–30]. We therefore conducted the current analysis. To the best of our knowledge, this is the first report linking skeletal muscle loss with liver damage in CLDs in a Japanese population using data for VTQ.

In our results, a significant inverse correlation between SMI and VTQ level in both males and females, and a significant difference of VTQ level between patients with and without D-SMI were found. Additionally, AUROC of VTQ for D-SMI was 0.706, and higher VTQ levels were revealed to be significantly associated with the development of D-SMI in the multivariate analysis ($p < 0.0001$). These results denote that VTQ level can be helpful for not only assessing the degree of liver fibrosis, but also for predicting D-SMI. A recent Korean study ($n = 309$) demonstrated that significant stratification was found in terms of the proportion of sarcopenia as evaluated by the appendicular skeletal muscle mass divided by body weight among subjects with normal livers, those with NAFLD, and those with NASH, which were in line with our current data [35].

Although LC-related muscle mass loss is defined as secondary sarcopenia as well as chronic inflammatory diseases and advanced malignancies, aging can cause D-SMI in CLDs at least in part [24,26]. The significant positive correlation between age and VTQ level ($r_s = 0.4418$, $p < 0.0001$) may be associated with our current results. The fact that FIB-4 index includes age may also well explain the statistical significance of FIB-4 index for predicting D-SMI in the multivariate analysis. As a greater number of Japanese CLD patients have been aging in recent years, this is a critical problem.

BTR had the second strongest correlation with VTQ level ($r_s = -0.6061$) and was revealed to be an independent predictor for the development of D-SMI ($p = 0.0031$). The liver is a central organ for the metabolism of three major classes of molecules: fats, proteins, and carbohydrates [37,38]. Deterioration in liver functional reserve can be accompanied by numerous nutritional disorders, and BTR reflects the nutritional state [39,40]. Poor nutritional status can cause muscle mass depletion. Branched-chain amino acid granules are promising for ameliorating muscle mass depletion [28]. In a sense, VTQ level may be helpful for assessing nutritional state in CLD patients. It is also of note that VTQ level had significant positive correlation with serum ammonia level ($r_s = 0.3191$, $p < 0.0001$). Elevated serum ammonia levels lead to the suppression of protein synthesis in the muscle [6,23,26].

In our results, lower BMI had strong impact on D-SMI, while in the Korean national study with large NAFLD cohort ($n = 2761$), the proportion of sarcopenia using dual-energy X-ray absorptiometry was prominent in obese patients [34]. The average BMIs in our study and their study were 22.8 kg/m^2

and 25.8 kg/m^2, respectively. In our cohort, 109 patients (23.3%) had BMI >25 kg/m^2 and only five patients (1.1%) had BMI >35 kg/m^2. The distribution of BMI in baseline characteristics between these studies may lead to such different results. The incidence of sarcopenic obesity has been increasing and the relation between muscle mass and BMI should be further examined in future studies [31,32].

We acknowledge several weak points to our study. First, this is a retrospective single center Japanese study. Thus, whether our data can be applied to other ethnic backgrounds remains unclear. Second, in this cross-sectional study, we are unable to interpret any causal relationship; in other words, an in-depth mechanism for the independent association between D-SMI and liver fibrosis was not clarified in our study. Third, liver biopsy has a significant limitation for sampling errors in evaluating the severity of liver fibrosis. Finally, patients with severe ascites who are expected to have D-SMI with higher rates were excluded from our analysis, potentially leading to bias. Caution should therefore be exercised when interpreting our results. However, our current results presented that VTQ can be useful for predicting D-SMI in CLD patients. In our previous investigation, we reported that a predictive model involving VTQ level is promising for assessing the risk of liver carcinogenesis [10]. Thus, we anticipate that VTQ involves various clinical significances for CLD patients.

In conclusion, VTQ level can provide useful insights for predicting D-SMI in patients with CLDs.

Acknowledgments: The authors would like to thank all medical staff in our nutritional guidance room and ultrasound center for data collection.

Author Contributions: Hiroki Nishikawa, Takashi Nishimura and Hirayuki Enomoto analyzed data and wrote the paper. Hiroko Iijima supervised this study. Other remaining authors collected data.

Abbreviations

CLDs: chronic liver diseases; ARFI: acoustic radiation force impulse; VTQ: virtual touch quantification; m/s: meters/second; LC: liver cirrhosis; AST: aspartate aminotransferase; BIA: bio-electronic impedance analysis; APRI: AST to platelet ratio index; NAFLD: non-alcoholic fatty liver disease; NASH: non-alcoholic steatohepatitis; BMI: body mass index; SMI: skeletal muscle mass; D-SMI: decreased skeletal muscle mass; ALT: alanine aminotransferase; ROC: receiver operating characteristic curve; AUROC: area under the ROC; HCV: hepatitis C virus; BTR: branched-chain amino acid to tyrosine ratio; ORs: odds ratios.

References

1. Van der Meer, A.J.; Berenguer, M. Reversion of disease manifestations after HCV eradication. *J. Hepatol.* **2016**, *65*, 95–108. [CrossRef] [PubMed]
2. Karanjia, R.N.; Crossey, M.M.; Cox, I.J.; Fye, H.K.; Njie, R.; Goldin, R.D.; Taylor-Robinson, S.D. Hepatic steatosis and fibrosis: Non-invasive assessment. *World J. Gastroenterol.* **2016**, *22*, 9880–9897. [CrossRef] [PubMed]
3. Friedrich-Rust, M.; Poynard, T.; Castera, L. Critical comparison of elastography methods to assess chronic liver disease. *Nat. Rev. Gastroenterol. Hepatol.* **2016**, *13*, 402–411. [CrossRef] [PubMed]
4. Westbrook, R.H.; Dusheiko, G. Natural history of hepatitis C. *J. Hepatol.* **2014**, *61*, 58–68. [CrossRef] [PubMed]
5. Yu, M.L. Hepatitis C Treatment from "Response-guided" to "Resource-guided" therapy in the transition era from IFN-containing to IFN-free regimens. *J. Gastroenterol. Hepatol.* **2017**. [CrossRef] [PubMed]
6. Majumdar, A.; Kitson, M.T.; Roberts, S.K. Systematic review: Current concepts and challenges for the direct-acting antiviral era in hepatitis C cirrhosis. *Aliment. Pharmacol. Ther.* **2016**, *43*, 1276–1292. [CrossRef] [PubMed]
7. Lupsor, M.; Badea, R.; Stefanescu, H.; Sparchez, Z.; Branda, H.; Serban, A.; Maniu, A. Performance of a new elastographic method (ARFI technology) compared to unidimensional transient elastography in the noninvasive assessment of chronic hepatitis C. Preliminary results. *J. Gastrointestin. Liver Dis.* **2009**, *18*, 303–310. [PubMed]
8. Takahashi, H.; Ono, N.; Eguchi, Y.; Eguchi, T.; Kitajima, Y.; Kawaguchi, Y.; Nakashita, S.; Ozaki, I.; Mizuta, T.; Toda, S.; et al. Evaluation of acoustic radiation force impulse elastography for fibrosis staging of chronic liver disease: A pilot study. *Liver Int.* **2010**, *30*, 538–545. [CrossRef] [PubMed]

9. Friedrich-Rust, M.; Wunder, K.; Kriener, S.; Sotoudeh, F.; Richter, S.; Bojunga, J.; Herrmann, E.; Poynard, T.; Dietrich, C.F.; Vermehren, J.; et al. Liver fibrosis in viral hepatitis: Noninvasive assessment with acoustic radiation force impulse imaging versus transient elastography. *Radiology* **2009**, *252*, 595–604. [CrossRef] [PubMed]
10. Aoki, T.; Iijima, H.; Tada, T.; Kumada, T.; Nishimura, T.; Nakano, C.; Kishino, K.; Shimono, Y; Yoh, K.; Takata, R.; et al. Prediction of development of hepatocellular carcinoma using a new scoring system involving virtual touch quantification in patients with chronic liver diseases. *J. Gastroenterol.* **2017**, *52*, 104–112. [CrossRef] [PubMed]
11. Friedrich-Rust, M.; Nierhoff, J.; Lupsor, M.; Sporea, I.; Fierbinteanu-Braticevici, C.; Strobel, D.; Takahashi, H.; Yoneda, M.; Suda, T.; Zeuzem, S.; et al. Performance of acoustic radiation force impulse imaging for the staging of liver fibrosis: A pooled meta-analysis. *J. Viral Hepat.* **2012**, *19*, 212–219. [CrossRef] [PubMed]
12. Bota, S.; Herkner, H.; Sporea, I.; Salzl, P.; Sirli, R.; Neghina, A.M.; Peck-Radosavljevic, M. Meta-analysis: ARFI elastography versus transient elastography for the evaluation of liver fibrosis. *Liver Int.* **2013**, *33*, 1138–1147. [CrossRef] [PubMed]
13. Takuma, Y.; Morimoto, Y.; Takabatake, H.; Toshikuni, N.; Tomokuni, J.; Sahara, A.; Matsueda, K.; Yamamoto, H. Measurement of spleen stiffness with acoustic radiation force impulse imaging predicts mortality and hepatic decompensation in patients with liver cirrhosis. *Clin. Gastroenterol. Hepatol.* **2016**. [CrossRef] [PubMed]
14. Lurie, Y.; Webb, M.; Cytter-Kuint, R.; Shteingart, S.; Lederkremer, G.Z. Non-invasive diagnosis of liver fibrosis and cirrhosis. *World J. Gastroenterol.* **2015**, *21*, 11567–11583. [CrossRef] [PubMed]
15. De Lucca Schiavon, L.; Narciso-Schiavon, J.L.; de Carvalho-Filho, R.J. Non-invasive diagnosis of liver fibrosis in chronic hepatitis C. *World J. Gastroenterol.* **2014**, *20*, 2854–2866. [CrossRef] [PubMed]
16. Castera, L.; Forns, X.; Alberti, A. Non-invasive evaluation of liver fibrosis using transient elastography. *J. Hepatol.* **2008**, *48*, 835–847. [CrossRef] [PubMed]
17. Lin, Z.H.; Xin, Y.N.; Dong, Q.J.; Wang, Q.; Jiang, X.J.; Zhan, S.H.; Sun, Y.; Xuan, S.Y. Performance of the aspartate aminotransferase-to-platelet ratio index for the staging of hepatitis C-related fibrosis: An updated meta-analysis. *Hepatology* **2011**, *53*, 726–736. [CrossRef] [PubMed]
18. Nishikawa, H.; Nishijima, N.; Enomoto, H.; Sakamoto, A.; Nasu, A.; Komekado, H.; Nishimura, T.; Kita, R.; Kimura, T.; Iijima, H.; et al. Comparison of FIB-4 index and aspartate aminotransferase to platelet ratio index on carcinogenesis in chronic hepatitis B treated with entecavir. *J. Cancer* **2017**, *8*, 152–161. [CrossRef] [PubMed]
19. Xiao, G.; Yang, J.; Yan, L. Comparison of diagnostic accuracy of aspartate aminotransferase to platelet ratio index and fibrosis-4 index for detecting liver fibrosis in adult patients with chronic hepatitis B virus infection: A systemic review and meta-analysis. *Hepatology* **2015**, *61*, 292–302. [CrossRef] [PubMed]
20. Kim, W.R.; Berg, T.; Asselah, T.; Flisiak, R.; Fung, S.; Gordon, S.C.; Janssen, H.L.A.; Lampertico, P.; Lau, D.; Bornstein, J.D.; et al. Evaluation of APRI and FIB-4 scoring systems for non-invasive assessment of hepatic fibrosis in chronic hepatitis B patients. *J. Hepatol.* **2016**, *64*, 773–780. [CrossRef] [PubMed]
21. Houot, M.; Ngo, Y.; Munteanu, M.; Marque, S.; Poynard, T. Systematic review with meta-analysis: Direct comparisons of biomarkers for the diagnosis of fibrosis in chronic hepatitis C and B. *Aliment. Pharmacol. Ther.* **2016**, *43*, 16–29. [CrossRef] [PubMed]
22. Cruz-Jentoft, A.J.; Baeyens, J.P.; Bauer, J.M.; Boirie, Y.; Cederholm, T.; Landi, F.; Martin, F.C.; Michel, J.P.; Rolland, Y.; Schneider, S.M.; et al. Sarcopenia: European consensus on definition and diagnosis: Report of the European Working Group on Sarcopenia in older people. *Age Ageing* **2010**, *39*, 412–423. [CrossRef] [PubMed]
23. Dasarathy, S. Consilience in sarcopenia of cirrhosis. *J. Cachexia Sarcopenia Muscle* **2012**, *3*, 225–237. [CrossRef] [PubMed]
24. Dasarathy, S.; Merli, M. Sarcopenia from mechanism to diagnosis and treatment in liver disease. *J. Hepatol.* **2016**, *65*, 1232–1244. [CrossRef] [PubMed]
25. Sinclair, M.; Gow, P.J.; Grossmann, M.; Angus, P.W. Review article: Sarcopenia in cirrhosis-aetiology, implications and potential therapeutic interventions. *Aliment. Pharmacol. Ther.* **2016**, *43*, 765–777. [CrossRef] [PubMed]

26. Nishikawa, H.; Shiraki, M.; Hiramatsu, A.; Moriya, K.; Hino, K.; Nishiguchi, S. Japan Society of Hepatology guidelines for sarcopenia in liver disease: Recommendation from the working group for creation of sarcopenia assessment criteria. *Hepatol. Res.* **2016**, *46*, 951–963. [CrossRef] [PubMed]
27. Carey, E.J.; Lai, J.C.; Wang, C.W.; Dasarathy, S.; Lobach, I.; Montano-Loza, A.J.; Dunn, M.A. A multi-center study to define sarcopenia in patients with end-stage liver disease. *Liver Transpl.* **2017**. [CrossRef] [PubMed]
28. Hanai, T.; Shiraki, M.; Nishimura, K.; Ohnishi, S.; Imai, K.; Suetsugu, A.; Takai, K.; Shimizu, M.; Moriwaki, H. Sarcopenia impairs prognosis of patients with liver cirrhosis. *Nutrition* **2015**, *31*, 193–199. [CrossRef] [PubMed]
29. Durand, F.; Buyse, S.; Francoz, C.; Laouénan, C.; Bruno, O.; Belghiti, J.; Moreau, R.; Vilgrain, V.; Valla, D. Prognostic value of muscle atrophy in cirrhosis using psoas muscle thickness on computed tomography. *J. Hepatol.* **2014**, *60*, 1151–1157. [CrossRef] [PubMed]
30. Hanai, T.; Shiraki, M.; Watanabe, S.; Kochi, T.; Imai, K.; Suetsugu, A.; Takai, K.; Moriwaki, H.; Shimizu, M. Sarcopenia predicts minimal hepatic encephalopathy in patients with liver cirrhosis. *Hepatol. Res.* **2017**. [CrossRef] [PubMed]
31. Itoh, S.; Yoshizumi, T.; Kimura, K.; Okabe, H.; Harimoto, N.; Ikegami, T.; Uchiyama, H.; Shirabe, K.; Nishie, A.; Maehara, Y. Effect of sarcopenic obesity on outcomes of living-donor liver transplantation for hepatocellular carcinoma. *Anticancer Res.* **2016**, *36*, 3029–3034. [PubMed]
32. Hara, N.; Iwasa, M.; Sugimoto, R.; Mifuji-Moroka, R.; Yoshikawa, K.; Terasaka, E.; Hattori, A.; Ishidome, M.; Kobayashi, Y.; Hasegawa, H.; et al. Sarcopenia and sarcopenic obesity are prognostic factors for overall survival in patients with cirrhosis. *Intern. Med.* **2016**, *55*, 863–870. [CrossRef] [PubMed]
33. Petta, S.; Ciminnisi, S.; Di Marco, V.; Cabibi, D.; Cammà, C.; Licata, A.; Marchesini, G.; Craxì, A. Sarcopenia is associated with severe liver fibrosis in patients with non-alcoholic fatty liver disease. *Aliment. Pharmacol. Ther.* **2017**, *45*, 510–518. [CrossRef] [PubMed]
34. Lee, Y.H.; Kim, S.U.; Song, K.; Park, J.Y.; Kim, D.Y.; Ahn, S.H.; Lee, B.W.; Kang, E.S.; Cha, B.S.; Han, K.H. Sarcopenia is associated with significant liver fibrosis independently of obesity and insulin resistance in nonalcoholic fatty liver disease: Nationwide surveys (KNHANES 2008–2011). *Hepatology* **2016**, *63*, 776–786. [CrossRef] [PubMed]
35. Koo, B.K.; Kim, D.; Joo, S.K.; Kim, J.H.; Chang, M.S.; Kim, B.G.; Lee, K.L.; Kim, W. Sarcopenia is an independent risk factor for non-alcoholic steatohepatitis and significant fibrosis. *J. Hepatol.* **2017**, *66*, 123–131. [CrossRef] [PubMed]
36. Bedossa, P. Intraobserver and interobserver variations in liver biopsy interpretation in patients with chronic hepatitis C. *Hepatology* **1994**, *20*, 15–20.
37. Charlton, M.R. Branched-chain amino acid enriched supplements as therapy for liver disease. *J. Nutr.* **2006**, *136*, 295–298. [CrossRef]
38. Kawaguchi, T.; Izumi, N.; Charlton, M.R.; Sata, M. Branched-chain amino acids as pharmacological nutrients in chronic liver disease. *Hepatology* **2011**, *54*, 1063–1070. [CrossRef] [PubMed]
39. Alberino, F.; Gatta, A.; Amodio, P.; Merkel, C.; Di Pascoli, L.; Boffo, G.; Caregaro, L. Nutrition and survival in patients with liver cirrhosis. *Nutrition* **2001**, *17*, 445–450. [CrossRef]
40. Suzuki, K.; Suzuki, K.; Koizumi, K.; Ichimura, H.; Oka, S.; Takada, H.; Kuwayama, H. Measurement of serum branched-chain amino acids to tyrosine ratio level is useful in a prediction of a change of serum albumin level in chronic liver disease. *Hepatol. Res.* **2008**, *38*, 267–272. [CrossRef] [PubMed]

10

Nutritional Needs and Support for Children with Chronic Liver Disease

Christine H. Yang [1], Brandon J. Perumpail [2], Eric R. Yoo [3], Aijaz Ahmed [4,*] and John A. Kerner Jr. [1]

1. Division of Pediatric Gastroenterology, Hepatology and Nutrition, Lucile Packard Children's Hospital, Palo Alto, Stanford, CA 94304, USA; christine.yang@stanford.edu (C.H.Y.); JKerner@stanfordhealthcare.org (J.A.K.J.)
2. Department of Medicine, Drexel University College of Medicine, Philadelphia, PA 19129, USA; bjp63@drexel.edu
3. Department of Medicine, Santa Clara Valley Medical Center, San Jose, CA 95128, USA; eric.r.yoo@gmail.com
4. Division of Gastroenterology and Hepatology, Stanford University School of Medicine, Stanford, CA 94305, USA

* Correspondence: aijazahmed@stanford.edu

Abstract: Malnutrition has become a dangerously common problem in children with chronic liver disease, negatively impacting neurocognitive development and growth. Furthermore, many children with chronic liver disease will eventually require liver transplantation. Thus, this association between malnourishment and chronic liver disease in children becomes increasingly alarming as malnutrition is a predictor of poorer outcomes in liver transplantation and is often associated with increased morbidity and mortality. Malnutrition requires aggressive and appropriate management to correct nutritional deficiencies. A comprehensive review of the literature has found that infants with chronic liver disease (CLD) are particularly susceptible to malnutrition given their low reserves. Children with CLD would benefit from early intervention by a multi-disciplinary team, to try to achieve nutritional rehabilitation as well as to optimize outcomes for liver transplant. This review explains the multifactorial nature of malnutrition in children with chronic liver disease, defines the nutritional needs of these children, and discusses ways to optimize their nutritional.

Keywords: nutrition; chronic liver disease; children

---

1. Introduction

The liver plays a crucial role in many of the body's metabolic processes, including regulating protein, fat, and carbohydrate metabolism; vitamin storage and activation; and detoxification and excretion of waste products [1]. In children with chronic liver disease (CLD), disruption of these processes results in improper nutrient digestion, absorption, and usage, and ultimately malnutrition. CLD is defined as progressive destruction and regeneration of liver parenchyma leading to fibrosis and cirrhosis, which has been present for at least six months [2]. It results from hepatic injury leading to irreversible impairment of liver function, with changes in architecture and blood supply [3]. This results in impaired synthesis of serum proteins and clotting factors, compromised glycemic control and ammonia metabolism, and impaired bile secretion and cholestasis [4]. The prevalence and etiologies for CLD in children can vary by country and age of onset. In the United States, the prevalence of liver disease in children is unclear; however, it is estimated that 15,000 children are hospitalized for liver disease annually [5]. The overall incidence of liver disease in neonates in the United States is approximately 1 in every 2500 live births [6] with extrahepatic biliary atresia, metabolic disorders, and neonatal hepatitis being the most common causes of CLD in neonates [7]. In older children in the United States, common causes of CLD include metabolic disorders, chronic intrahepatic cholestasis, obesity-related steatohepatitis, drug- and toxin-induced disorders, and viral hepatitis [5]. In Australia, the most common cause of CLD starting in the neonatal age in children is biliary atresia, occurring in approximately 1 in 8000 live births, with other common causes being alpha-1-antitrypsin deficiency and Alagille's syndrome [8,9]. Similarly, in Brazil, biliary atresia is the most common cause of CLD in children [10]. In contrast, a study in Pakistan found viral hepatitis to be the most common cause of neonatal onset CLD, followed by metabolic disorders and biliary atresia [11] while a study in India found metabolic disorders to be the most common cause of CLD in children [12].

Children are particularly susceptible to malnutrition due to their high energy needs for growth [13]. Approximately 25% of children diagnosed with CLD worldwide are undernourished, with the incidence being higher in developing countries [14]. Furthermore, many children with chronic liver disease will eventually require liver transplantation, and studies have noted that malnourishment during liver transplantation is associated with poorer outcomes, including increased risks for morbidity and mortality [15–17] as well as compromised neurocognitive development [18,19] and growth [20]. Otherwise unexplained clinical or laboratory nutritional deficiencies (such as iron deficiency, vitamin D deficiency/rickets, vitamin K deficiency/coagulopathy) should raise suspicion for CLD potentially complicating another diagnosis, such as celiac disease, inflammatory bowel disease, or chronic cholestasis [21]. This review discusses the multi-factorial mechanisms behind malnutrition in children with CLD, as well as strategies to optimize nutritional support in children with CLD.

2. Mechanisms of Malnutrition in Children with Cld

2.1. Decreased Energy Intake

Children with CLD are often unable to consume adequate calories for their energy needs (Figure 1) [22]. Contributing factors include anorexia, changes in taste perception, early satiety, and nausea and vomiting [13]. Anorexia is attributed to changes in amino acid metabolism, which results in increased tryptophan levels and subsequent increases in brain serotonergic activity. Tryptophan is the amino acid precursor to serotonin, which regulates eating behavior. Increased cerebrospinal concentrations of tryptophan have been associated with anorexia in patients with CLD [23]. Deficiency in zinc or magnesium contributes to changes in taste perception, which may be aggravated by supplementation with unpalatable formulas and also discourages intake [13]. Furthermore, pediatric CLD patients have decreased stomach volume and discomfort from ascites and organomegaly that result in early satiety [24]. Increased pro-inflammatory cytokines, common in children with CLD, results in nausea and vomiting [25]. Together, these factors lead to decreased consumption and reduced energy intake.

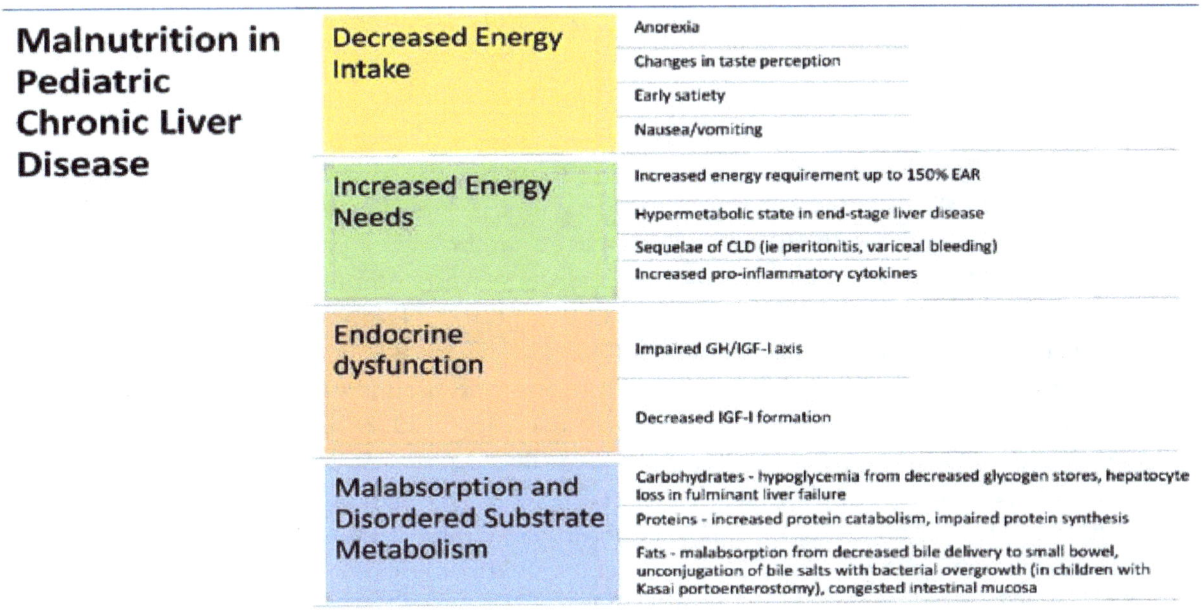

Figure 1. Mechanisms of malnutrition in children with CLD.

EAR: estimated average requirements; GH: growth hormone; IGF: insulin-like growth factor.

2.2. Increased Energy Needs

Children with CLD can have an increase in energy requirements of up to 140% compared to children without CLD [26–28]. Children with end-stage liver disease in particular are in a hypermetabolic state, in which there is increased metabolic activity and excess lipid oxidation [29]. Moreover, this is further aggravated by the sequelae of CLD, including episodes of sepsis from peritonitis or cholangitis, as well as variceal bleeding [13,30]. Children with CLD can also have higher levels of pro-inflammatory cytokines, which have been correlated with malnutrition due to increased energy consumption [31].

2.3. Endocrine Dysfunction

In addition to decreased energy intake and increased metabolism, growth failure in children with CLD is further aggravated by an impaired growth hormone (GH)/insulin-like growth factor (IGF-I) axis. IGF-I and its major circulating binding protein, IGF Binding Protein 3 (IGF-BP3), are synthesized in the liver, and protein malnutrition decreases IGF-I formation, as well as increases its serum clearance and degradation [32]. IGF-I levels are decreased further due to GH resistance in children with CLD caused by downregulation of the GH receptor [30].

2.4. Malabsorption and Disordered Substrate Metabolism

2.4.1. Carbohydrates

The liver receives glucose-rich blood via the portal vein, from which it creates glycogen to be stored in the liver. Glucose is also circulated from the liver to the muscles where lactate, pyruvate, and alanine are generated via glycolysis [33,34]. However, in children with CLD, glycogen stores are depleted from their longstanding condition, resulting in hypoglycemia. Significant hepatocyte loss, such as that in fulminant liver failure, can also cause hypoglycemia [35]. Infants and small children are particularly susceptible due to their lower reserve [13]. In contrast, adults with cirrhosis have increased insulin levels and can develop diabetes mellitus due to increased insulin secretion by the pancreas, decreased insulin degradation by the liver [36] and decreased glucose uptake by tissues [37].

These processes may also occur in children, but unlike adults, few children with CLD (aside from those with cystic fibrosis) develop diabetes mellitus [38].

2.4.2. Proteins

With reduced glycogen stores in CLD, proteins are increasingly utilized for gluconeogenesis [39]. However, the liver's capacity for protein synthesis in CLD is limited due to reduced substrate availability, decreased hepatocyte function, and increased catabolism. Consequently, hypoalbuminemia can develop, leading to peripheral edema, ascites, and decreased enteral intake due to discomfort [13]. Additionally, the liver is the site of synthesis for all coagulation factors with the exception of factor VIII, thus coagulopathy is also a consequence of CLD [30]. Increased protein catabolism also results in increased nitrogenous waste products such as ammonia, which is normally converted to urea by the liver for excretion. This conversion is compromised in CLD, resulting in increased ammonia levels. Abnormal protein use by the liver in CLD results in increased aromatic amino acids (AAAs) and decreased branched-chain amino acids (BCAAs) [40]. An abnormal ratio of BCAAs to AAAs correlates with both histologic damage and encephalopathy [40]. Increased cerebral uptake of AAAs results in formation of false neurotransmitters and causes neurologic dysfunction, along with increased ammonia levels [41]. That said, children with CLD usually do not require protein restriction due to their increased growth needs [42].

2.4.3. Fats

Cholestasis in CLD results in compromised absorption of fats due to decreased delivery of bile salts to the small bowel [43]. This can further be aggravated by small bowel bacterial overgrowth, such as in children who have undergone a Kasai portoenterostomy for biliary atresia, as the bacteria unconjugate bile salts [44]. Congested gastric and intestinal mucosa from portal hypertension further worsen fat malabsorption, and medications, such as cholestyramine to treat pruritus, bind bile salts, decreasing micellar solubilization and thus absorption of di- and monoglycerides from long-chain triglycerides (LCTs) [30]. Children with Alagille syndrome can also have pancreatic insufficiency and decreased lipase, which compromises the hydrolysis of triglycerides [45]. Due to these mechanisms, up to 50% of LCTs, fat-soluble vitamins, and essential polyunsaturated fatty acids (PUFAs) may not be absorbed well in children with CLD [46–48] and deficiencies in long-chain polyunsaturated fatty acids (LCPs) critical to neurologic growth and development, such as arachidonic acid and docosahexaenoic acid (DHA), can develop within 8–12 weeks [30]. Furthermore, children with CLD have increased fat oxidation, likely due to decreased carbohydrate stores. This increased oxidation further decreases fat stores, which then are difficult to replete given the presence of fat malabsorption [13,29]. Lastly, impaired bile flow from cholestasis can result in increased plasma concentration of triglycerides and cholesterol, which may then deposit in the hands, elbows, knees, ankles, and corneas as xanthomas [49].

2.5. Fat-Soluble Vitamins

CLD affects absorption, metabolism, and storage of fat-soluble vitamins. Decreased delivery of bile salts to the small bowel results in malabsorption of fat, as well as the fat-soluble vitamins A, D, E, and K. Without supplementation, fat-soluble vitamin deficiency can develop within 6–12 weeks of birth [30] and even after supplementation up to 30% of severely cholestatic children will remain deficient in all fat-soluble vitamins [50,51].

2.5.1. Vitamin A

Vitamin A has the activity of all-*trans* retinol. Retinol is required for rhodopsin formation (a pigment required for retina rod cell function and dark adaptation), as well as normal cell differentiation. In the diet, vitamin A is available as retinyl palmitate from animal sources (dairy, eggs, fish oils) and as carotenoids from plants (leafy green vegetables, orange-colored fruits, vegetables). Decreased bile salts in the intestine results in decreased hydrolysis of retinyl esters to retinol, as well as decreased formation of micelles, which are required for absorption. Retinol-binding protein (RBP), which is synthesized by the liver and transports vitamin A to peripheral tissues, is also decreased in CLD, thus impairing utilization. Vitamin A deficiency can result in night blindness, xerophthalmia, and keratomalacia [13].

2.5.2. Vitamin D

Vitamin D consists of a group of fat-soluble prohormones and their metabolites, the chief of which are vitamin D_2 (ergocalciferol) and vitamin D_3 (cholecalciferol). These must first undergo hydroxylation in the liver and kidney before they can be utilized by the body. Vitamin D helps regulate calcium and phosphorus, and is critical in bone homeostasis. It can be synthesized in the skin when exposed to sunlight, and can be consumed in the diet from fish oils and fortified dairy products. In CLD, vitamin D deficiency develops from malabsorption, decreased dietary intake and sunlight exposure, and compromised liver hydroxylation. Deficiency results in defective bone mineralization, and if untreated, rickets and fractures [13]. Infants are particularly susceptible, as their bone mineral content can decrease rapidly over the first two years of life [52]. Breastfed infants with CLD are at even higher risk, as breastmilk contains low amounts of vitamin D [53].

2.5.3. Vitamin E

Vitamin E, which consists of tocopherols and tocotrienols, has important anti-oxidant properties. Vitamin E is found in leafy green vegetables, vegetable oils, and nuts. Deficiency in vitamin E in CLD results from malabsorption, and consequences thereof include problems with nerve conduction, including peripheral neuropathy, myopathy, and spinocerebellar dysfunction. Vitamin E deficiency can also result in hemolytic anemia due to oxidative damage to the membranes of red blood cells [54].

2.5.4. Vitamin K

Vitamin K is necessary for carboxylation of glutamic residues on coagulation factors II, VII, IX, and X, as well as proteins C and S, within the liver. Vitamin K_1 [phylloquinone] is found in leafy green vegetables and dairy products, and vitamin K_2 [menaquinone] is synthesized by intestinal bacterial flora. Deficiency in vitamin K in CLD results from malabsorption and manifests as coagulopathy, with easy bleeding and bruising [13]. Due to limited ability of the body to store vitamin K, vitamin K deficiency is one of the earliest fat-soluble vitamin deficiencies to develop in children with CLD [55].

2.6. Trace Elements and Metals

Derangements in trace elements and metals can occur with CLD. Calcium and magnesium are often depleted in CLD, as vitamin D stimulates their absorption from the intestines. They also bind to unabsorbed fatty acids, which further decreases their absorption in children with CLD. Iron deficiency can occur from recurrent gastrointestinal bleeds [13]. Iron deficiency can result in compromised neurologic development in children [56] and multiple studies have found that children with CLD demonstrate delays in mental (−1 standard deviation) and motor (−2 standard deviations) function [6]. Zinc deficiency can develop due to malabsorption as well as increased urinary losses, as zinc is retained in the body by being bound to albumin [57]. Deficiency in zinc results in acrodermatitis, immunodeficiency, and altered protein metabolism; in addition, zinc deficiency, as well as selenium deficiency, can exacerbate growth failure and poor protein synthesis [22,58]. In contrast, copper and manganese levels may be increased in children with cholestasis and CLD, as they are excreted in the bile [59,60]. Thus, in children with CLD who are receiving total parenteral nutrition (TPN), the amount of manganese they receive should be closely monitored, as manganese toxicity in the form of deposition in the basal ganglia can develop [61,62].

3. Strategies to Manage Malnutrition in Cld

3.1. Nutritional Assessment

Accurate nutritional assessment is critical to the management of children with CLD. Standard weight and height measurements may be inaccurate in children with CLD, as they can be confounded by fluid overload, ascites, and organomegaly [30]. Body weight alone may underestimate the incidence of malnutrition in adults and children with CLD by up to 50% [63]. Linear growth is a more sensitive parameter, but stunting and growth deceleration do not occur until late in growth failure. Thus, other measurements, such as triceps or subscapular skinfolds, midarm circumference, and arm muscle measurements (midarm muscle area), should be used. Triceps, skinfolds, and midarm circumference are indicators of body fat and protein, and can reveal early loss in fat stores before height and weight are affected. In children with CLD, triceps skinfold thickness has been shown to be more sensitive for malnutrition compared to weight-for-height *z* scores [14,16]. Furthermore, these upper limb measurements are less affected by edema compared to truncal or lower limb measurements [13]. When growth data are documented, they should be charted as standard deviation scores related to the median value for the child's age and sex, where a *z*-score of 0 is equivalent to the 50th percentile. This will assist in evaluating whether nutritional interventions are effective. Children who are particularly at risk for developing malnutrition include those younger than two years in age with severe cholestasis (bilirubin > 4 mg/dL), progressive liver diseases (biliary atresia and severe familial intrahepatic cholestasis), end-stage liver disease awaiting liver transplantation, and recurrent complications of liver disease (ascites, bleeding varices) [30].

Protein markers, such as albumin and prealbumin, are of limited utility in children with CLD. Albumin may be depressed due to hepatic synthetic dysfunction, inflammation, or acute physiologic stress [64]. Prealbumin is a more sensitive marker of malnutrition compared to albumin, as it has a shorter half-life (2 days compared to 18–20 days); that said, prealbumin levels can be normal in chronic malnutrition [65]. On the other hand, essential fatty acid deficiency can be diagnosed with an increased serum triene to tetraene ratio (greater than 0.4). Essential fatty acid deficiency may exist in up to a third of children with end-stage liver disease awaiting liver transplant [22]. Although there are drawbacks to each of the individual assessment tools, a combination of the tools described can be used to more clearly evaluate malnutrition.

3.2. Supplementation of Specific Macronutrients and Micronutrients

Because of the increased energy needs of children with CLD, energy intake should be increased to 140–200% of estimated average requirements (EARs). In infants, this can be achieved by concentrating medium-chain triglyceride (MCT)-containing formulas (an example being Pregestimil by Mead Johnson Nutrition), so as to increase the number of kilocalories per ounce. Older children can be supplemented with high-calorie, nutrient-dense drinks (examples including Pediasure Peptide by Abbott Nutrition, Peptamen by Nestle Healthcare Nutrition). If a sufficient amount cannot be consumed orally, nasogastric (NG) feedings may be needed [30]. Despite disruption to the GH/IGF-I axis, GH therapy has not been found to have benefits in children with end-stage liver disease [66,67].

3.2.1. Carbohydrates

Carbohydrates are a major source of energy, and can be particularly useful for increasing caloric intake. They can be given as monomers, polymers, and starch. Complex carbohydrates such as maltodextrin and glucose polymers can be particularly useful, as their use restricts the osmolality of feeds, while maintaining a high-energy density greater than 1 kcal/mL. In infants, glucose polymers can be added to feeds, while in older children, a supplemental drink can be given, or mixed with fluids and foods [30].

3.2.2. Proteins

Protein restriction is rarely needed in children or adults with CLD [68]. Children with CLD require 2–3 g/kg/day of protein, but can tolerate up to 4 g/kg/day without developing encephalopathy [42]. Severe protein restriction (<2 g/kg/day) may be temporarily required in the context of acute encephalopathy, but should not be continued long-term, as this can lead to endogenous muscle protein consumption [27].

Given the abnormal AAA to BCAA ratio in children with CLD, there has been interest in whether BCAA-enriched formulas can have nutritional benefit. Specific hypercaloric formulas with low salt and lactose, high MCT and BCAA are available [27]. Thus far there is insufficient evidence to recommend routine use of BCAA-enriched formulas, though there have been studies showing potential benefit. One study which compared children receiving 32% BCAA formula compared to standard formula showed improved lean body mass, though no improvement in amino acid levels [69]. Another study evaluated infants receiving 50% BCAA formula compared to 22% BCAA formula, and demonstrated that infants receiving the 50% BCAA formula had improved protein retention due to suppressed endogenous protein catabolism and normalization of the plasma amino acid profile [28]. Animal models of biliary obstruction have increased weight gain, protein and muscle mass, body composition, and bone mineral density if given BCAAs [70]. That said, numerous studies in adults have not demonstrated a clear benefit to BCAA supplementation [71].

3.2.3. Fats

MCTs, unlike LCTs, do not require micellar solubilization to be transported into the enterocyte, and are transferred directly into the enterocyte and to the portal circulation without reesterification [72]. 95% of MCTs are absorbed even in very cholestatic children, thus MCTs are critical in managing nutrition in children with CLD, where absorption of LCTs is highly compromised [73]. Although 30–50% of total fat should be provided as MCTs [13], care should be taken to ensure LCTs are not eliminated from the diet, as they provide essential fatty acids. Thus, it is necessary to increase overall total fat intake, in both LCTs and MCTs. For older children, MCT oil and emulsions can be added to meals, and should be balanced by fats high in LCP content [30]. For infants, formulas containing up to 75% fat as MCT can be given, but formulas with >80% MCTs can lead to essential fatty acid deficiency. Increased MCT content can also worsen steatorrhea [74]. The minimal linoleic acid intake recommended for infants is 1–2% of total energy intake, with a ratio of linoleic to linolenic acid of 5:15.1 [75]. They can be supplemented in the form of walnut or fish oils, as well as dietary products rich in PUFAs, such as egg yolks [30].

3.3. Fat-Soluble Vitamins

In the presence of direct-reacting serum bilirubin levels greater than 2 mg/dL, the diet should be adequately supplemented with fat-soluble vitamins [76]. The role of serum bile acid as a surrogate marker to guide the monitoring of fat-soluble vitamin deficiency is still undefined. In infants with biliary atresia, total serum bilirubin appears to be a better predictor of fat-soluble vitamin deficiency compared to serum bile acids, though neither are perfect [77]. Serum vitamin and prothrombin levels should be monitored to allow proper adjustment of dosages to the specific needs of the patient [78].

3.3.1. Vitamin A

Serum retinol level is the most convenient and practical means of measuring vitamin A status, though retinol dose response (RDR) is believed to be more reliable but is not widely available (Figure 2). It is important to monitor levels in children receiving supplementation, as hypervitaminosis A can lead to potentially fatal hepatotoxicity [13]. Supplementation with 5000–10,000 IU/day may be needed in children with CLD [30].

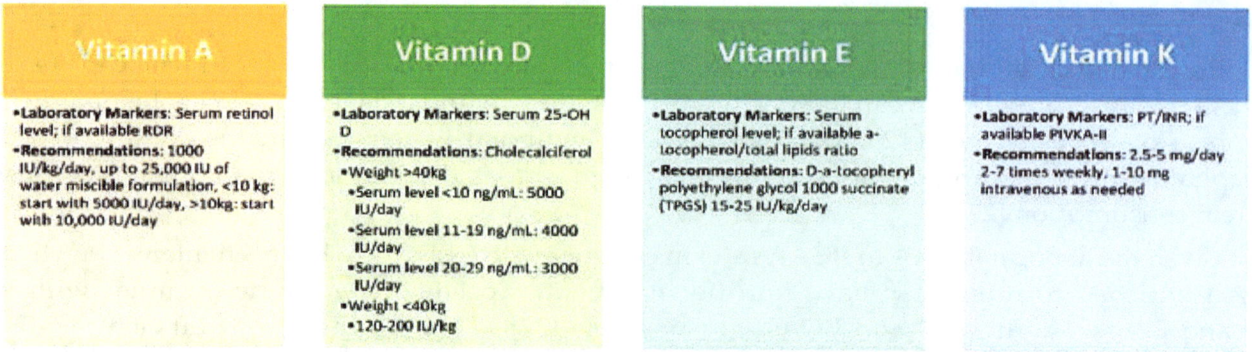

Figure 2. Management of fat-soluble vitamin deficiency in CLD. INR: international normalized ratio; IU: international unit; PIVKA-II: protein induced in vitamin K absence; PT: prothrombin time; RDR: retinol dose response.

3.3.2. Vitamin D

Serum 25-OH D is the most abundant vitamin D metabolite in the body, and can be used to monitor vitamin D status. Low levels of 25-OH D are associated with reduced bone mineral density in children with CLD [52]. It is important to optimize vitamin D levels before liver transplantation due to the use of corticosteroids post-transplant, which can compromise bone density [79]. Co-supplementation with a micellar vitamin E formulation can improve vitamin D absorption in children with cholestatic liver disease [80] and 25-OH D_3 is more water-soluble and thus better absorbed compared to vitamin D_2 [81]. 25-OH D levels, along with calcium and phosphorus, should be monitored to prevent vitamin D overdose. Up to 400 IU/day can be given as supplementation; however, children who are deficient may need substantially higher doses [13].

3.3.3. Vitamin E

The serum tocopherol level is commonly used to measure vitamin E status, though the alpha tocopherol/total lipids ratio is more specific [82]. D-alpha-tocopheryl polyethylene glycol 1000 succinate (TPGS) is the most readily absorbed form of vitamin E in cholestatic patients, as it can form micelles without the need for bile salts [13]. Unfortunately, correction of vitamin E deficiency may not reverse severe spinocerebellar degeneration [83], but it can reverse most other neurologic complications [84]. Supplementation with 50–400 IU/day of TPGS may be needed in children with CLD [30].

3.3.4. Vitamin K

The PIVKA-II [protein induced in vitamin K absence] assay is the most sensitive for measuring vitamin K deficiency, but it is not widely available [50,85]. Therefore, vitamin K status is usually evaluated by checking coagulation values, including prothrombin time (PT) and international normalized ratio (INR). Deficiency can be diagnosed if these values improve after a dose of parenteral vitamin K [13]. Supplementation with 2.5–5 mg/day of vitamin K may be needed [30], though oral vitamin K, even in micellar form, is poorly absorbed in children with CLD [86]. This is further exacerbated by medications commonly used to treat encephalopathy, such as lactulose, which reduces intestinal bacterial production of vitamin K. Thus, intermittent parenteral repletion may be required [13].

3.4. Water-Soluble Vitamins and Minerals

Water-soluble vitamins should also be supplemented in children with CLD in the form of a multivitamin. For minerals, including selenium, zinc, calcium, and magnesium, supplementation should be based from plasma levels. Iron may need to be supplemented in children with chronic blood loss from gastrointestinal bleeds [30]. Repletion of zinc and magnesium in particular may be helpful, as zinc plays a role in immune function and tissue repair [13], while magnesium may help improve bone status [87].

3.5. Mode of Delivery

Nutritional supplementation should be given enterally whenever possible. Enteral nutrition has numerous advantages over parenteral nutrition: it is cheaper, more physiologic, does not come with the risk of catheter-associated bloodstream infections, maintains gastrointestinal tract immunity as well as gut barrier integrity, and reduces bacterial overgrowth. However, as discussed in a previous section, many children with CLD are unable to orally consume sufficient calories to treat or prevent malnutrition. Therefore, NG tube feedings are often required. Gastrostomy tubes are generally avoided in children with CLD due to portal hypertension and the potential for stomal varices to develop, placement difficulty due to organomegaly, and risk of peritoneal infection with ascites [8,68]; they may be helpful in children with stable compensated liver disease such as cystic fibrosis [30]. With modern soft Silastic™ (Dow Corning Corporation, Midland, MI, USA) NG tubes, NG feeds are safe even in patients with esophageal varices [42,88–90]. Using a NG tube for nocturnal feeds is usually the first choice, as it allows for normal oral feeding during the day while supplementing overnight. Nocturnal feeding is also helpful in infants with severe CLD, as it prevents fasting hypoglycemia and reduces protein catabolism. Children with severe malabsorption or feeding intolerance may require continuous feeds [30]. Intensive enteral NG feeding can successfully reverse malnutrition in children with CLD, as well as decrease parental anxiety [42,73,91]. However, feeding aversion can also develop, especially in infants who have received long-term NG feeds. This is further aggravated by the need for often unpalatable medication and formulas. Thus, involvement of a multidisciplinary care team including dieticians, psychologists, and speech and occupational therapists is critical. Strategies to prevent feeding aversion include promoting daytime oral intake, as well as encouraging children to experiment with various age-appropriate flavors and textures [73].

Some children with CLD will require parenteral nutrition. These include children who cannot tolerate enteral nutrition due to feeding intolerance, or those with recurrent variceal bleeding. In the short-term, parenteral nutrition is not associated with hepatobiliary dysfunction or worsened cholestasis, though these certainly do occur with long-term use [92]. Standard amino acid and lipid formulations are well tolerated in patients with stable CLD, though triglyceride levels should be closely monitored in children with severe liver disease, hepatic encephalopathy, and sepsis. Amino acid levels should also be monitored. If encephalopathy does develop, the amino acid content can be decreased to 1–2 g/kg/day [30]. Manganese levels also need to be monitored given the potential for manganese toxicity to exacerbate CLD [93,94]. Parenteral nutrition is particularly helpful in children with acute fulminant liver failure, as these children are in a hypercatabolic state. In these children, standard formulations can be used, but the total volume should be restricted to 75% of maintenance, and concentration may need to be further increased to prevent hypoglycemia. Protein restriction should not be needed, especially if the patient is being electively ventilated [30].

4. Effect of Liver Transplantation on Nutritional Status [Figure 3]

Malnutrition is a significant risk factor for both morbidity and mortality related to liver transplantation, thus nutritional support is of utmost importance in children with CLD prior to undergoing transplant (Figure 3) [15,95,96]. Children who were malnourished prior to transplant may require support with parenteral nutrition peri-operatively, while children with normal nutritional status prior to transplant can start enteral feedings with rapid buildup of calories within 3–5 days postoperatively. Children after liver transplant require at least 120% of EAR post-operatively, which can be administered in the form of high-energy pediatric and infant formulas, either orally or via nasogastric tube [30]. Children with oral aversion pre-operatively will likely require nasogastric supplementation post-operatively for up to two months; regular diet for age is usually achieved by six months [97]. Energy intake should include 6–8 g/kg/day of carbohydrates, 2.5–3 g/kg/day of protein, and 5–6 g/kg/day of fat [30].

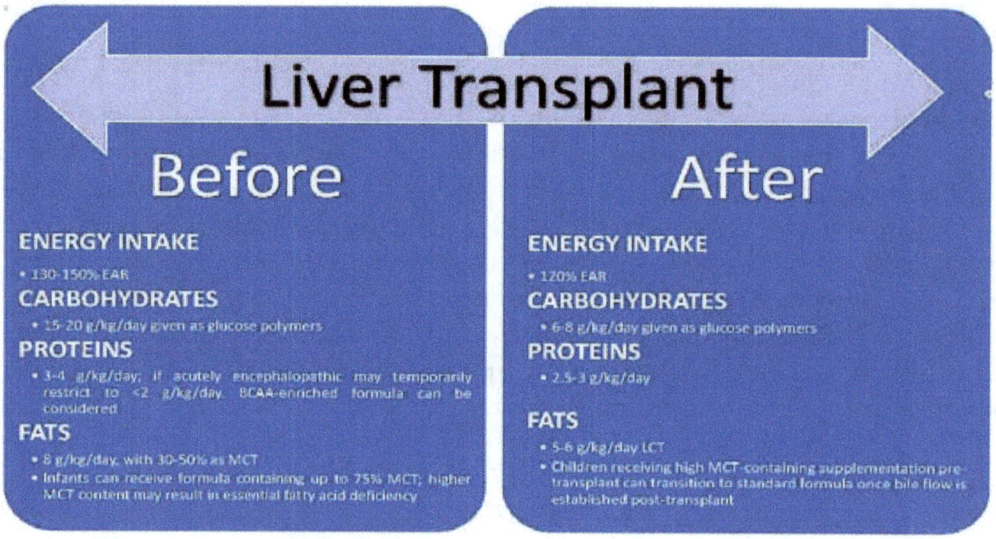

Figure 3. Nutritional needs of children with CLD before and after liver transplant. EAR: estimated average requirements; LCT: long-chain triglycerides; MCT: medium-chain triglycerides.

Preoperative nutritional status also affects postoperative growth. Children who are more stunted, with a height standard deviation score (SDS) >-2, grow more rapidly after a transplant, but may not achieve normal height. This is in contrast to children who are less stunted: while their initial growth velocity post-operatively is slower, they ultimately achieve normal growth velocity [98]. There is no difference in catch-up growth between genders or pre-transplantation liver disease; the exception being Alagille syndrome, which is associated with growth failure, both before and after a transplant, in up to 50% of patients [99,100]. Recombinant GH has been trialed in eight growth-retarded children after a transplant, and while there were increases in both median growth rate and height SDS, growth velocity was not maintained beyond the first year [101].

Ultimately, nutritional rehabilitation can be achieved with liver transplantation [73,102,103]. After transplantation, there is a rapid return to normal midarm muscle area and midarm fat within 3–6 months [103,104] and catch-up growth is usually achieved within 18 months [15]. However, it can take months to years for bone density to return to normal. Osteoporosis and fractures have been described within 3–6 months after a transplant, and can be exacerbated by glucocorticoid therapy required after a transplant [67]. Long-chain PUFA and BCAA metabolism also take time to normalize after a transplant [71,105] and abnormalities in IGF-binding proteins BP1, BP2, and BP3 persist for several months [106].

5. Conclusions

Malnutrition is common in children with CLD, and requires aggressive and appropriate management to correct nutritional deficiencies. Infants with CLD are particularly susceptible to malnutrition given their low reserves. Children with CLD would benefit from early intervention by a multi-disciplinary team, to try to achieve nutritional rehabilitation, as well as to optimize outcomes for liver transplantation.

Acknowledgments: No sources of funding were used for this work.

References

1. Pratt, C.A.; Garcia, M.G.; Kerner, J.A., Jr. Nutritional management of neonatal and infant liver disease. *NeoReviews* **2001**, *2*, e215–e222. [CrossRef]
2. Widodo, A.D.; Soelaeman, E.J.; Dwinanda, N.; Narendraswari, P.P.; Purnomo, B. Chronic liver disease is a risk factor for malnutrition and growth retardation in children. *Asia Pac. J. Clin. Nutr.* **2017**, *26* (Suppl. 1), S57–S60. [PubMed]
3. Young, S.; Kwarta, E.; Azzam, R.; Sentongo, T. Nutrition assessment and support in children with end-stage liver disease. *Nutr. Clin. Pract.* **2013**, *28*, 317–329. [CrossRef] [PubMed]
4. Sokal, E.M.; Goldstein, D.; Ciocca, M.; Lewindon, P.; Ni, Y.H.; Silveira, T.; Sibal, A.; Dhawan, A.; Mack, C.; Bucuvalas, J.; et al. End-stage liver disease and liver transplant: Current situation and key issues. *J. Pediatr. Gastroenterol. Nutr.* **2008**, *47*, 239–246. [CrossRef] [PubMed]
5. Arya, G.; Balistreri, W.F. Pediatric liver disease in the United States: Epidemiology and impact. *J. Gastroenterol. Hepatol.* **2002**, *17*, 521–525. [CrossRef] [PubMed]
6. Rodriguez-Baez, N.; Wayman, K.I.; Cox, K.L. Growth and development in chronic liver disease. *NeoReviews* **2001**, *2*, e211–e214. [CrossRef]
7. Danks, D.M.; Campbell, P.E.; Jack, I.; Rogers, J.; Smith, A.L. Studies of the aetiology of neonatal hepatitis and biliary atresia. *Arch. Dis. Child.* **1977**, *52*, 360–367. [CrossRef] [PubMed]
8. Baker, A.; Stevenson, R.; Dhawan, A.; Goncalves, I.; Socha, P.; Sokal, E. Guidelines for nutritional care for infants with cholestatic liver disease before liver transplantation. *Pediatr. Transplant.* **2007**, *11*, 825–834. [CrossRef] [PubMed]
9. Smart, K.M.; Alex, G.; Hardikar, W. Feeding the child with liver disease: A review and practical clinical guide. *J. Gastroenterol. Hepatol.* **2011**, *26*, 810–815. [CrossRef] [PubMed]
10. Pinto, R.B.; Schneider, A.C.; da Silveira, T.R. Cirrhosis in children and adolescents: An overview. *World J. Hepatol.* **2015**, *7*, 392–405. [CrossRef] [PubMed]
11. Tahir, A.; Malik, F.R.; Ahmad, I.; Akhtar, P. Aetiological factors of chronic liver disease in children. *J. Ayub Med. Coll. Abbottabad* **2011**, *23*, 12–14. [PubMed]
12. Dhole, S.D.; Kher, A.S.; Ghildiyal, R.G.; Tambse, M.P. Chronic Liver Diseases in Children: Clinical Profile and Histology. *J. Clin. Diagn. Res.* **2015**, *9*, SC04–SC07. [CrossRef] [PubMed]
13. Nightingale, S.; Ng, V.L. Optimizing nutritional management in children with chronic liver disease. *Pediatr. Clin. N. Am.* **2009**, *56*, 1161–1183. [CrossRef] [PubMed]
14. Sokol, R.J.; Stall, C. Anthropometric evaluation of children with chronic liver disease. *Am. J. Clin. Nutr.* **1990**, *52*, 203–208. [PubMed]
15. Chin, S.; Shepherd, R.; Cleghorn, G.; Patrick, M.; Javorsky, G.; Frangoulis, E.; Ong, T.H.; Balderson, G.; Koido, Y.; Matsunami, H.; et al. Survival, growth and quality of life in children after orthotopic liver transplantation: A 5 year experience. *J. Paediatr. Child Health* **1991**, *27*, 380–385. [CrossRef] [PubMed]
16. Shepherd, R.; Chin, S.; Cleghorn, G.; Patrick, M.; Ong, T.; Lynch, S.; Balderson, G.; Strong, R. Malnutrition in children with chronic liver disease accepted for liver transplanation: Clinical profile and effect on outcome. *J. Paediatr. Child Health* **1991**, *27*, 295–299. [CrossRef] [PubMed]
17. DeRusso, P.; Ye, W.; Shepherd, R.; Haber, B.; Shneider, B.; Whitington, P.; Schwarz, K.B.; Bezerra, J.A.; Rosenthal, P.; Karpen, S.; et al. Growth failure and outcomes in infants with biliary atresia: A report from the Biliary Atresia Research Consortium. *Hepatology* **2007**, *46*, 1632–1638. [CrossRef] [PubMed]
18. Wayman, K.; Cox, K.; Esquivel, C. Neurodevelopmental outcome of young children with extrahepatic biliary atresia 1 year after liver transplantation. *J. Pediatr.* **1997**, *131*, 894–898. [CrossRef]
19. Stewart, S.; Uauy, R.; Waller, D.; Kennard, B.; Benser, M.; Andrews, W. Mental and motor development, social competence, and growth one year after successful pediatric liver transplantation. *J. Pediatr.* **1989**, *114 (4 Pt 1)*, 574–581. [CrossRef]
20. Moukarzel, A.; Najm, I.; Vargas, J.; McDiarmid, S.; Busuttil, R.; Ament, M. Effect of nutritional status on outcome of orthotopic liver transplantation in pediatric patients. *Transplant. Proc.* **1990**, *22*, 1560–1563. [PubMed]
21. Vajro, P.; Maddaluno, S.; Veropalumbo, C. Persistent hypertransaminasemia in asymptomatic children: A stepwise approach. *World J. Gastroenterol.* **2013**, *19*, 2740–2751. [CrossRef] [PubMed]

22. Chin, S.; Shepherd, R.; Thomas, B.; Cleghorn, G.; Patrick, M.; Wilcox, J.; Ong, T.H.; Lynch, S.V.; Strong, R. The nature of malnutrition in children with end-stage liver disease awaiting orthotopic liver transplantation. *Am. J. Clin. Nutr.* **1992**, *56*, 164–168. [PubMed]
23. Laviano, A.; Cangiano, C.; Preziosa, I. Plasma tryptophan levels and anorexia in liver cirrhosis. *Int. J. Eat. Disord.* **1997**, *21*, 181–186. [CrossRef]
24. Aqel, B.; Scolapio, J.; Dickson, R.; Burton, D.; Bouras, E. Contribution of ascites to impaired gastric function and nutritonal intake in patients with cirrhosis and ascites. *Clin. Gastroenterol. Hepatol.* **2005**, *3*, 1095–1100. [CrossRef]
25. Aranda-Michel, J. Nutrition in hepatic failure and liver transplantation. *Curr. Gastroenterol. Rep.* **2001**, *3*, 362–370. [CrossRef] [PubMed]
26. Cortez, A.; de Morais, M.; Speridiao, P.G.; da Motta, M.R.; Calanca, F.; Neto, U. Food intake, growth and body composition of children and adolescents with autoimmune hepatitis. *J. Clin. Gastroenterol.* **2010**, *44*, 200–207. [CrossRef] [PubMed]
27. Pierro, A.K.; Carnielli, V.; Superina, R.; Roberts, E.; Filler, R.; Smith, J.; Heim, T. Resting energy expenditure is increased in infants and children with extrahepatic biliary atresia. *J. Pediatr. Surg.* **1989**, *24*, 534–538. [CrossRef]
28. Protheroe, S.; McKieran, P.; Kelly, D. Can measurement of dietary-induced thermogenesis (DIT) predict response to nutritional intervention in infants with liver disease? *Clin. Nutr.* **1996**, *15*, 39. [CrossRef]
29. Greer, R.; Lehnert, M.; Lewindon, P.; Cleghorn, G.; Shepherd, R. Body composition and components of energy expenditure in children with end-stage liver disease. *J. Pediatr. Gastroenterol. Nutr.* **2003**, *36*, 358–363. [CrossRef] [PubMed]
30. Kelly, D.A.; Proteroe, S.; Clarke, S. Acute and chronic liver disease. In *Nutrition in Pediatrics*, 5th ed.; Duggan, C., Watkins, J.B., Koletzko, B., Walker, W.A., Eds.; People's Medical Publishing House-USA: Shelton, CT, USA, 2016; pp. 851–863.
31. Santetti, D.; Wilasco, M.I.d.A.; Dornelles, C.T.L.; Werlang, I.C.R.; Fontella, F.U.; Kieling, C.O.; Luiz dos Santos, J.; Gonçalves Vieira, S.M.; Sueno Goldani, H.A. Serum proinflammatory cytokines and nutritional status in pediatric chronic liver disease. *World J. Gastroenterol.* **2015**, *21*, 8927–8934. [CrossRef] [PubMed]
32. Zamboni, G.; Dufillot, D.; Antoniazzi, F.; Valentini, R.; Gendrel, D.; Tato, L. Growth hormone-binding proteins and insulin-like grwoth factor-binding proteins in protein-energy malnutrition, before and after nutritonal rehabilitation. *Pediatr. Res.* **1996**, *39*, 410–414. [CrossRef] [PubMed]
33. Romjin, J.; Endert, E.; Suerwein, H. Glucose and fat metablism during short-term starvation in cirrhosis. *Gastroenterology* **1991**, *100*, 731–737. [CrossRef]
34. Hellerstein, M.; Munro, H. Interaction of liver, muscle and adipose tissue in the regulation of metabolism in response to nutritional and other factors. In *The Liver: Biology and Pathobiology*, 3rd ed.; Arias, I., Boyer, J., Fausto, N., Eds.; Raven Press: New York, NY, USA, 1994; pp. 1169–1191.
35. Changani, K.; Jalan, R.; Cox, I.; Ala-Korpela, M.; Bhakoo, K.; Taylor-Robinson, S.; Bell, J.D. Evidence for altered hepatic gluconeogenesis in patients with cirrhosis using in vivo 31-phosphorus magnetic resonance spectroscopy. *Gut* **2001**, *49*, 557–564. [CrossRef] [PubMed]
36. Petrides, A.; DeFronzo, R. Glucose and insulin metabolism in cirrhosis. *J. Hepatol.* **1989**, *8*, 107–114. [CrossRef]
37. Nielsen, M.; Caumo, A.; Aagaard, N.; Chandramouli, V.; Schumann, W.; Landau, B.; Schmitz, O.; Vilstrup, H. Contribution of defects in glucose uptake to carbohydrate intolerance in liver cirrhosis: Assessment during physiological glucose and insulin concentrations. *Am. J. Physiol. Gastrointest. Liver Physiol.* **2005**, *288*, G1135–G1143. [CrossRef] [PubMed]
38. Cleghorn, G. The role of basic nutritional research in pediatric liver disease: A historical perspective. *Gastroenterol. Hepatol.* **2009**, *24*, S93–S96. [CrossRef] [PubMed]
39. Swart, G.R.; van den Berg, J.W.; Wattimena, J.L.; Rietveld, T.; van Vuure, J.K.; Frenkel, M. Elevated protein requirements in cirrhosis of the liver investigated by whole body protein turnover studies. *Clin. Sci.* **1988**, *75*, 101–107. [CrossRef] [PubMed]
40. Protheroe, S.; Jones, R.; Kelly, D. Evaluation of the role of branched chain amino acids in the treatment of protein malnutrition in infants with liver disease. *Gut* **1995**, *37*, A350.
41. Munro, H.N.; Fernstrom, J.D.; Wurtman, R.J. Insulin, plasma amino acid imbalance, and hepatic coma. *Lancet* **1975**, *1*, 722–724. [CrossRef]

42. Charlton, C.P.; Buchanan, E.; Holden, C.E.; Preece, M.A.; Green, A.; Booth, I.W.; Tarlow, M.J. Intensive enteral feeding in advanced cirrhosis: Reversal of malnutrition without precipitation of hepatic encephalopathy. *Arch. Dis. Child.* **1992**, *67*, 603–607. [CrossRef] [PubMed]
43. Dietschy, J. The biology of bile acids. *Arch. Intern. Med.* **1972**, *130*, 473–474. [CrossRef] [PubMed]
44. Yamamoto, T.; Hamanak, Y.; Suzuki, T. Intestinal microflora and bile acids following biliary tract reconstruction. *Nippon Geka Gakkai Zasshi* **1991**, *92*, 1288–1291. [PubMed]
45. Emerick, K.; Rand, E.; Goldmuntz, E.; Krantz, I.; Spinner, N.; Piccoli, D. Features of Alagille syndrome in 92 patients: Frequency and relation to prognosis. *Hepatology* **1999**, *29*, 822–829. [CrossRef] [PubMed]
46. Greenberger, N.; Skillman, T. Medium-chain triglycerides. *N. Engl. J. Med.* **1969**, *280*, 1045–1058. [CrossRef] [PubMed]
47. Glasgow, J.; Hamilton, J.; Sass-Kortsak, A. Fat absorption in congenital obstructive liver disease. *Arch. Dis. Child.* **1973**, *48*, 601–607. [CrossRef] [PubMed]
48. Phan, C.; Tso, P. Intestinal lipid absorption and transport. *Front. Biosci.* **2001**, *6*, D299–D319. [CrossRef] [PubMed]
49. Sabesin, S.M. Cholestatic lipoproteins—Their pathogenesis and significance. *Gastroenterology* **1982**, *83*, 704–709. [PubMed]
50. Mager, D.R.; McGee, P.L.; Furuya, K.N.; Roberts, E.A. Prevalence of vitamin K deficiency in children with mild to moderate chronic liver disease. *J. Pediatr. Gastroenterol. Nutr.* **2006**, *42*, 71–76. [CrossRef] [PubMed]
51. Shneider, B.L.; Magee, J.C.; Bezerra, J.A.; Haber, B.; Karpen, S.J.; Raghunathan, T.; Rosenthal, P.; Schwarz, K.; Suchy, F.J.; Kerkar, N. Efficacy of fat-soluble vitamin supplementation in infants with biliary atresia. *Pediatrics* **2012**, *130*, e607–e614. [CrossRef] [PubMed]
52. Argao, E.A.; Specker, B.L.; Heubi, J.E. Bone mineral content in infants and children with chronic cholestatic liver disease. *Pediatrics* **1993**, *91*, 1151–1154. [PubMed]
53. Leerbeck, E.; Sondergaard, H. The total content of vitamin D in human milk and cow's milk. *Br. J. Nutr.* **1980**, *44*, 7–12. [CrossRef] [PubMed]
54. Sokol, R.J.; Heubi, J.E.; Iannaccone, S.; Bove, K.E.; Balistreri, W.F. Mechanism causing vitamin E deficiency during chronic childhood cholestasis. *Gastroenterology* **1983**, *85*, 1172–1182. [PubMed]
55. Usui, Y.; Tanimura, H.; Nishimura, N.; Kobayashi, N.; Okanoue, T.; Ozawa, K. Vitamin K concentrations in the plasma and liver of surgical patients. *Am. J. Clin. Nutr.* **1990**, *51*, 846–852. [PubMed]
56. Grantham-McGregor, S.; Ani, C. A review of studies on the effect of iron deficiency on cognitive development in children. *J. Nutr.* **2001**, *131*, 649S–666S. [PubMed]
57. Stamoulis, I.; Kouraklis, G.; Theocharis, S. Zinc and the liver: An active interaction. *Dig. Dis. Sci.* **2007**, *52*, 1595–1612. [CrossRef] [PubMed]
58. Umusig-Quitain, P.; Gregorio, G.V. High incidence of zinc deficiency among Filipino children with compensated and decompensated liver disease. *J. Gastroenterol. Hepatol.* **2010**, *25*, 387–390. [CrossRef] [PubMed]
59. Goksu, N.; Ozsoylu, S. Hepatic and serum levels of zinc, copper, and magnesium in childhood cirrhosis. *J. Pediatr. Gastroenterol. Nutr.* **1986**, *5*, 459–462. [CrossRef] [PubMed]
60. Bayliss, E.A.; Hambidge, K.M.; Sokol, R.J.; Stewart, B.; Lilly, J.R. Hepatic concentrations of zinc, copper and manganese in infants with extrahepatic biliary atresia. *J. Trace Elem. Med. Biol.* **1995**, *9*, 40–43. [CrossRef]
61. Fitzgerald, K.; Mikalunas, V.; Rubin, H.; McCarthey, R.; Vanagunas, A.; Craig, R.M. Hypermanganesemia in patients receiving total parenteral nutrition. *JPEN J. Parenter. Enter. Nutr.* **1999**, *23*, 333–336. [CrossRef] [PubMed]
62. Ikeda, S.; Yamaguchi, Y.; Sera, Y.; Ohshiro, H.; Uchino, S.; Yamashita, Y.; Ogawa, M. Manganese deposition in the globus pallidus in patients with biliary atresia. *Transplantation* **2000**, *69*, 2339–2343. [CrossRef] [PubMed]
63. Trocki, O.; Wotton, M.J.; Cleghorn, G.J.; Shepherd, R.W. Value of total body potassium in assessing the nutritional status of children with end-stage liver disease. *Ann. N. Y. Acad. Sci.* **2000**, *904*, 400–405. [CrossRef] [PubMed]
64. Klein, S. The myth of serum albumin as a measure of nutritional status. *Gastroenterology* **1990**, *99*, 1845–1846. [CrossRef]
65. Myron Johnson, A.; Merlini, G.; Sheldon, J.; Ichihara, K. Scientific Division Committee on Plasma Proteins IFoCC, Laboratory M. Clinical indications for plasma protein assays: Transthyretin (prealbumin) in inflammation and malnutrition. *Clin. Chem. Lab. Med.* **2007**, *45*, 419–426. [CrossRef] [PubMed]

66. Bucuvalas, J.C.; Horn, J.A.; Chernausek, S.D. Resistance to growth hormone in children with chronic liver disease. *Pediatr. Transplant.* **1997**, *1*, 73–79. [PubMed]
67. Hogler, W.; Baumann, U.; Kelly, D. Endocrine and bone metabolic complications in chronic liver disease and after liver transplantation in children. *J. Pediatr. Gastroenterol. Nutr.* **2012**, *54*, 313–321. [CrossRef] [PubMed]
68. Protheroe, S.M. Feeding the child with chronic liver disease. *Nutrition* **1998**, *14*, 796–800. [CrossRef]
69. Chin, S.E.; Shepherd, R.W.; Thomas, B.J.; Cleghorn, G.J.; Patrick, M.K.; Wilcox, J.A.; Ong, T.H.; Lynch, S.V.; Strong, R. Nutritional support in children with end-stage liver disease: A randomized crossover trial of a branched-chain amino acid supplement. *Am. J. Clin. Nutr.* **1992**, *56*, 158–163. [PubMed]
70. Sokal, E.M.; Baudoux, M.C.; Collette, E.; Hausleithner, V.; Lambotte, L.; Buts, J.P. Branched chain amino acids improve body composition and nitrogen balance in a rat model of extra hepatic biliary atresia. *Pediatr. Res.* **1996**, *40*, 66–71. [CrossRef] [PubMed]
71. Platell, C.; Kong, S.E.; McCauley, R.; Hall, J.C. Branched-chain amino acids. *J. Gastroenterol. Hepatol.* **2000**, *15*, 706–717. [CrossRef] [PubMed]
72. Carey, M.C.; Small, D.M.; Bliss, C.M. Lipid digestion and absorption. *Annu. Rev. Physiol.* **1983**, *45*, 651–677. [CrossRef] [PubMed]
73. Beath, S.V.; Booth, I.W.; Kelly, D.A. Nutritional support in liver disease. *Arch. Dis. Child.* **1993**, *69*, 545–547. [CrossRef] [PubMed]
74. Kaufman, S.S.; Scrivner, D.J.; Murray, N.D.; Vanderhoof, J.A.; Hart, M.H.; Antonson, D.L. Influence of portagen and pregestimil on essential fatty acid status in infantile liver disease. *Pediatrics* **1992**, *89*, 151–154. [PubMed]
75. Koletzko, B.; Agostoni, C.; Carlson, S.E.; Clandinin, T.; Hornstra, G.; Neuringer, M.; Uauy, R.; Yamashiro, Y.; Willatts, P. Long chain polyunsaturated fatty acids (LC-PUFA) and perinatal development. *Acta Paediatr.* **2001**, *90*, 460–464. [CrossRef] [PubMed]
76. Shneider, B.L.; Magee, J.C.; Karpen, S.J.; Rand, E.B.; Narkewicz, M.R.; Bass, L.M.; Schwarz, K.; Whitington, P.F.; Bezerra, J.A.; Kerkar, N.; et al. Total Serum Bilirubin within 3 Months of Hepatoportoenterostomy Predicts Short-Term Outcomes in Biliary Atresia. *J. Pediatr.* **2016**, *170*. [CrossRef] [PubMed]
77. Venkat, V.L.; Shneider, B.L.; Magee, J.C.; Turmelle, Y.; Arnon, R.; Bezerra, J.A.; Hertel, P.M.; Karpen, S.J.; Kerkar, N.; Loomes, K.M. Total serum bilirubin predicts fat-soluble vitamin deficiency better than serum bile acids in infants with biliary atresia. *J. Pediatr. Gastroenterol. Nutr.* **2014**, *59*, 702–707. [CrossRef] [PubMed]
78. Catzola, A.; Vajro, P. Management options for cholestatic liver disease in children. *Expert Rev. Gastroenterol. Hepatol.* **2017**, *11*, 1019–1030. [CrossRef] [PubMed]
79. Guichelaar, M.M.; Kendall, R.; Malinchoc, M.; Hay, J.E. Bone mineral density before and after OLT: Long-term follow-up and predictive factors. *Liver Transpl.* **2006**, *12*, 1390–1402. [CrossRef] [PubMed]
80. Argao, E.A.; Heubi, J.E.; Hollis, B.W.; Tsang, R.C. D-Alpha-tocopheryl polyethylene glycol-1000 succinate enhances the absorption of vitamin D in chronic cholestatic liver disease of infancy and childhood. *Pediatr. Res.* **1992**, *31*, 146–150. [CrossRef] [PubMed]
81. Heubi, J.E.; Hollis, B.W.; Specker, B.; Tsang, R.C. Bone disease in chronic childhood cholestasis. I. Vitamin D absorption and metabolism. *Hepatology* **1989**, *9*, 258–264. [CrossRef] [PubMed]
82. Sokol, R.J.; Heubi, J.E.; Iannaccone, S.T.; Bove, K.E.; Balistreri, W.F. Vitamin E deficiency with normal serum vitamin E concentrations in children with chronic cholestasis. *N. Engl. J. Med.* **1984**, *310*, 1209–1212. [CrossRef] [PubMed]
83. Perlmutter, D.H.; Gross, P.; Jones, H.R.; Fulton, A.; Grand, R.J. Intramuscular vitamin E repletion in children with chronic cholestasis. *Am. J. Dis. Child.* **1987**, *141*, 170–174. [CrossRef] [PubMed]
84. Sokol, R.J.; Butler-Simon, N.; Conner, C.; Heubi, J.E.; Sinatra, F.R.; Suchy, F.J.; Heyman, M.B.; Perrault, J.; Rothbaum, R.J.; Levy, J. Multicenter trial of D-alpha-tocopheryl polyethylene glycol 1000 succinate for treatment of vitamin E deficiency in children with chronic cholestasis. *Gastroenterology* **1993**, *104*, 1727–1735. [CrossRef]
85. Ferland, G.; Sadowski, J.A.; O'Brien, M.E. Dietary induced subclinical vitamin K deficiency in normal human subjects. *J. Clin. Invest.* **1993**, *91*, 1761–1768. [CrossRef] [PubMed]
86. Pereira, S.P.; Shearer, M.J.; Williams, R.; Mieli-Vergani, G. Intestinal absorption of mixed micellar phylloquinone [vitamin K1] is unreliable in infants with conjugated hyperbilirubinaemia: Implications

for oral prophylaxis of vitamin K deficiency bleeding. *Arch. Dis. Child Fetal Neonatal Ed.* **2003**, *88*, F113–F118. [CrossRef] [PubMed]

87. Heubi, J.E.; Higgins, J.V.; Argao, E.A.; Sierra, R.I.; Specker, B.L. The role of magnesium in the pathogenesis of bone disease in childhood cholestatic liver disease: A preliminary report. *J. Pediatr. Gastroenterol. Nutr.* **1997**, *25*, 301–306. [CrossRef] [PubMed]
88. Cabre, E.; Gonzalez-Huix, F.; Abad-Lacruz, A.; Esteve, M.; Acero, D.; Fernandez-Banares, F.; Xiol, X.; Gassull, M.A. Effect of total enteral nutrition on the short-term outcome of severely malnourished cirrhotics. A randomized controlled trial. *Gastroenterology* **1990**, *98*, 715–720. [CrossRef]
89. Kearns, P.J.; Young, H.; Garcia, G.; Blaschke, T.; O'Hanlon, G.; Rinki, M.; Sucher, K.; Gregory, P. Accelerated improvement of alcoholic liver disease with enteral nutrition. *Gastroenterology* **1992**, *102*, 200–205. [CrossRef]
90. Cabre, E.; Rodriguez-Iglesias, P.; Caballeria, J.; Quer, J.C.; Sanchez-Lombrana, J.L.; Pares, A.; Papo, M.; Planas, R.; Gassull, M.A. Short- and long-term outcome of severe alcohol-induced hepatitis treated with steroids or enteral nutrition: A multicenter randomized trial. *Hepatology* **2000**, *32*, 36–42. [CrossRef] [PubMed]
91. Moreno, L.A.; Gottrand, F.; Hoden, S.; Turck, D.; Loeuille, G.A.; Farriaux, J.P. Improvement of nutritional status in cholestatic children with supplemental nocturnal enteral nutrition. *J. Pediatr. Gastroenterol. Nutr.* **1991**, *12*, 213–216. [CrossRef] [PubMed]
92. Kelly, D.; Tong, C. Neonatal and paediatric infection. In *Viral Hepatitis*, 4th ed.; Wiley Blackwell: Hoboken, NJ, USA, 2012.
93. Fell, J.M.; Reynolds, A.P.; Meadows, N.; Khan, K.; Long, S.G.; Quaghebeur, G.; Taylor, W.J.; Milla, P.J. Manganese toxicity in children receiving long-term parenteral nutrition. *Lancet* **1996**, *347*, 1218–1221. [CrossRef]
94. Huang, C.C.; Chu, N.S.; Lu, C.S.; Wang, J.D.; Tsai, J.L.; Tzeng, J.L.; Wolters, E.C.; Calne, D.B. Chronic manganese intoxication. *Arch. Neurol.* **1989**, *46*, 1104–1106. [CrossRef] [PubMed]
95. Barshes, N.R.; Chang, I.F.; Karpen, S.J.; Carter, B.A.; Goss, J.A. Impact of pretransplant growth retardation in pediatric liver transplantation. *J. Pediatr. Gastroenterol. Nutr.* **2006**, *43*, 89–94. [CrossRef] [PubMed]
96. Rodeck, B.; Melter, M.; Kardorff, R.; Hoyer, P.F.; Ringe, B.; Burdelski, M.; Oldhafer, K.J.; Pichlmayr, R.; Brodehl, J. Liver transplantation in children with chronic end stage liver disease: Factors influencing survival after transplantation. *Transplantation* **1996**, *62*, 1071–1076. [CrossRef] [PubMed]
97. SM F, R.J. Feeding patterns in infants post liver transplant. *J. Pediatr. Gastroenterol.* **2004**, *39*, S94.
98. Bartosh, S.M.; Thomas, S.E.; Sutton, M.M.; Brady, L.M.; Whitington, P.F. Linear growth after pediatric liver transplantation. *J. Pediatr.* **1999**, *135*, 624–631. [CrossRef]
99. Cardona, J.; Houssin, D.; Gauthier, F.; Devictor, D.; Losay, J.; Hadchouel, M.; Bernard, O. Liver transplantation in children with Alagille syndrome—A study of twelve cases. *Transplantation* **1995**, *60*, 339–342. [CrossRef] [PubMed]
100. Kamath, B.M.; Yin, W.; Miller, H.; Anand, R.; Rand, E.B.; Alonso, E.; Bucuvalas, J. Outcomes of liver transplantation for patients with Alagille syndrome: The studies of pediatric liver transplantation experience. *Liver Transpl.* **2012**, *18*, 940–948. [CrossRef] [PubMed]
101. Kelly, D.A. Posttransplant growth failure in children. *Liver Transpl. Surg.* **1997**, *3* (5 Suppl. 1), S32–S39. [PubMed]
102. Van Mourik, I.D.; Beath, S.V.; Brook, G.A.; Cash, A.J.; Mayer, A.D.; Buckels, J.A.; Kelly, D.A. Long-term nutritional and neurodevelopmental outcome of liver transplantation in infants aged less than 12 months. *J. Pediatr. Gastroenterol. Nutr.* **2000**, *30*, 269–275. [CrossRef] [PubMed]
103. Holt, R.I.; Broide, E.; Buchanan, C.R.; Miell, J.P.; Baker, A.J.; Mowat, A.P.; Mieli-Vergani, G. Orthotopic liver transplantation reverses the adverse nutritional changes of end-stage liver disease in children. *Am. J. Clin. Nutr.* **1997**, *65*, 534–542. [PubMed]
104. Amedee-Manesme, O.; Furr, H.C.; Alvarez, F.; Hadchouel, M.; Alagille, D.; Olson, J.A. Biochemical indicators of vitamin A depletion in children with cholestasis. *Hepatology* **1985**, *5*, 1143–1148. [CrossRef] [PubMed]
105. Lapillonne, A.; Hakme, C.; Mamoux, V.; Chambon, M.; Fournier, V.; Chirouze, V.; Lachaux, A. Effects of liver transplantation on long-chain polyunsaturated fatty acid status in infants with biliary atresia. *J. Pediatr. Gastroenterol. Nutr.* **2000**, *30*, 528–532. [CrossRef] [PubMed]
106. Holt, R.I.; Jones, J.S.; Stone, N.M.; Baker, A.J.; Miell, J.P. Sequential changes in insulin-like growth factor I (IGF-I) and IGF-binding proteins in children with end-stage liver disease before and after successful orthotopic liver transplantation. *J. Clin. Endocrinol. Metab.* **1996**, *81*, 160–168. [PubMed]

11

Parenteral Nutrition-Associated Liver Disease: The Role of the Gut Microbiota

Monika Cahova [1,*], Miriam Bratova [1] and Petr Wohl [2]

[1] Centre for Experimental Medicine, Institute for Clinical and Experimental Medicine, Department of Metabolism and Diabetes, Videnska 1958/9, 14021 Prague 4, Czech Republic; miriam.bratova@ikem.cz
[2] Centre of Diabetology, Institute for Clinical and Experimental Medicine, Department of Metabolism and Diabetes, Videnska 1958/9, 14021 Prague 4, Czech Republic; petr.wohl@ikem.cz
* Correspondence: monika.cahova@ikem.cz

Abstract: Parenteral nutrition (PN) provides life-saving nutritional support in situations where caloric supply via the enteral route cannot cover the necessary needs of the organism. However, it does have serious adverse effects, including parenteral nutrition-associated liver disease (PNALD). The development of liver injury associated with PN is multifactorial, including non-specific intestine inflammation, compromised intestinal permeability, and barrier function associated with increased bacterial translocation, primary and secondary cholangitis, cholelithiasis, short bowel syndrome, disturbance of hepatobiliary circulation, lack of enteral nutrition, shortage of some nutrients (proteins, essential fatty acids, choline, glycine, taurine, carnitine, etc.), and toxicity of components within the nutrition mixture itself (glucose, phytosterols, manganese, aluminium, etc.). Recently, an increasing number of studies have provided evidence that some of these factors are directly or indirectly associated with microbial dysbiosis in the intestine. In this review, we focus on PN-induced changes in the taxonomic and functional composition of the microbiome. We also discuss immune cell and microbial crosstalk during parenteral nutrition, and the implications for the onset and progression of PNALD. Finally, we provide an overview of recent advances in the therapeutic utilisation of pro- and prebiotics for the mitigation of PN-associated liver complications.

Keywords: Parenteral nutrition; microbiota; PNALD; intestinal permeability; gut-associated immune system; bile acids; FXR signalling; pre/probiotics

---

1. Introduction

Parenteral nutrition (PN) provides life-saving nutritional support in situations where caloric supply via the enteral route is either not possible or cannot cover the necessary needs of the organism, e.g., preterm neonates with immature gut, perioperatively in patients requiring massive intestinal surgery, or in patients with short bowel syndrome (SBS). PN preserves lean body mass, supports immune functions, and reduces metabolic complications in patients who are otherwise unable to feed [1]. Nevertheless, PN does have serious adverse effects, one of which is the deterioration of liver function. PN-induced cholestasis generally refers to the onset of liver disease in the context of the administration of intravenous nutrition in patients with temporary or permanent intestinal failure. Other terms commonly used to describe the condition are parenteral nutrition-associated cholestasis (PNAC) and intestinal failure-associated liver disease (IFALD), but the most frequently used is parenteral nutrition-associated liver disease (PNALD) [2]. PNALD clinical manifestations—which range from steatosis, cholestasis, gallbladder sludge/stones, fibrosis, and cirrhosis—can occur separately or in combination [3,4]. Steatosis (defined as fat accumulation in hepatocytes) can present as mild to moderate elevations in liver function tests and is usually benign. Cholestasis results from impaired secretion or obstruction of bile, and is associated with elevations in alkaline phosphatase, gamma-glutamyl transferase, and conjugated bilirubin [5].

There are some differences between child and adult patients totally dependent on parenteral nutrition (TPN) with regard to the pathogenesis of PNALD. Cholestasis occurs in 40–60% of infants, steatosis in 40–55% of adults, while biliary sludge and cholelithiasis occur in both adults and children. Child TPN patients (premature infants) typically exhibit prematurity (impaired transsulfuration, lack of cystathionase, etc.) and bowel lengths <25 cm, while necrotising enterocolitis is frequently the cause of intestinal failure. In addition, the high-energy requirements (80–100 kcal/kg per day) for growth are associated with the rapid onset of PNALD within months. All of these factors make children patients significantly more susceptible to PNALD/IFALD. In adults, a history of PNALD is characterised by elevated liver enzymes and associated steatosis, which can last for years. Ensuing complications include steatohepatitis, cholestatic hepatitis, as well as fibrosis and cirrhosis. In contrast, histology findings in child-type PNALD are defined by cholestasis, portal fibrosis, peri-cellular fibrosis, bile duct proliferation, pigmented Kupffer cells and non-progressive cirrhosis. Risk factors in children include lack of taurine, excess of calories, excess of lipids (>3.5 g/kg/day, mainly omega-6 fatty acids), phytosterols, bowel inflammation, catheter infections, and an absence of the ileo-caecal valve. In adults, risk factors include lack of choline, excess of calories, excess of lipids >1 g/kg/day, phytosterols, bowel inflammation, small bowel bacterial overgrowth, and absence of the ileo-caecal valve. In both groups, sepsis is a significant complication. The detailed differences of the pathomechanisms that underlie liver damage in both PN-dependent paediatric and adult patients are beyond the scope of this paper. More information is available in some excellent recent reviews [6,7].

Although the pathogenesis of PNALD is undoubtedly a multifactorial phenomenon, the privileged role may be attributed to the impaired function of the intestine. It harbours most of the immune cells in the body and represents the largest area for contact with antigens from the environment. The gut microbiome plays an essential role in intestinal development and homeostasis maintenance [8]. In humans, the gut microbiome is composed of approximate 1000 species and it is estimated that their genomes exceed the human genome by more than one hundred-fold. This represents a major stimulus to the immune system and facilitates the performance of many physiological functions [9]. The gut microbiota is the most abundant cohort of antigen-presenting cells. Based on the above facts, it is conceivable that the radical alteration of gut microbiome composition and function as a result of switching to total parenteral nutrition could lead to detrimental effects on the intestine and significantly contribute to PNALD development.

2. PN and the Gut Microbiota

Data on the gut microbiota in the context of PN have been obtained under three different group settings: animal models (mouse, rat, piglet), neonate babies (most of them premature), and adult patients who have lost a substantial portion of functional gut tissue and cannot feed themselves via the enteral route. Although PN is present in all cases, each of these groups has specific features that strongly influence microbiome composition (Table 1).

Table 1. The effect of parenteral nutrition on gut microbiome composition.

Model	Bowel Resection	TPN Duration	Enteral Feeding		References
Rat-adult	No	14 days	No	*Firmicutes/Bacteroidetes* ratio; shift in favour of Bacteroidetes	[10]
Mouse-adult	No	5 days	No	Shift from *Firmicutes* to *Proteobactoria* and *Bacteroidetes*, i.e., *Salmonella, Proteus, Escherichia, Bacteroides*	[11]
Mouse-adult	No	5 days	No	Shift from *Firmicutes* to *Bacteroidetes* and *Proteobacteria*	[12]
Piglet-newborn	Yes	6 weeks	No	Changes in the composition of the *Firmicutes* phylum (decrease of *Anaerotruncus, Clostridium, Ruminococcus, Peptostreptococcus;* increase in *Acidaminococcus* and *Mitsuokella*)	[13]
Piglet-newborn	No	7 days	No	Lower total bacterial counts and reduced bacterial diversity, enriched in *Clostridium difficile*	[14]
Piglet-newborn	No	7 days	No	Enriched in *C. perfringens* and sulphated monosaccharide-degrading bacteria	[15]
Piglet-newborn	No	14 days	No	PN + ω-3: increased *Parabacteroides*	[16]
				PN + ω-6: increased *Enterobacteriaceae*	
Human-pre-term newborn	Yes	Long-term	Yes	Higher diversity, higher abundance of Gram-negative bacteria, lower odds of death and late-onset sepsis cases	[17]
			No	Less diversity, lower abundance of Gram-negative bacteria, increased odds of death and late-onset sepsis cases	
Human-paediatric/adult	Yes	Long-term	Yes	Increased *Staphylococcus, Pseudomonas, Campylobacter, Propionibacterium, Chryseomonas*	[18]
			No	Increased *Enterobacter, Shigella, Klebsiella, Fusobacterium*	
Human-adult	Yes	Long-term	Yes	Enrichment in *Lactobacillus/Leuconostoc*; depletion of anaerobes, especially *Clostridiaceae*	[19,20]
Human-adult	Yes	Long-term	Yes	High abundance of *Proteobacteria*, especially *Enterobacteriaceae* and *Fusobacteria*; changes in the *Firmicutes* spectrum, depletion of *Lachnospiraceae* and *Ruminococcaceae*	[21]

2.1. Adult Animal Models

In rats, Hodin et al. demonstrated that after 14 days of PN, total bacterial numbers per gram of luminal content did not differ between PN-fed and control rats; however, the composition of the bacterial population significantly changed. *Firmicutes* abundance dropped while the abundance of *Bacteroidetes* did not differ between groups. Consequently, the proportional representation of these two phyla in PN rats significantly shifted in favour of *Bacteroidetes* [10]. In a mouse model (5 days of PN), Miyasaka demonstrated that at the phylum level, the vast majority of mucosa-associated bacteria in the small bowels of control mice were *Firmicutes*. However, in the PN group, the dominant phyla were *Proteobacteria* and *Bacteroidetes*. At the genus level, PN mice had more bacteria in the genera *Salmonella, Escherichia, Proteus,* and *Bacteroides*. These genera are often associated with clinical infections, potentially indicating the development of a pathological state within the intestinal microbial community. Furthermore, enteral nutrient deprivation resulted in a loss of diversity in the large and small intestines [11]. Similar results indicating a shift from *Firmicutes* to *Bacteroides* have also been reported by an independent group [12]. A common feature of all these models is the overall deprivation of enteral nutrition for the entire duration of the experiments.

2.2. Neonates: Humans

In preterm neonates, the immature gut is much more prone to insults resulting from reduced intestinal motility, inappropriate immune responses, decreased protective gastrointestinal secretions, reduced digestive and absorptive function, and increased intestinal epithelial permeability [22]. In a prospective two-centre study, Parm et al. compared the effect of enteral-versus-parenteral feeding on the pattern of gut colonisation in preterm neonates at risk of late-onset sepsis and necrotising enterocolitis. PN was associated with the reduced acquisition of both Gram-positive and Gram-negative colonising microorganisms. *Candida albicans* colonisation was more frequent in neonates receiving PN. Despite greater mucosal colonisation by potentially pathogenic microorganisms (e.g., *Enterobacteriaceae* and *Enterococcus*), an enteral feeding regimen was associated with lower odds of late-onset sepsis and mortality in premature neonates than a PN regimen [17]. *Enterococcus faecalis* is the main immune modulator among human intestinal lactic acid bacteria, and is able to downregulate the expression of the host immune genes that participate in inflammation [23]. Thus, in the context of the naïve gut, colonisation with some *Enterococci* may be beneficial due to the suppression of specific toll-like receptors (TLR)-signalling pathways. Nevertheless, the conclusions drawn by Parm et al. are limited in that their study only included individuals under third-level neonatal intensive care, with all participants receiving at least one but usually more antibiotics, all of which may have significantly influenced gut microflora composition.

2.3. Neonates: Animal Models

In controlled animal model experiments that investigate the effect of PN on gut colonisation in neonates, enterally fed piglets exhibited a higher bacterial diversity, higher concentrations of bacteria (CFU/g), and increased colonisation of all segments of the intestinal tract compared to PN pigs. Translocation of bacteria from the intestinal tract to tissues or blood was similar in both groups. PN-treated piglets were at higher risk of colonisation by toxin-expressing strains of *C. difficile* [14]. Using the same model but a different method of bacterial taxa identification (16S rRNA NGS sequencing versus DGGE analysis), Deplancke found that the bacterial community structure was equally complex in the ilea of enterally and parenterally fed piglets; however, profiles clustered according to the mode of nutrition. The opportunistic pathogen *C. perfringens,* as well as mucus-associated bacteria, were specifically enriched in the guts of animals dependent on PN [15]. Bacteria capable of using sulphated monosaccharides were also more abundant in PN samples.

A recently published study by Lavallee et al. demonstrated that not only PN *per se* but also the type of lipid constituent affects microbiome composition in newborns. As expected, the gut microbial composition of PN-dependent piglets differed from those fed with sow milk, but the microbiota further clustered according to ω-3 or ω-6 PUFA content in the nutrition mixture. Piglets fed with ω-3 PUFA-rich PN were more similar to the sow milk-fed group than those administered ω-6 PUFA. The group with prevailing ω-6 PUFA on PN showed a specific and significant increase in *Parabacteroides,* while the ω-3 group showed an increase in *Enterobacteriaceae* [16]. The limitation of this study is that the antibiotic treatment was administered only to piglets exhibiting signs of sepsis, but not globally to the whole cohort. Nevertheless, this innovative study points out an unexpected aspect of PN, namely the interplay of the gut microbiota and lipid components of the nutrition mixture.

2.4. Patients with Small Intestinal Resections: Fed vs. Enterally Deprived Portions of the Intestine

The common denominator for all of the above therapeutic or experimental settings is the absence of enteral nutrition, which leaves the intestinal microbiota in a state of acute nutrient withdrawal. No animal study comparing the effect of PN alone or PN in combination with enteral nutrition has been carried out. Ralls et al. published an interesting study comparing microbial diversity and differences in microbial characteristics in enterally fed and enterally deprived portions of the small bowel obtained after surgical resection [18]. The restraint of this study was the low number of samples used and the highly heterogeneous population of the patients. However, some valuable implications can be derived. Although only a partial stratification of microbial communities between fed and enterally deprived groups was found, some groups tended to expand in the fed group (*Staphylococcus, Pseudomonas, Campylobacter, Propionibacterium, Chryseomonas*) in comparison to others in the enterally deprived group (*Enterobacter, Shigella, Klebsiella and Fusobacterium*). A close correlation was identified in patients with low levels of enteric microbial diversity and those who developed post-operative enteric-derived infections.

2.5. Adult SBS Patients: The Specific Intestinal Environment

Patients diagnosed with short bowel syndrome (SBS) represent a specific group that are dependent on total parenteral nutrition. SBS occurs in patients with an extensive resection of the short bowel, leaving less than 150 cm. These patients suffer from severely decreased absorption capacity for water, electrolytes, and nutrients, while intravenous supplementation is required to maintain vital functions [24]. General adaptations following intestinal resection include compensatory hyperphagia, mucosal remodelling of the remaining part of the intestine and major modifications of the microbiota [25]. In contrast to previously described patient groups and animal models, these subjects do intake food per os, whereby the residual lumen of the gut is supplied with abundant but poorly digested substrates. In addition to the excessive nutrient delivery, the gut ecological system of SBS patients is altered in several other ways. Faecal pH has been shown to be lower in patients than in controls, with mean faecal pH at approx. 5.6 in type II SBS patients in comparison to the normal laboratory range of pH (pH = 6 to pH = 7) [19]. Acidic pH creates a specific environment that favours low pH-tolerant microorganisms [26]. In SBS patients, it is possible that because of the short length of the remnant small intestine and colon, the level of oxygen becomes too high, and thus anaerobic bacteria are discriminated in favour of more tolerant facultative anaerobes. The disruption of enterohepatic circulation may result in disturbed bile acid metabolism and a preference for microbiota that are tolerant to bile acids.

2.6. Adult SBS Patients: Microbiota Composition

Original studies that describe the microbiome in SBS patients are remarkably consistent in their findings. The common feature of the SBS microbiota is significantly reduced α-diversity when compared with healthy controls [21,27,28], which positively correlates with remaining small bowel length [21] and PN dependence duration [28]. SBS patients harbour a specific faecal microbiota that is enriched in the *Lactobacillus/Leuconostoc* group and depleted in anaerobic microorganisms, especially those of the *Clostridiaceae* family [19,20]. A characteristic feature of this microbiota is its high abundance of *Proteobacteria*, especially *Enterobacteriaceae* [21,28]. The expansion of *Proteobacteria* may be linked to altered nutrition supply, as *Proteobacteria* can metabolise broader classes of substrates (including amino acids) and are therefore more flexible than other phyla. The decrease of *Bacteroidetes* has been reported both for mucosa [19] and luminal content [28]. The important feature of the SBS microbiome is the alteration of the *Firmicutes* community. *Firmicutes* is a dominant phylum of the healthy gut microbiota. In SBS patients, this phylum is still highly abundant but some important families of butyrate-producers, such as *Lachnospiraceae, Ruminococcaceae* and others, are almost entirely absent [21].

The severe dysbiosis found in SBS patients has a significant impact on the faecal metabolome and seriously affects the host metabolism. The bioconversion of macromolecules into metabolites is carried out by the bacteria of various functional groups, resulting in metabolic trophic chains. In SBS, the trophic chains and fermentation end-products are produced by the lactobiota, and are thus different from those produced by the healthy microbiota. The dominance of the carbohydrate-fermenting *Lactobacillus/Leuconostoc* taxa and the depletion of lactate-consuming anaerobic bacteria result in the excessive formation of both D- and L-lactate. Mayeur et al. [27] demonstrated that the individual lactic acid bacteria composition predicts whether or not a particular SBS patient will accumulate D-lactate in stools. In healthy humans, the lactate produced by the gut microbiota is not accumulated in faeces but it is readily absorbed by intestinal cells or converted to other metabolites, particularly the short-chain fatty acids (SCFA) [29,30]. Furthermore, in healthy humans, D-lactate is efficiently metabolised in the liver, and is thus eliminated from circulation. SBS patients who often suffer from compromised liver function are at an increased risk of lactate acidosis and D-lactate encephalopathy. Another consequence of the profound shift in microbiota composition, particularly the elimination of butyrate-producing anaerobes, is the significant decrease in SCFA production. This SCFA shortage may have multiple impacts on the gut immune system, intestinal wall integrity, and endocrine signalling.

3. PN and the Immune System

The gut microbiota profoundly influences the host immune system [31]. Numerous microbial products—including proteins, polysaccharides, and molecules that activate pattern recognition receptors—activate Toll-like receptors (TLRs) and NOD-like receptors (NODs) and stimulate the mucosal immune system [32]. The gut microbiota has an irreplaceable role in mucosal and systemic immunity maturation [33–35]. It also promotes a tolerogenic state in the intestinal mucosa (stimulation of Treg lymphocytes, attenuation of NF-κB signalling, etc.) [36–40], and instigates mechanisms that prevent bacterial overgrowth (induction of IgA secretion) [41–44]. Some commensals even produce targeted antimicrobial peptides themselves [45]. The healthy gut microbiota provides its host with a physical barrier to incoming pathogens and stimulates it to produce various antimicrobial compounds [31].

3.1. The Microbiota and TLR Signalling

The loss of diversity associated with prolonged PN administration has several adverse impacts on immune functions. The extinction of normally robust commensals facilitates the expansion of pathogenic strains due to the alleviation of competitive exclusion. For instance, the *Proteobacteria* found in the intestines of PN patients includes the opportunistic pathogens *E. coli*, *Salmonella*, *Yersinia*, *Helicobacter*, and *Vibrio*, all of which are commonly associated with infection [46]. Concurrently, some beneficial commensals that normally stimulate immunotolerance are underrepresented in the PN-associated microbiota. The shift in the intestinal microbiota (particularly the enrichment in *Proteobacteria* expressing many TLR ligands) and the activation of MyD88-dependent TLR signalling are suspected as causes of pro-inflammatory status in the PN-associated intestinal mucosa. Nevertheless, results obtained from mice models deficient in TLR signalling in intestinal epithelial cells are contradictory. Several authors have shown the protective effects of MyD88-targeted deletion in intestinal epithelial cells. MyD88 deletion inhibited colitis development in a model of spontaneous colitis (SHP-2 IEC-KO mice), rescued the goblet/intermediate cell ratio and prevented NFκB hyperactivation and inflammation [47]. In a model of diet-induced obesity, MyD88 KO mice exhibited increased anti-inflammatory endocannabinoids, antimicrobial peptide production, and intestinal regulatory T cells, and were partially protected against diet-induced obesity, diabetes, and inflammation [48]. Accordingly, enhanced MyD88 signalling (C57Bl/6 mice expressing a constitutively active form of TLR4 in the intestinal epithelium) resulted in an elevated bacterial translocation, impaired epithelial barrier function, different expression of antimicrobial peptide genes, and altered epithelial cell differentiation [49]. In contrast, Frantz et al. reported that a loss of epithelial MyD88 signalling caused the following effects: increased numbers of mucus-associated bacteria; the translocation of bacteria to mesenteric lymph nodes; reduced transmucosal electrical resistance; impaired mucus-associated antimicrobial activity; and, downregulated expression of polymeric immunoglobulin receptor (the epithelial IgA transporter), mucin-2 and the antimicrobial peptides RegIII and Defa-rs1. These mice were also more susceptible to experimental colitis [50]. MyD88 signalling has also been shown to stimulate gastrointestinal motility [51] and promote the differentiation of intestinal epithelial cells [52]. These rather contradictory outcomes suggest that (i) both low and excessive TLR4 signalling can promote intestinal inflammation and (ii) the interaction between the intestinal microbiota and the immune system is complex. Further research is needed in order to better understand these causal relationships.

3.2. The Microbiota and Intestinal Macrophages

An important population of innate immune cells are intestinal resident macrophages, which play a central role in the maintenance of homeostasis in the gastrointestinal tract [53]. Intestinal macrophages constitutively produce IL-10, one of the major anti-inflammatory cytokines that promotes differentiation and maintenance of Treg cells. They are also hyporesponsive to TLR stimulation [54] and are less prone to the secretion of pro-inflammatory cytokines after LPS stimulation [55]. Resident intestinal macrophages contribute to the attenuation of the immune response to various bacterial and food antigens, while maintaining anti-inflammatory tone in the intestine [56,57]. Recent studies have shown that circulating and tissue-resident macrophages (lung, brain, skin, liver) consist of populations of different embryonic origin, and are also independently maintained in a steady state in adulthood [58,59]. Intestinal macrophages seem to be the only exception to this rule. During the neonatal period, intestinal macrophages are derived from embryonic precursors (the yolk sac and foetal liver), but are gradually replaced by the progeny of conventional haematopoiesis (i.e., Ly6C^{hi} blood monocytes) in adulthood [54]. This process occurs in both the small intestine and the colon, but is regulated by different mechanisms. In the colon, the establishment of the gut microbiota and commensal-derived signals [54,57] drives the replenishment of resident macrophages. Consequently, the microbiota can stimulate macrophages to produce tolerogenic IL-10 either via TLR-signalling [60,61] or via activation of intestinal macrophage receptor GPR109a by microbial metabolites (butyrate, niacin). This setting helps to establish an "immunotolerogenic" feedback loop, whereby the gut microbiota actively promotes the recruitment of circulating macrophages into the intestinal mucosa. These macrophages in turn create a tolerant environment that facilitates the growth of these bacteria. In contrast to the colon, replenishment and IL-10 production of small intestine macrophages are not regulated by the gut microbiota but directly by dietary amino acids [62]. PN administration leads to a profound decline in the number of IL-10-producing macrophages in the small intestine [62]. The compromised replenishment of IL-10-producing macrophages together with the shift in microbial composition towards a more immunogenic phenotype (TLR ligand-rich *Proteobacteria*) may act in synergy towards generating a pro-inflammatory state in the PN-dependent small intestine. To our knowledge, no data are available regarding the direct effect of PN on colon macrophages. However, the facts we do have at our disposal, namely the shift in microbiota composition and the increase in the pro-inflammatory cytokine production, at least suggest a similar scenario.

3.3. The Microbiota and Paneth Cells

Paneth cells are important components of mucosal immunity. They occur at the base of small intestinal crypts and are the primary source of small peptides that exhibit antimicrobial activity (AMPs), such as secretory phospholipase A2 (sPLA2), lysozyme, and α and β-defensins [63–65]. Paneth cells sense bacteria via MyD88-dependent toll-like receptor (TLR) activation, which triggers antimicrobial action [66]. In the PN mouse model, the attenuated expression of Paneth cell antimicrobial proteins was associated with a compositional shift in the microbiome (decreased *Firmicutes;* increased *Bacteroidetes* and *Proteobacteria*), weaker bactericidal activity of mucosal secretions and greater susceptibility to enteroinvasion by *E. coli* [14]. Omata et al. demonstrated that PN feeding resulted in the suppressed secretion of sPLA2 and increased bacterial survival. Taking these data together, PN significantly impairs the innate immune response by suppressing Paneth cell function [67].

3.4. The Microbiota and B-Lymphocytes

The current paradigm supposes that the antibody response is directly or indirectly mediated through TLR signalling, and that it depends on the interaction of bacterial DNA, proteins, and cell wall components with TLR receptors [68,69]. Quite recently, Kim et al. reported a new mechanism whereby the gut microbiota affects host antibody responses via their fermentation products (SCFA) [70]. A positive correlation between dietary fibre intake and intestinal IgAs levels was shown previously [71]. Kim et al. tested the hypothesis that SCFA, the main fermentation product of dietary fibre, affects antibody production. They showed that in isolated mice spleen B-cells in vitro, SCFA increased acetyl-CoA and regulated metabolic sensors to increase oxidative phosphorylation, glycolysis and fatty acid synthesis. This in turn produced energy and building blocks that supported antibody production. In parallel, SCFA controlled gene expression and expressed molecules necessary for plasma B cell differentiation. The effects of all major SCFA (C2, C3 and C4) were comparable. In vivo, mice fed a low dietary fibre (DF) diet were more susceptible to *Citrobacter rodentium* infection compared with mice fed a high DF diet. In susceptible animals, supplementation with DF or propionate (C3) increased host resistance and the IgA response to *C. rodentium* [70].

4. PNALD and Bile Acid Metabolism

4.1. Bile Acid Metabolism and Function

Bile acids (BAs) are synthesised from cholesterol in the liver as primary BAs, which are represented by chenodeoxycholic (CDCA) acid and cholic (CA) acid in humans. Primary BAs are conjugated to taurine or glycine in the liver and as bile salts secreted into bile through bile-salt export proteins (BSEP, ABCB11). Approximately 95% of BAs are reabsorbed in the small intestine via enterohepatic circulation, while a minor fraction escapes before being further metabolised by the gut microbiota in the colon to the secondary BAs, such as deoxycholic (DCA), urodeoxycholic (UDCA), and lithocholic (LCA) acids in humans [72]. In rodents, muricholic (MCA) acid is synthesised as well [73]. Primary and secondary BAs fulfil multiple functions. First, they serve as physiological emulsifiers that facilitate enteral absorption of dietary fat and fat-soluble vitamins [74]. Second, they have direct antibacterial effects. Third, BAs are potent signalling molecules that regulate the host glucose and lipid metabolism as well as energy homeostasis [75,76]. This regulatory function depends on the interaction of BAs with specific receptors, predominantly farnesoid-X receptor (FXR) and G-protein-coupled receptor (TGR5) [77]. However, FXR and TGR5 have different affinities to individual BAs, as FXR is activated by CDCA > DCA > LCA >> CA and TGR5 is activated by LCA > DCA > CDCA > CA [78].

4.2. Interplay Between Bile Acids and the Gut Microbiota

Because the transformation of BAs is solely dependent on the gut microbiota, the extent of BA receptor activation is largely dependent on microbiota composition [79]. FXR is a key regulator of BA metabolism. Activated FXR inhibits CYP7A1, a rate-limiting enzyme of BA synthesis in hepatocytes, by two mechanisms. In hepatocytes, FXR forms a heterodimer with SHP (small heterodimer partner) to suppress the transcription of CYP7A1 [80]. In enterocytes, activated FXR stimulates production of FGF15/19. This cytokine binds to FGFR4 receptor on the hepatocyte surface, thus suppressing CYP7A1 and BA synthesis [81]. Myiata et al. showed that antibiotic treatment elevates hepatic BA synthesis in mice via the suppression of FGF15 expression in the ileum [82], which confirms the potent effect of the gut microbiome on BA metabolism. FXR also regulates enterohepatic BA circulation by regulating the expression of BA transporters. Bacterial modifications of BAs start with primary BA deconjugation by bacteria that exhibit bile salt hydrolase (BSH) activity, followed by the formation of secondary BAs by microbes that exhibit 7α-dehydroxylase and 7α-dehydrogense activity [83]. A wide array of bacteria exhibit BSH activity, enabling them to deconjugate BAs. However, there are a few bacteria belonging to the *Clostridium* clusters XI and XVIa (exhibiting 7α-dehydroxylase activity), which may catalyse the dehydrogenation of deconjugated BAs [84]. As mentioned above, BAs are themselves toxic to bacteria. First, they have direct antibacterial effects. BAs may cause damage to the bacterial membrane because of their detergent properties [85], promote bacterial protein unfolding and aggregation [86], and trigger oxidative/nitrosative stress [87]. Second, they may influence bacterial growth indirectly via FXR activation. Among other genes, FXR controls expression of Ang1, iNos and IL18, which either counteract microbial overgrowth or protect the intestinal mucosa [88]. Activated FXR stimulates the expression of cathelicidin, an antimicrobial peptide that is active in bile ducts [89]. Nevertheless, the sensitivity of bacteria to BAs varies significantly. The growth of bacteria such as *Alistipes, Bilophila wadsworthia, Escherichia coli, Listeria monocytogenes* and *Bacteroides* is even facilitated by BAs, which handicap other symbiotic microbes [84]. Some bacteria are at least BA-tolerant, such as some *Lactobacillus, Bifidobacteria* and *Clostridium* species [87].

4.3. Bile Acids and PNALD

In the 1990s, Ohkohchi et al. reported that SBS children patients suffering from intractable diarrhoea exhibited a significantly increased faecal BA excretion and altered bile acid composition. They also observed that primary bile acids accounted for more than 95% of total BAs, while taurine- and glycine-conjugated BAs accounted for only 10%. In these children, the loss of bile acids was strongly associated with a decrease in the actual absorptive surface area of the residual small intestine, while growth of the normal bacterial flora was disturbed in the residual intestine [90]. The relationships between parenteral nutrition, PNALD and BA dysmetabolism were recently studied using animal models. In one SBS-PNALD model, newborn piglets were subjected to a 75% proximal small bowl resection and fed solely via the parenteral route [13]. Two and six weeks post-resection, a significant alteration in microbiota composition was observed, particularly the loss of *Clostridiales*. This was coupled with a decrease in the overall bacterial diversity in the colon as well as a shift to a primary BA-dominant profile in bile, portal serum, and colonic content. The animals also exhibited hepatic fibrosis, steatosis and inflammation. These changes were associated with a blunted FXR activation response in the intestine, altered FXR signalling in the liver and upregulated hepatic BA synthesis [83,91]. Taken together, these data suggest that the altered BA composition following microbial dysbiosis may contribute to PNALD due to the direct physiological effects of toxic BAs and altered FXR signalling.

5. PN and Intestinal Barrier Permeability

Epithelial barrier function is essential in order for the intestine to maintain an effective defence against intraluminal toxins, foreign antigens, and bacteria, and also for enabling the epithelium to effectively absorb nutrients. Such a defence mechanism requires an intact epithelial layer [92]. Increased incidence of sepsis is a common complication in patients dependent on long-term parenteral nutrition, and it is acknowledged that organisms arising from enteric flora constitute a large percentage of these infections [93]. In 1988, Alverdy showed that PN administration in rats significantly increased bacterial translocation to the mesenteric lymph nodes by increasing caecal bacterial counts and impairing the intestinal defence [94]. In subsequent years, the loss of epithelial barrier function was identified as one of the key factors in the development of septic complications associated with long-term PN dependence [95]. PN-associated loss of the epithelial barrier function is probably the result of several underlying mechanisms. First, the morphology of the intestinal wall is altered and the functionality of epithelial cells is compromised. Studies performed using PN mouse models have revealed structural changes, including the atrophy of small bowel villi, an increase in epithelial cell apoptosis and a decrease in epithelial cell proliferation [96–98]. Second, PN administration is associated with increased production of pro-inflammatory cytokines [99,100], while in vitro studies have demonstrated that cytokines produced by immune cells can result in increased permeability of the intestinal mucosa [101]. In particular, the upregulation of IFNγ and TNFα expression in intraepithelial lymphocytes together with decreased production of IL-10 have been identified as the main factors contributing to this pathology [92,102]. Finally, tight junction proteins have an essential role in the maintenance of epithelial barrier function. Among them, ZO (1 and 2), claudins and occludins are the most important and critical components in the structural and functional organisation of tight junctions [103–105]. These proteins regulate the transport of ions and small proteins across the intestinal wall, while their expression is downregulated with PN [92]. Increased TNFα signalling due to PN-associated pro-inflammatory status results in the dissociation of structural protein ZO-1 from tight junctions and worsens barrier function [106]. The exact mechanism underlying the aggravation of epithelial barrier function has not been fully elucidated yet, but there is strong evidence to suggest that an alteration in TLR signalling may represent a link between PN-induced changes in intestinal permeability and changes in microbiota composition.

It is important to stress that all of the above results have been obtained using PN models combined with complete enteral nutrient deprivation. The deprivation of enteral nutrients available to the intraluminal bacteria alters the selection pressure for determining the dominant species in the microbiota. In environments of relative starvation, *Proteobacteria* tend to dominate [107], while *Firmicutes* are usually the predominant group in enterally fed states [108]. Wildhaber et al. [97] showed that limited enteral feeding (covering only 25% of total caloric requirements), completely reversed the unfavourable phenotype associated with parenteral nutrition (increased bacterial translocation, elevated production of pro-inflammatory cytokines, T-subpopulation representation in the intestinal epithelium). Unfortunately, the authors did not determine microbiota composition, so it is not possible to discern whether the beneficial effect arose only from the provision of nutrients to intestinal epithelial cells or whether it was co-associated with a shift in microbiota composition.

6. PN and Pro/Prebiotic Treatment

We recently showed that the microbiota of adult SBS patients dependent on total parenteral nutrition is depleted of anaerobic butyrate producers and that the amount of SCFA (particularly propionate and butyrate) in luminal content is accordingly very low [32]. Intestinal dysbiosis is often treated with probiotics, which are defined as live microorganisms that confer a health benefit on the host when administered in adequate amounts [108]. Positive results have been reported for probiotic use in the management of postsurgical inflammatory bowel disease [109,110], antibiotic-associated diarrhoea [111], and necrotising enterocolitis [112]. The most popular components of probiotic preparations are the members of the *Lactobacillus* and *Bifidobacterium* genera, and their usage is usually safe. Nevertheless, in cases where probiotics have been administered to SBS children patients, positive as well as adverse effects have been reported. The only available double-blind, placebo-controlled randomised crossover clinical trial focusing on the effects of probiotics (*Lactobacillus rhamnosus* LCG) on intestinal permeability in SBS children was unable to prove any beneficial or negative effects [113]. A case-control study performed by Uchida et al. [114] evaluated the effects of treatment on *Bifidobacterium breve*, *Lactobacillus casei* and galacto-oligosaccharides. They proved elevation of stool SCFA in 3 out of 4 patients as well as a trend for increases in height and weight velocity. Five of the nine case studies delivered evidence on the positive effects of probiotic supplementation, while the remaining four reported adverse effects, such as *Lactobacillus* sepsis and D-lactic acidosis [115]. The variable outcomes of probiotic intervention are not surprising, bearing in mind the prevalence of *Lactobacilli* in the SBS microbiome. SBS patients suffer, not because of the lack of lactate-producers, but because of the virtual absence of butyrate-producers that use lactate in the healthy gut. In this setting, further supplementation with lactate-producing bacteria or their substrates (indigestible oligosaccharides) would not provide any benefit, and, with respect to microbiota composition in some cases, could even be detrimental. Supplementation of strictly anaerobic butyrate producers such as *Lachnospiraceae*, *Ruminococcaceae* and others could be theoretically more effective, but because of the significantly altered short-bowel environment (higher oxygen levels, more acidic pH, shorter transit time) the effectiveness of this treatment would be questionable. An interesting option for bypassing all of these obstacles is to supplement SCFA directly to the nutrition mixture. Using neonatal piglets that had undergone 80% proximal jejunoileal resection, Bartholome et al. demonstrated that the supplementation of a mixture with SCFA (acetate, propionate, and butyrate) or butyrate alone enhanced structural adaptations in the developing intestine [116]. In a mouse model, PN enriched with butyric acid partially reversed the parenteral nutrition-associated atrophy of gut-associated lymphoid tissue and improved IgA secretion in the intestinal and extraintestinal mucosae. In addition, it moderately recovered mucosal atrophy [117]. Other studies report that the intravenous butyrate improves the mechanical strength of colonic anastomosis [118], moderately increases mucosal protein synthesis [119] and ameliorates small-intestinal mucosal atrophy (PN rat model) [120]. Taken together, these data advocate intravenous SCFA (particularly butyrate) supplementation as a new option for the treatment of PN-associated intestinal complications.

7. Role of the Microbiota in PNALD Development

In the previous sections, we discussed the essential role of the gut microbiota in the maintenance of homeostasis in the intestinal environment and the adverse effects of dysbiosis (Figure 1). Recent results suggest that the overall decrease in microbial diversity and the overgrowth of the specific bacterial groups in the colonic microbiota are associated with PNALD. Wang et al. [121] showed that gut microbiota composition in SBS infant patients reflects the occurrence of complications like PNALD or central line-associated bloodstream infection (CLABSI). Although the overall diversity and number of bacterial species in samples from the asymptomatic group was similar to those from healthy control infants, there were striking differences in children suffering from PNALD and CLABSI. In addition to the decrease in diversity and the number of bacterial species, there was a shift from Gram-positive *Firmicutes* to Gram-negative *Proteobacteria* (mainly *Enterobacteriaceae*). Many *Proteobacteria* produce bacterial lipopolysaccharide (LPS), a potent hepatotoxic compound, and prolonged exposure to higher LPS concentrations may result in liver injury. Furthermore, the microbiome, when enriched in *Proteobacteria,* was demonstrated to accelerate liver fibrogenesis, which may contribute to PNALD development [122]. El Kasmi et al. demonstrated the interplay between intestinal injury and the intestinal microbiota in the development of PNALD. In mice, intestinal injury and increased permeability were induced by short-term (4 days) oral treatment with low doses of dextran sulphate sodium (DSS), followed by the continuous infusion of a soy lipid-based PN solution for 7 or 28 days. After 7 days on PN, the mice showed an increased intestinal permeability, elevated portal vein LPS levels, evidence of hepatocyte injury (elevated serum aspartate aminotransferase, alanine aminotransferase), cholestasis (elevated serum bile acids, total bilirubin), and an increased expression of interleukin-6, tumour necrosis factor alpha and transforming growth factor beta in Kupffer cells. Markers of liver injury remained elevated and were associated with lobular inflammation, hepatocyte apoptosis, peliosis and Kupffer cell hypertrophy and hyperplasia after 28 days on PN [123]. Interestingly, PN infusion without DSS pretreatment or DSS pretreatment alone did not result in liver injury or Kupffer cell activation. Suppression of the intestinal microbiota with broad-spectrum antibiotics and ablation of TLR4 signalling in *Tlr4* mutant mice prevented PNALD development, which strongly suggests the role of the microbiota in its etiopathogenesis. In a subsequent study, Harris et al. identified the specific microbial taxa associated with PNALD development in this model. Among those, members of the *Erysipelotrichaceae* family and representatives of the Gram-negative S24-7 lineage of *Bacteroidetes* were identified as candidates that might play a causal role in the pathogenesis of PNALD [124]. Interestingly, mice treated only with PN without intestinal injury did not develop PNALD, despite the similar composition of their intestinal microbiota. Taken together, these experiments suggest that at least two independent conditions must be met concurrently; (i) overgrowth of specific bacteria due to PN administration and (ii) increased intestinal permeability allowing MAMPs (microbe-associated molecular pattern) derived from these taxa to reach the liver and subsequently activate Kupffer cells [124,125].

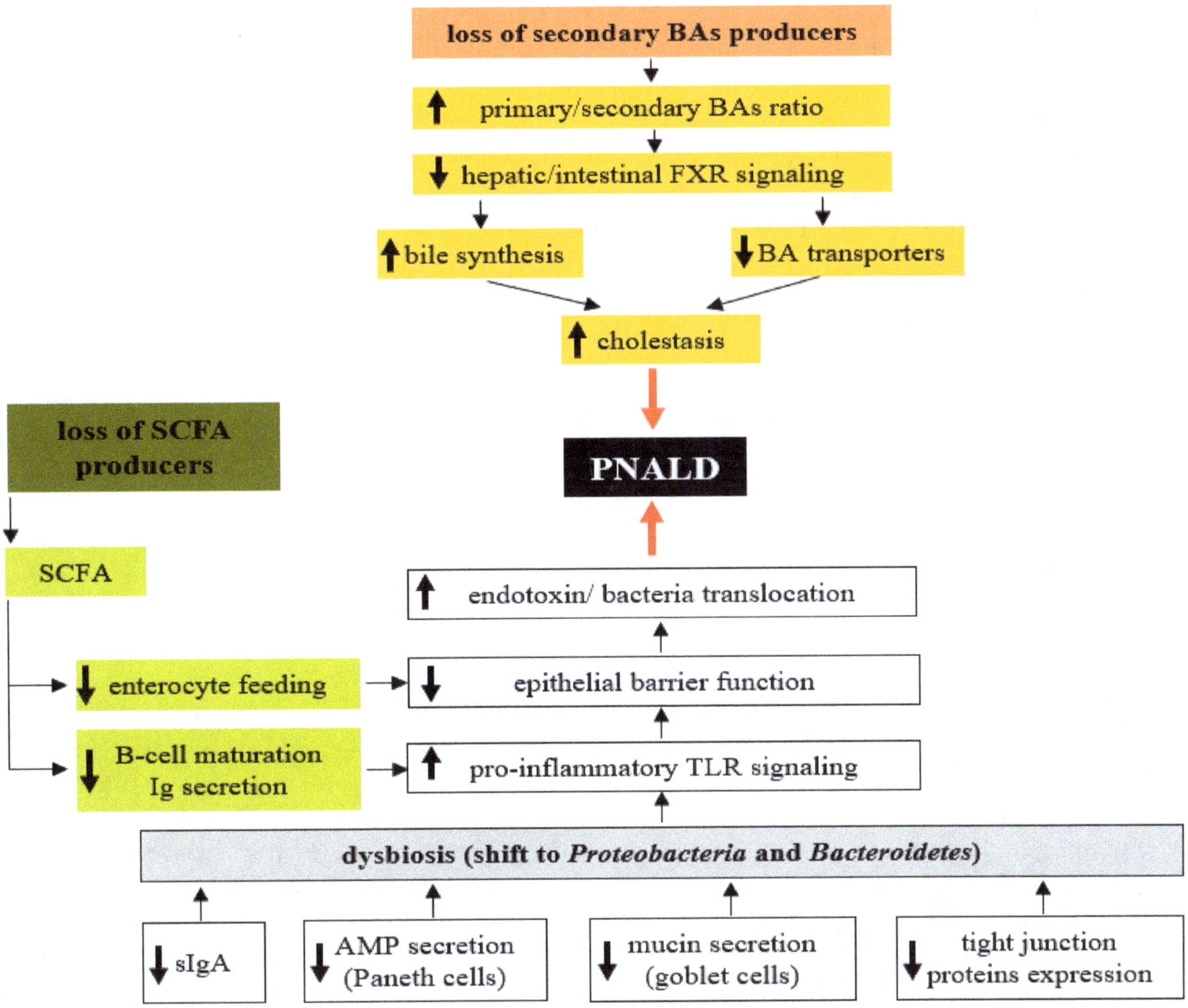

Figure 1. Gut microbiota-related factors contributing to PNALD development. Administration of parenteral nutrition (PN) is associated with decreased production of sIgA, reduced mucin synthesis in goblet cells and impaired antimicrobial function of Paneth cells. All these factors favour the growth of pathogenic bacteria (mostly from *Proteobacteria*) at the expense of beneficial commensals. In addition, the reduction in sIgA enables greater microbial access to the host epithelium and triggers an inflammatory response in the lamina propria. Enhanced toll-like receptors (TLR)-signalling due to the increased presence of potential pathogens stimulates the synthesis of pro-inflammatory cytokines in immune cells. Altogether, these factors contribute toward compromised epithelial barrier function (EBF) and increased translocation of endotoxins and even whole bacteria to the portal circulation and the liver, thereby inducing the inflammatory response. The lower abundance of SCFA producers results in decreased short-chain fatty acids (SCFA) availability, which attenuates B-cell maturation, specific antibody production and increased susceptibility to pathogens. The specific loss of secondary bile acids (BA) producers (*Clostridiales*) results in a significant shift towards primary BAs in faeces and impaired hepatic and intestinal farnesoid-X receptor (FXR) signalling. Consequently, bile acid synthesis in the liver becomes upregulated and expression of bile acid transporters becomes downregulated, resulting in the attenuation of BA transport to bile and the development of cholestasis.

8. Conclusions

A growing amount of evidence suggests that the deterioration of hepatic function in conjunction with long-term PN dependence is not the consequence of PN administration *per se* but because of intestinal failure and associated complications. The prominent factors seem to be increased permeability of the intestinal barrier, which facilitates massive translocation of bacterial toxins and even microorganisms into the portal circulation, mesenteric lymph nodes and liver, and overall pro-inflammatory status in the compromised intestine. The gut microbiota plays a profound role in the maintenance of intestinal barrier function and the establishment of either an immunotolerant or inflammatory setting of intestinal immunity. Therapeutic strategies focus on microbiota composition itself through the targeted delivery of beneficial microbiota products or by supplementation with immunomodulators. Nevertheless, understanding the complex interactions between the gut microbiota and the modified intestinal environment in PN patients is a crucial condition for efficient treatment.

Acknowledgments: This study was supported by the Ministry of Health of the Czech Republic, grant No. 15-28745A AZV CR.

Author Contributions: Monika Cahova: manuscript design, manuscript writing, critical review of the manuscript; Miriam Bratova: material collection, critical review; Petr Wohl: critical review. All authors discussed and agreed upon the final manuscript.

References

1. Mizock, B.A. Immunonutrition and critical illness: An update. *Nutrition* **2010**, *26*, 701–707. [CrossRef] [PubMed]
2. Beath, S.V.; Kelly, D.A. Total Parenteral Nutrition-Induced Cholestasis: Prevention and Management. *Clin. Liver Dis.* **2016**, *20*, 159–176. [CrossRef] [PubMed]
3. Drongowski, R.A.; Coran, A.G. An analysis of factors contributing to the development of total parenteral nutrition-induced cholestasis. *J. Parenter. Enter. Nutr.* **1989**, *13*, 586–589. [CrossRef] [PubMed]
4. Luman, W.; Shaffer, J.L. Prevalence, outcome and associated factors of deranged liver function tests in patients on home parenteral nutrition. *Clin. Nutr.* **2002**, *21*, 337–343. [CrossRef] [PubMed]
5. Bharadwaj, S.; Gohel, T.; Deen, O.J.; DeChicco, R.; Shatnawei, A. Fish oil-based lipid emulsion: Current updates on a promising novel therapy for the management of parenteral nutrition-associated liver disease. *Gastroenterol. Rep.* **2015**, *3*, 110–114. [CrossRef] [PubMed]
6. Orso, G.; Mandato, C.; Veropalumbo, C.; Cecchi, N.; Garzi, A.; Vajro, P. Pediatric parenteral nutrition-associated liver disease and cholestasis: Novel advances in pathomechanisms-based prevention and treatment. *Dig. Liver Dis.* **2016**, *48*, 215–222. [CrossRef] [PubMed]
7. Mateu de Antonio, J.; Florit-Sureda, M. Effects unrelated to anti-inflammation of lipid emulsions containing fish oil in parenteral nutrition for adult patients. *Nutr. Hosp.* **2017**, *34*, 193–203. [CrossRef] [PubMed]
8. Burcelin, R.; Serino, M.; Chabo, C.; Garidou, L.; Pomie, C.; Courtney, M.; Amar, J.; Bouloumié, A. Metagenome and metabolism: The tissue microbiota hypothesis. *Diabetes Obes. Metab.* **2013**, *15*, 61–70. [CrossRef] [PubMed]
9. Kverka, M.; Tlaskalova-Hogenova, H. Intestinal Microbiota: Facts and Fiction. *Dig. Dis.* **2017**, *35*, 139–147. [CrossRef] [PubMed]
10. Hodin, C.M.; Visschers, R.G.; Rensen, S.S.; Boonen, B.; Olde Damink, S.W.; Lenaerts, K.; Buurman, W.A. Total parenteral nutrition induces a shift in the Firmicutes to Bacteroidetes ratio in association with Paneth cell activation in rats. *J. Nutr.* **2012**, *142*, 2141–2147. [CrossRef] [PubMed]
11. Miyasaka, E.A.; Feng, Y.; Poroyko, V.; Falkowski, N.R.; Erb-Downward, J.; Gillilland, M.G.; Mason, K.L.; Huffnagle, G.B.; Teitelbaum, D.H. Total parenteral nutrition-associated lamina propria inflammation in mice is mediated by a MyD88-dependent mechanism. *J. Immunol.* **2013**, *190*, 6607–6615. [CrossRef] [PubMed]
12. Heneghan, A.F.; Pierre, J.F.; Tandee, K.; Shanmuganayagam, D.; Wang, X.; Reed, J.D.; Steele, J.L.; Kudsk, K.A. Parenteral nutrition decreases paneth cell function and intestinal bactericidal activity while increasing susceptibility to bacterial enteroinvasion. *J. Parenter. Enter. Nutr.* **2014**, *38*, 817–824. [CrossRef] [PubMed]
13. Lapthorne, S.; Pereira-Fantini, P.M.; Fouhy, F.; Wilson, G.; Thomas, S.L.; Dellios, N.L.; Scurr, M.; O'Sullivan, O.; Ross, R.P.; Stanton, C.; et al. Gut microbial diversity is reduced and is associated with colonic inflammation in a piglet model of short bowel syndrome. *Gut Microbes* **2013**, *4*, 212–221. [CrossRef] [PubMed]
14. Harvey, R.B.; Andrews, K.; Droleskey, R.E.; Kansagra, K.V.; Stoll, B.; Burrin, D.G.; Sheffield, C.L.; Anderson, R.C.; Nisbet, D.J. Qualitative and quantitative comparison of gut bacterial colonization in enterally and parenterally fed neonatal pigs. *Curr. Issues Intest. Microbiol.* **2006**, *7*, 61–64. [PubMed]

15. Deplancke, B.; Vidal, O.; Ganessunker, D.; Donovan, S.M.; Mackie, R.I.; Gaskins, H.R. Selective growth of mucolytic bacteria including Clostridium perfringens in a neonatal piglet model of total parenteral nutrition. *Am. J. Clin. Nutr.* **2002**, *76*, 1117–1125. [PubMed]
16. Lavallee, C.M.; MacPherson, J.A.; Zhou, M.; Gao, Y.; Wizzard, P.R.; Wales, P.W.; Turner, J.M.; Willing, B.P. Lipid Emulsion Formulation of Parenteral Nutrition Affects Intestinal Microbiota and Host Responses in Neonatal Piglets. *J. Parent. Enteral. Nutr.* **2016**. [CrossRef] [PubMed]
17. Parm, U.; Metsvaht, T.; Ilmoja, M.L.; Lutsar, I. Gut colonization by aerobic microorganisms is associated with route and type of nutrition in premature neonates. *Nutr. Res.* **2015**, *35*, 496–503. [CrossRef] [PubMed]
18. Ralls, M.W.; Miyasaka, E.; Teitelbaum, D.H. Intestinal microbial diversity and perioperative complications. *J. Parenter. Enter. Nutr.* **2014**, *38*, 392–399. [CrossRef] [PubMed]
19. Joly, F.; Mayeur, C.; Bruneau, A.; Noordine, M.L.; Meylheuc, T.; Langella, P.; Messing, B.; Duée, P.H.; Cherbuy, C.; Thomas, M. Drastic changes in fecal and mucosa-associated microbiota in adult patients with short bowel syndrome. *Biochimie* **2010**, *92*, 753–761. [CrossRef] [PubMed]
20. Dibaise, J.K.; Young, R.J.; Vanderhoof, J.A. Enteric microbial flora, bacterial overgrowth, and short-bowel syndrome. *Clin. Gastroenterol. Hepatol.* **2006**, *4*, 11–20. [CrossRef] [PubMed]
21. Huang, Y.; Guo, F.; Li, Y.; Wang, J.; Li, J. Fecal microbiota signatures of adult patients with different types of short bowel syndrome. *J. Gastroenterol. Hepatol.* **2017**. [CrossRef] [PubMed]
22. Siggers, R.H.; Siggers, J.; Thymann, T.; Boye, M.; Sangild, P.T. Nutritional modulation of the gut microbiota and immune system in preterm neonates susceptible to necrotizing enterocolitis. *J. Nutr. Biochem.* **2011**, *22*, 511–521. [CrossRef] [PubMed]
23. Wang, S.; Ng, L.H.; Chow, W.L.; Lee, Y.K. Infant intestinal Enterococcus faecalis down-regulates inflammatory responses in human intestinal cell lines. *World J. Gastroenterol.* **2008**, *14*, 1067–1076. [CrossRef] [PubMed]
24. Messing, B.; Lémann, M.; Landais, P.; Gouttebel, M.C.; Gérard-Boncompain, M.; Saudin, F.; Vangossum, A.; Beau, P.; Guédon, C.; Barnoud, D.; et al. Prognosis of patients with nonmalignant chronic intestinal failure receiving long-term home parenteral nutrition. *Gastroenterology* **1995**, *108*, 1005–1010. [CrossRef]
25. Mayeur, C.; Gillard, L.; Le Beyec, J.; Bado, A.; Joly, F.; Thomas, M. Extensive Intestinal Resection Triggers Behavioral Adaptation, Intestinal Remodeling and Microbiota Transition in Short Bowel Syndrome. *Microorganisms* **2016**, *4*, 1. [CrossRef] [PubMed]
26. Duncan, S.H.; Louis, P.; Thomson, J.M.; Flint, H.J. The role of pH in determining the species composition of the human colonic microbiota. *Environ. Microbiol.* **2009**, *11*, 2112–2122. [CrossRef] [PubMed]
27. Mayeur, C.; Gratadoux, J.J.; Bridonneau, C.; Chegdani, F.; Larroque, B.; Kapel, N.; Corcos, O.; Thomas, M.; Joly, F. Faecal D/L lactate ratio is a metabolic signature of microbiota imbalance in patients with short bowel syndrome. *PLoS ONE* **2013**, *8*, e54335. [CrossRef] [PubMed]
28. Lilja, H.E.; Wefer, H.; Nystrom, N.; Finkel, Y.; Engstrand, L. Intestinal dysbiosis in children with short bowel syndrome is associated with impaired outcome. *Microbiome* **2015**, *3*, 18. [CrossRef] [PubMed]
29. Belenguer, A.; Holtrop, G.; Duncan, S.H.; Anderson, S.E.; Calder, A.G.; Flint, H.J.; Lobley, G.E. Rates of production and utilization of lactate by microbial communities from the human colon. *FEMS Microbiol. Ecol.* **2011**, *77*, 107–119. [CrossRef] [PubMed]
30. Bourriaud, C.; Robins, R.J.; Martin, L.; Kozlowski, F.; Tenailleau, E.; Cherbut, C.; Michel, C. Lactate is mainly fermented to butyrate by human intestinal microfloras but inter-individual variation is evident. *J. Appl. Microbiol.* **2005**, *99*, 201–212. [CrossRef] [PubMed]
31. Sekirov, I.; Russell, S.L.; Antunes, L.C.; Finlay, B.B. Gut microbiota in health and disease. *Physiol. Rev.* **2010**, *90*, 859–904. [CrossRef] [PubMed]
32. Abreu, M.T. Toll-like receptor signalling in the intestinal epithelium: How bacterial recognition shapes intestinal function. *Nat. Rev. Immunol.* **2010**, *10*, 131–144. [CrossRef] [PubMed]
33. Mazmanian, S.K.; Liu, C.H.; Tzianabos, A.O.; Kasper, D.L. An immunomodulatory molecule of symbiotic bacteria directs maturation of the host immune system. *Cell* **2005**, *122*, 107–118. [CrossRef] [PubMed]
34. Christensen, H.R.; Frokiaer, H.; Pestka, J.J. Lactobacilli differentially modulate expression of cytokines and maturation surface markers in murine dendritic cells. *J. Immunol.* **2002**, *168*, 171–178. [CrossRef] [PubMed]
35. Ivanov, I.I.; de Llanos Frutos, R.; Manel, N.; Yoshinaga, K.; Rifkin, D.B.; Sartor, R.B.; Finlay, B.B.; Littman, D.R. Specific microbiota direct the differentiation of IL-17-producing T-helper cells in the mucosa of the small intestine. *Cell Host Microbe* **2008**, *4*, 337–349. [CrossRef] [PubMed]

36. Beutler, B.; Rietschel, E.T. Innate immune sensing and its roots: The story of endotoxin. *Nat. Rev. Immunol.* **2003**, *3*, 169. [CrossRef] [PubMed]
37. Kelsall, B.L.; Leon, F. Involvement of intestinal dendritic cells in oral tolerance, immunity to pathogens, and inflammatory bowel disease. *Immunol. Rev.* **2005**, *206*, 132–148. [CrossRef] [PubMed]
38. Kelly, D.; Campbell, J.I.; King, T.P.; Grant, G.; Jansson, E.A.; Coutts, A.G.; Pettersson, S.; Conway, S. Commensal anaerobic gut bacteria attenuate inflammation by regulating nuclear-cytoplasmic shuttling of PPAR-gamma and RelA. *Nat. Immunol.* **2004**, *5*, 104. [CrossRef] [PubMed]
39. Lee, J.; Mo, J.H.; Katakura, K.; Alkalay, I.; Rucker, A.N.; Liu, Y.T.; Hyun-Ku, L.; Shen, C.; Cojocaru, G.; Shenouda, S.; et al. Maintenance of colonic homeostasis by distinctive apical TLR9 signalling in intestinal epithelial cells. *Nat. Cell Biol.* **2006**, *8*, 1327. [CrossRef] [PubMed]
40. Iwasaki, A.; Kelsall, B.L. Freshly isolated Peyer's patch, but not spleen, dendritic cells produce interleukin 10 and induce the differentiation of T helper type 2 cells. *J. Exp. Med.* **1999**, *190*, 229–239. [CrossRef] [PubMed]
41. Macpherson, A.J.; Uhr, T. Induction of protective IgA by intestinal dendritic cells carrying commensal bacteria. *Science* **2004**, *303*, 1662–1665. [CrossRef] [PubMed]
42. Peterson, D.A.; McNulty, N.P.; Guruge, J.L.; Gordon, J.I. IgA response to symbiotic bacteria as a mediator of gut homeostasis. *Cell Host Microbe* **2007**, *2*, 328–339. [CrossRef] [PubMed]
43. Suzuki, K.; Meek, B.; Doi, Y.; Muramatsu, M.; Chiba, T.; Honjo, T.; Fagarasan, S. Aberrant expansion of segmented filamentous bacteria in IgA-deficient gut. *Proc. Natl. Acad. Sci. USA* **2004**, *101*, 1981–1986. [CrossRef] [PubMed]
44. Yanagibashi, T.; Hosono, A.; Oyama, A.; Tsuda, M.; Hachimura, S.; Takahashi, Y.; Itoh, K.; Hirayama, K.; Takahashi, K.; Kaminogawa, S. Bacteroides induce higher IgA production than Lactobacillus by increasing activation-induced cytidine deaminase expression in B cells in murine Peyer's patches. *Biosci. Biotechnol. Biochem.* **2009**, *73*, 372–377. [CrossRef] [PubMed]
45. Zipperer, A.; Konnerth, M.C.; Laux, C.; Berscheid, A.; Janek, D.; Weidenmaier, C.; Burian, M.; Schilling, N.A.; Slavetinsky, C.; Marschal, M.; et al. Human commensals producing a novel antibiotic impair pathogen colonization. *Nature* **2016**, *535*, 511–516. [CrossRef] [PubMed]
46. Pierre, J.F. Gastrointestinal immune and microbiome changes during parenteral nutrition. *Am. J. Physiol. Gastrointest. Liver Physiol.* **2017**, *312*, G246–G256. [CrossRef] [PubMed]
47. Coulombe, G.; Langlois, A.; De Palma, G.; Langlois, M.J.; McCarville, J.L.; Gagné-Sanfaçon, J.; Perreault, N.; Feng, G.S.; Bercik, P.; Boudreau, F.; et al. SHP-2 Phosphatase Prevents Colonic Inflammation by Controlling Secretory Cell Differentiation and Maintaining Host-Microbiota Homeostasis. *J. Cell. Physiol.* **2016**, *231*, 2529–2540. [CrossRef] [PubMed]
48. Everard, A.; Geurts, L.; Caesar, R.; van Hul, M.; Matamoros, S.; Duparc, T.; Denis, R.G.; Cochez, P.; Pierard, F.; Castel, J.; et al. Intestinal epithelial MyD88 is a sensor switching host metabolism towards obesity according to nutritional status. *Nat. Commun.* **2014**, *5*, 5648. [CrossRef] [PubMed]
49. Dheer, R.; Santaolalla, R.; Davies, J.M.; Lang, J.K.; Phillips, M.C.; Pastorini, C.; Vazquez-Pertejo, M.T.; Abreu, M.T. Intestinal Epithelial Toll-Like Receptor 4 Signalling Affects Epithelial Function and Colonic Microbiota and Promotes a Risk for Transmissible Colitis. *Infect. Immun.* **2016**, *84*, 798–810. [CrossRef] [PubMed]
50. Frantz, A.L.; Rogier, E.W.; Weber, C.R.; Shen, L.; Cohen, D.A.; Fenton, L.A.; Bruno, M.E.C.; Kaetzel, C.S. Targeted deletion of MyD88 in intestinal epithelial cells results in compromised antibacterial immunity associated with downregulation of polymeric immunoglobulin receptor, mucin-2, and antibacterial peptides. *Mucosal Immunol.* **2012**, *5*, 501. [CrossRef] [PubMed]
51. Anitha, M.; Vijay-Kumar, M.; Sitaraman, S.V.; Gewirtz, A.T.; Srinivasan, S. Gut microbial products regulate murine gastrointestinal motility via Toll-like receptor 4 signalling. *Gastroenterology* **2012**, *143*, 1006–1016. [CrossRef] [PubMed]
52. Cheesman, S.E.; Neal, J.T.; Mittge, E.; Seredick, B.M.; Guillemin, K. Epithelial cell proliferation in the developing zebrafish intestine is regulated by the Wnt pathway and microbial signalling via Myd88. *Proc. Natl. Acad. Sci. USA* **2011**, *108*, 4570–4577. [CrossRef] [PubMed]
53. Cerovic, V.; Bain, C.C.; Mowat, A.M.; Milling, S.W. Intestinal macrophages and dendritic cells: What's the difference? *Trends Immunol.* **2014**, *35*, 270–277. [CrossRef] [PubMed]

54. Bain, C.C.; Bravo-Blas, A.; Scott, C.L.; Perdiguero, E.G.; Geissmann, F.; Henri, S.; Malissen, B.; Osborne, L.C.; Artis, D.; Mowat, A.M. Constant replenishment from circulating monocytes maintains the macrophage pool in the intestine of adult mice. *Nat. Immunol.* **2014**, *15*, 929–937. [CrossRef] [PubMed]
55. Smith, P.D.; Smythies, L.E.; Shen, R.; Greenwell-Wild, T.; Gliozzi, M.; Wahl, S.M. Intestinal macrophages and response to microbial encroachment. *Mucosal Immunol.* **2011**, *4*, 31–42. [CrossRef] [PubMed]
56. Denning, T.L.; Norris, B.A.; Medina-Contreras, O.; Manicassamy, S.; Geem, D.; Madan, R.; Karp, C.L.; Pulendran, B. Functional specializations of intestinal dendritic cell and macrophage subsets that control Th17 and regulatory T cell responses are dependent on the T cell/APC ratio, source of mouse strain, and regional localization. *J. Immunol.* **2011**, *187*, 733–747. [CrossRef] [PubMed]
57. Rivollier, A.; He, J.; Kole, A.; Valatas, V.; Kelsall, B.L. Inflammation switches the differentiation program of Ly6Chi monocytes from antiinflammatory macrophages to inflammatory dendritic cells in the colon. *J. Exp. Med.* **2012**, *209*, 139–155. [CrossRef] [PubMed]
58. Schulz, C.; Perdiguero, E.G.; Chorro, L.; Szabo-Rogers, H.; Cagnard, N.; Kierdorf, K.; Prinz, M.; Wu, B.; Jacobsen, S.E.W.; Pollard, J.W.; et al. A lineage of myeloid cells independent of Myb and hematopoietic stem cells. *Science* **2012**, *336*, 86–90. [CrossRef] [PubMed]
59. Hashimoto, D.; Chow, A.; Noizat, C.; Teo, P.; Beasley, M.B.; Leboeuf, M.; Becker, C.D.; See, P.; Price, J.; Lucas, D.; et al. Tissue-resident macrophages self-maintain locally throughout adult life with minimal contribution from circulating monocytes. *Immunity* **2013**, *38*, 792–804. [CrossRef] [PubMed]
60. Ueda, Y.; Kayama, H.; Jeon, S.G.; Kusu, T.; Isaka, Y.; Rakugi, H.; Yamamoto, M.; Takeda, K. Commensal microbiota induce LPS hyporesponsiveness in colonic macrophages via the production of IL-10. *Int. Immunol.* **2010**, *22*, 953–962. [CrossRef] [PubMed]
61. Hayashi, A.; Sato, T.; Kamada, N.; Mikami, Y.; Matsuoka, K.; Hisamatsu, T.; Hibi, T.; Roers, A.; Yagita, H.; Ohteki, T.; et al. A single strain of Clostridium butyricum induces intestinal IL-10-producing macrophages to suppress acute experimental colitis in mice. *Cell Host Microbe* **2013**, *13*, 711–722. [CrossRef] [PubMed]
62. Ochi, T.; Feng, Y.; Kitamoto, S.; Nagao-Kitamoto, H.; Kuffa, P.; Atarashi, K.; Honda, K.; Teitelbaum, D.H.; Kamada, N. Diet-dependent, microbiota-independent regulation of IL-10-producing lamina propria macrophages in the small intestine. *Sci. Rep.* **2016**, *6*, 27634. [CrossRef] [PubMed]
63. Bevins, C.L. Paneth cell defensins: key effector molecules of innate immunity. *Biochem. Soc. Trans.* **2006**, *34*, 263–266. [CrossRef] [PubMed]
64. Porter, E.M.; Bevins, C.L.; Ghosh, D.; Ganz, T. The multifaceted Paneth cell. *Cell Mol. Life Sci.* **2002**, *59*, 156–170. [CrossRef] [PubMed]
65. Ouellette, A.J. Defensin-mediated innate immunity in the small intestine. *Best Pract. Res. Clin. Gastroenterol.* **2004**, *18*, 405–419. [CrossRef] [PubMed]
66. Vaishnava, S.; Behrendt, C.L.; Ismail, A.S.; Eckmann, L.; Hooper, L.V. Paneth cells directly sense gut commensals and maintain homeostasis at the intestinal host-microbial interface. *Proc. Natl. Acad. Sci. USA* **2008**, *105*, 20858–20863. [CrossRef] [PubMed]
67. Omata, J.; Pierre, J.F.; Heneghan, A.F.; Tsao, F.H.; Sano, Y.; Jonker, M.A.; Kudsk, K.A. Parenteral nutrition suppresses the bactericidal response of the small intestine. *Surgery* **2013**, *153*, 17–24. [CrossRef] [PubMed]
68. Kirkland, D.; Benson, A.; Mirpuri, J.; Pifer, R.; Hou, B.; DeFranco, A.L.; Yarovinsky, F. B cell-intrinsic MyD88 signalling prevents the lethal dissemination of commensal bacteria during colonic damage. *Immunity* **2012**, *36*, 228–238. [CrossRef] [PubMed]
69. Teng, F.; Klinger, C.N.; Felix, K.M.; Bradley, C.P.; Wu, E.; Tran, N.L.; Umesaki, Y.; Wu, H.J.J. Gut Microbiota Drive Autoimmune Arthritis by Promoting Differentiation and Migration of Peyer's Patch T Follicular Helper Cells. *Immunity* **2016**, *44*, 875–888. [CrossRef] [PubMed]
70. Kim, M.; Qie, Y.; Park, J.; Kim, C.H. Gut Microbial Metabolites Fuel Host Antibody Responses. *Cell Host Microbe* **2016**, *20*, 202–214. [CrossRef] [PubMed]
71. Kudoh, K.; Shimizu, J.; Wada, M.; Takita, T.; Kanke, Y.; Innami, S. Effect of indigestible saccharides on B lymphocyte response of intestinal mucosa and cecal fermentation in rats. *J. Nutr. Sci. Vitaminol.* **1998**, *44*, 103–112. [CrossRef] [PubMed]
72. Bjorkhem, I. Mechanism of degradation of the steroid side chain in the formation of bile acids. *J. Lipid Res.* **1992**, *33*, 455–471. [PubMed]
73. Zhang, Y.; Limaye, P.B.; Renaud, H.J.; Klaassen, C.D. Effect of various antibiotics on modulation of intestinal microbiota and bile acid profile in mice. *Toxicol. Appl. Pharmacol.* **2014**, *277*, 138–145. [CrossRef] [PubMed]

74. Chiang, J.Y. Bile acid regulation of gene expression: Roles of nuclear hormone receptors. *Endocr. Rev.* **2002**, *23*, 443–463. [CrossRef] [PubMed]
75. Fan, M.; Wang, X.; Xu, G.; Yan, Q.; Huang, W. Bile acid signalling and liver regeneration. *Biochim. Biophys. Acta* **2015**, *1849*, 196–200. [CrossRef] [PubMed]
76. Duboc, H.; Tache, Y.; Hofmann, A.F. The bile acid TGR5 membrane receptor: From basic research to clinical application. *Dig. Liver Dis.* **2014**, *46*, 302–312. [CrossRef] [PubMed]
77. Li, T.; Chiang, J.Y. Bile acids as metabolic regulators. *Curr. Opin. Gastroenterol.* **2015**, *31*, 159–165. [CrossRef] [PubMed]
78. Jones, M.L.; Martoni, C.J.; Ganopolsky, J.G.; Labbe, A.; Prakash, S. The human microbiome and bile acid metabolism: Dysbiosis, dysmetabolism, disease and intervention. *Expert Opin. Biol. Ther.* **2014**, *14*, 467–482. [CrossRef] [PubMed]
79. Ridlon, J.M.; Kang, D.J.; Hylemon, P.B. Bile salt biotransformations by human intestinal bacteria. *J. Lipid Res.* **2006**, *47*, 241–259. [CrossRef] [PubMed]
80. Goodwin, B.; Jones, S.A.; Price, R.R.; Watson, M.A.; McKee, D.D.; Moore, L.B.; Galardi, C.; Wilson, J.G.; Lewis, M.C.; Roth, M.E.; et al. A regulatory cascade of the nuclear receptors FXR, SHP-1, and LRH-1 represses bile acid biosynthesis. *Mol. Cell* **2000**, *6*, 517–526. [CrossRef]
81. Holt, M.P.; Cheng, L.; Ju, C. Identification and characterization of infiltrating macrophages in acetaminophen-induced liver injury. *J. Leukoc. Biol.* **2008**, *84*, 1410–1421. [CrossRef] [PubMed]
82. Miyata, M.; Takamatsu, Y.; Kuribayashi, H.; Yamazoe, Y. Administration of ampicillin elevates hepatic primary bile acid synthesis through suppression of ileal fibroblast growth factor 15 expression. *J. Pharmacol. Exp. Ther.* **2009**, *331*, 1079–1085. [CrossRef] [PubMed]
83. Pereira-Fantini, P.M.; Lapthorne, S.; Joyce, S.A.; Dellios, N.L.; Wilson, G.; Fouhy, F.; Thomas, S.L.; Scurr, M.; Hill, C.; Gahan, C.G.; et al. Altered FXR signalling is associated with bile acid dysmetabolism in short bowel syndrome-associated liver disease. *J. Hepatol.* **2014**, *61*, 1115–1125. [CrossRef] [PubMed]
84. Nie, Y.F.; Hu, J.; Yan, X.H. Cross-talk between bile acids and intestinal microbiota in host metabolism and health. *J. Zhejiang Univ. Sci. B* **2015**, *16*, 436–446. (In Chinese) [CrossRef] [PubMed]
85. Islam, K.S.; Fukiya, S.; Hagio, M.; Fujii, N.; Ishizuka, S.; Ooka, T.; Ogura, Y.; Hayashi, T.; Yokota, A. Bile acid is a host factor that regulates the composition of the cecal microbiota in rats. *Gastroenterology* **2011**, *141*, 1773–1781. [CrossRef] [PubMed]
86. Cremers, C.M.; Knoefler, D.; Vitvitsky, V.; Banerjee, R.; Jakob, U. Bile salts act as effective protein-unfolding agents and instigators of disulfide stress in vivo. *Proc. Natl. Acad. Sci. USA* **2014**, *111*, E1610–E1619. [CrossRef] [PubMed]
87. Begley, M.; Gahan, C.G.; Hill, C. The interaction between bacteria and bile. *FEMS Microbiol. Rev.* **2005**, *29*, 625–651. [CrossRef] [PubMed]
88. Inagaki, T.; Moschetta, A.; Lee, Y.K.; Peng, L.; Zhao, G.; Downes, M.; Ruth, T.Y.; Shelton, J.M.; Richardson, J.A.; Repa, J.J.; et al. Regulation of antibacterial defense in the small intestine by the nuclear bile acid receptor. *Proc. Natl. Acad. Sci. USA* **2006**, *103*, 3920–3925. [CrossRef] [PubMed]
89. D'Aldebert, E.; Mve, M.J.B.B.; Mergey, M.; Wendum, D.; Firrincieli, D.; Coilly, A.; Fouassier, L.; Corpechot, C.; Poupon, R.; Housset, C.; et al. Bile salts control the antimicrobial peptide cathelicidin through nuclear receptors in the human biliary epithelium. *Gastroenterology* **2009**, *136*, 1435–1443. [CrossRef] [PubMed]
90. Ohkohchi, N.; Andoh, T.; Izumi, U.; Igarashi, Y.; Ohi, R. Disorder of bile acid metabolism in children with short bowel syndrome. *J. Gastroenterol.* **1997**, *32*, 472–479. [CrossRef] [PubMed]
91. Pereira-Fantini, P.M.; Bines, J.E.; Lapthorne, S.; Fouhy, F.; Scurr, M.; Cotter, P.D.; Gahan, C.G.; Joyce, S.A. Short bowel syndrome (SBS)-associated alterations within the gut-liver axis evolve early and persist long-term in the piglet model of short bowel syndrome. *J. Gastroenterol. Hepatol.* **2016**, *31*, 1946–1955. [CrossRef] [PubMed]
92. Sun, X.; Yang, H.; Nose, K.; Nose, S.; Haxhija, E.Q.; Koga, H.; Feng, Y.; Teitelbaum, D.H. Decline in intestinal mucosal IL-10 expression and decreased intestinal barrier function in a mouse model of total parenteral nutrition. *Am. J. Physiol. Gastrointest. Liver Physiol.* **2008**, *294*, G139–G147. [CrossRef] [PubMed]
93. Deitch, E.A. Gut-origin sepsis: Evolution of a concept. *Surgeon* **2012**, *10*, 350–356. [CrossRef] [PubMed]
94. Alverdy, J.C.; Aoys, E.; Moss, G.S. Total parenteral nutrition promotes bacterial translocation from the gut. *Surgery* **1988**, *104*, 185–190. [PubMed]

95. Demehri, F.R.; Barrett, M.; Ralls, M.W.; Miyasaka, E.A.; Feng, Y.; Teitelbaum, D.H. Intestinal epithelial cell apoptosis and loss of barrier function in the setting of altered microbiota with enteral nutrient deprivation. *Front. Cell. Infect. Microbiol.* **2013**, *3*, 105. [CrossRef] [PubMed]
96. Feng, Y.; Sun, X.; Yang, H.; Teitelbaum, D.H. Dissociation of E-cadherin and beta-catenin in a mouse model of total parenteral nutrition: A mechanism for the loss of epithelial cell proliferation and villus atrophy. *J. Physiol.* **2009**, *587*, 641–654. [CrossRef] [PubMed]
97. Wildhaber, B.E.; Yang, H.; Spencer, A.U.; Drongowski, R.A.; Teitelbaum, D.H. Lack of enteral nutrition—Effects on the intestinal immune system. *J. Surg. Res.* **2005**, *123*, 8–16. [CrossRef] [PubMed]
98. Demehri, F.R.; Barrett, M.; Teitelbaum, D.H. Changes to the Intestinal Microbiome With Parenteral Nutrition: Review of a Murine Model and Potential Clinical Implications. *Nutr. Clin. Pract.* **2015**, *30*, 798–806. [CrossRef] [PubMed]
99. Feng, Y.; Teitelbaum, D.H. Tumour necrosis factor—Induced loss of intestinal barrier function requires TNFR1 and TNFR2 signalling in a mouse model of total parenteral nutrition. *J. Physiol.* **2013**, *591*, 3709–3723. [CrossRef] [PubMed]
100. Yang, H.; Fan, Y.; Teitelbaum, D.H. Intraepithelial lymphocyte-derived interferon-gamma evokes enterocyte apoptosis with parenteral nutrition in mice. *Am. J. Physiol. Gastrointest. Liver Physiol.* **2003**, *284*, G629–G637. [CrossRef] [PubMed]
101. Clayburgh, D.R.; Shen, L.; Turner, J.R. A porous defense: The leaky epithelial barrier in intestinal disease. *Lab. Investig.* **2004**, *84*, 282–291. [CrossRef] [PubMed]
102. Yang, H.; Kiristioglu, I.; Fan, Y.; Forbush, B.; Bishop, D.K.; Antony, P.A.; Zhou, H.; Teitelbaum, D.H. Interferon-gamma expression by intraepithelial lymphocytes results in a loss of epithelial barrier function in a mouse model of total parenteral nutrition. *Ann. Surg.* **2002**, *236*, 226–234. [CrossRef] [PubMed]
103. Mitic, L.L.; Anderson, J.M. Molecular architecture of tight junctions. *Annu. Rev. Physiol.* **1998**, *60*, 121–142. [CrossRef] [PubMed]
104. Prasad, S.; Mingrino, R.; Kaukinen, K.; Hayes, K.L.; Powell, R.M.; MacDonald, T.T.; Collins, J.E. Inflammatory processes have differential effects on claudins 2, 3 and 4 in colonic epithelial cells. *Lab. Investig.* **2005**, *85*, 1139–1162. [CrossRef] [PubMed]
105. Fanning, A.S.; Jameson, B.J.; Jesaitis, L.A.; Anderson, J.M. The tight junction protein ZO-1 establishes a link between the transmembrane protein occludin and the actin cytoskeleton. *J. Biol. Chem.* **1998**, *273*, 29745–29753. [CrossRef] [PubMed]
106. Chen, C.; Wang, P.; Su, Q.; Wang, S.; Wang, F. Myosin light chain kinase mediates intestinal barrier disruption following burn injury. *PLoS ONE* **2012**, *7*, e34946. [CrossRef] [PubMed]
107. Sinclair, J.L.; Alexander, M. Role of resistance to starvation in bacterial survival in sewage and lake water. *Appl. Environ. Microbiol.* **1984**, *48*, 410–415. [PubMed]
108. Costello, E.K.; Gordon, J.I.; Secor, S.M.; Knight, R. Postprandial remodeling of the gut microbiota in Burmese pythons. *ISME J.* **2010**, *4*, 1375–1385. [CrossRef] [PubMed]
109. Gionchetti, P.; Rizzello, F.; Helwig, U.; Venturi, A.; Lammers, K.M.; Brigidi, P.; Vitali, B.; Poggioli, G.; Miglioli, M.; Campieri, M. Prophylaxis of pouchitis onset with probiotic therapy: A double-blind, placebo-controlled trial. *Gastroenterology* **2003**, *124*, 1202–1209. [CrossRef]
110. Mimura, T.; Rizzello, F.; Helwig, U.; Poggioli, G.; Schreiber, S.; Talbot, I.C.; Nicholls, R.J.; Gionchetti, P.; Campieri, M.; Kamm, M.A. Once daily high dose probiotic therapy (VSL#3) for maintaining remission in recurrent or refractory pouchitis. *Gut* **2004**, *53*, 108–114. [PubMed]
111. Szajewska, H.; Ruszczynski, M.; Radzikowski, A. Probiotics in the prevention of antibiotic-associated diarrhea in children: A meta-analysis of randomized controlled trials. *J. Pediatr.* **2006**, *149*, 367–372. [CrossRef] [PubMed]
112. Barclay, A.R.; Stenson, B.; Simpson, J.H.; Weaver, L.T.; Wilson, D.C. Probiotics for necrotizing enterocolitis: A systematic review. *J. Pediatr. Gastroenterol. Nutr.* **2007**, *45*, 569–576. [CrossRef] [PubMed]
113. Sentongo, T.A.; Cohran, V.; Korff, S.; Sullivan, C.; Iyer, K.; Zheng, X. Intestinal permeability and effects of Lactobacillus rhamnosus therapy in children with short bowel syndrome. *J. Pediatr. Gastroenterol. Nutr.* **2008**, *46*, 41–47. [CrossRef] [PubMed]
114. Uchida, K.; Takahashi, T.; Inoue, M.; Morotomi, M.; Otake, K.; Nakazawa, M.; Tsukamoto, Y.; Miki, C.; Kusunoki, M. Immunonutritional effects during synbiotics therapy in pediatric patients with short bowel syndrome. *Pediatr. Surg. Int.* **2007**, *23*, 243–248. [CrossRef] [PubMed]

115. Reddy, V.S.; Patole, S.K.; Rao, S. Role of probiotics in short bowel syndrome in infants and children—A systematic review. *Nutrients* **2013**, *5*, 679–699. [CrossRef] [PubMed]
116. Bartholome, A.L.; Albin, D.M.; Baker, D.H.; Holst, J.J.; Tappenden, K.A. Supplementation of total parenteral nutrition with butyrate acutely increases structural aspects of intestinal adaptation after an 80% jejunoileal resection in neonatal piglets. *J. Parenter. Enter. Nutr.* **2004**, *28*, 210–222. [CrossRef] [PubMed]
117. Murakoshi, S.; Fukatsu, K.; Omata, J.; Moriya, T.; Noguchi, M.; Saitoh, D.; Koyama, I. Effects of adding butyric acid to PN on gut-associated lymphoid tissue and mucosal immunoglobulin A levels. *J. Parenter. Enter. Nutr.* **2011**, *35*, 465–472. [CrossRef] [PubMed]
118. Rolandelli, R.H.; Buckmire, M.A.; Bernstein, K.A. Intravenous butyrate and healing of colonic anastomoses in the rat. *Dis. Colon Rectum* **1997**, *40*, 67–70. [CrossRef] [PubMed]
119. Stein, T.P.; Yoshida, S.; Schluter, M.D.; Drews, D.; Assimon, S.A.; Leskiw, M.J. Comparison of intravenous nutrients on gut mucosal proteins synthesis. *J. Parenter. Enter. Nutr.* **1994**, *18*, 447–452. [CrossRef] [PubMed]
120. Koruda, M.J.; Rolandelli, R.H.; Bliss, D.Z.; Hastings, J.; Rombeau, J.L.; Settle, R.G. Parenteral nutrition supplemented with short-chain fatty acids: Effect on the small-bowel mucosa in normal rats. *Am. J. Clin. Nutr.* **1990**, *51*, 685–689. [PubMed]
121. Wang, P.; Wang, Y.; Lu, L.; Yan, W.; Tao, Y.; Zhou, K.; Jie, J.; Wei, C. Alterations in intestinal microbiota relate to intestinal failure-associated liver disease and central line infections. *J. Pediatr. Surg.* **2017**, *52*, 1318–1326. [CrossRef] [PubMed]
122. De Minicis, S.; Rychlicki, C.; Agostinelli, L.; Saccomanno, S.; Candelaresi, C.; Trozzi, L.; Mingarelli, E.; Facinelli, B.; Magi, G.; Palmieri, C.; et al. Dysbiosis contributes to fibrogenesis in the course of chronic liver injury in mice. *Hepatology* **2014**, *59*, 1738–1749. [CrossRef] [PubMed]
123. El Kasmi, K.C.; Anderson, A.L.; Devereaux, M.W.; Fillon, S.A.; Harris, J.K.; Lovell, M.A.; Finegold, M.J.; Sokol, R.J. Toll-like receptor 4-dependent Kupffer cell activation and liver injury in a novel mouse model of parenteral nutrition and intestinal injury. *Hepatology* **2012**, *55*, 1518–1528. [CrossRef] [PubMed]
124. Harris, J.K.; El Kasmi, K.C.; Anderson, A.L.; Devereaux, M.W.; Fillon, S.A.; Robertson, C.E.; Wagner, B.D.; Stevens, M.J.; Pace, N.R.; Sokol, R.J. Specific microbiome changes in a mouse model of parenteral nutrition associated liver injury and intestinal inflammation. *PLoS ONE* **2014**, *9*, e110396. [CrossRef] [PubMed]
125. Lee, W.S.; Sokol, R.J. Intestinal Microbiota, Lipids, and the Pathogenesis of Intestinal Failure-Associated Liver Disease. *J. Pediatr.* **2015**, *167*, 519–526. [CrossRef] [PubMed]

12

Predictors Associated with Increase in Skeletal Muscle Mass after Sustained Virological Response in Chronic Hepatitis C Treated with Direct Acting Antivirals

Kazunori Yoh, Hiroki Nishikawa, Hirayuki Enomoto *, Akio Ishii, Yoshinori Iwata, Yuho Miyamoto, Noriko Ishii, Yukihisa Yuri, Kunihiro Hasegawa, Chikage Nakano, Takashi Nishimura, Nobuhiro Aizawa, Yoshiyuki Sakai, Naoto Ikeda, Tomoyuki Takashima, Ryo Takata, Hiroko Iijima and Shuhei Nishiguchi

Division of Hepatobiliary and Pancreatic Disease, Department of Internal Medicine, Hyogo College of Medicine, Hyogo 663-8501, Japan; mm2wintwin@ybb.ne.jp (K.Y.); hi-nishikawa@hyo-med.ac.jp (H.N.); akio0010@yahoo.co.jp (A.I.); yo-iwata@hyo-med.ac.jp (Y.I.); yuho.0818.1989@gmail.com (Y.M.); ishinori1985@yahoo.co.jp (N.I.); gyma27ijo04td@gmail.com (Y.Y.); hiro.red1230@gmail.com (K.H.); chikage@hyo-med.ac.jp (C.N.); tk-nishimura@hyo-med.ac.jp (T.N.); nobu23hiro@yahoo.co.jp (N.A.); sakai429@hyo-med.ac.jp (Y.S.); nikeneko@hyo-med.ac.jp (N.I.); tomo0204@yahoo.co.jp (T.T.); chano_chano_rt@yahoo.co.jp (R.T.); hiroko-i@hyo-med.ac.jp (H.I.); nishiguc@hyo-med.ac.jp (S.N.)

* Correspondence: enomoto@hyo-med.ac.jp

Abstract: Aims: We aimed to examine changes in skeletal muscle mass in chronic hepatitis C (CHC) patients undergoing interferon (IFN)-free direct acting antivirals (DAAs) therapy who achieved sustained virological response (SVR). Patients and methods: A total of 69 CHC patients treated with DAAs were analyzed. We compared the changes in skeletal muscle index (SMI) using bio-impedance analysis at baseline and SMI at SVR. SMI was calculated as the sum of skeletal muscle mass in upper and lower extremities divided by height squared (cm^2/m^2). Further, we identified pretreatment parameters contributing to the increased SMI at SVR. Results: SMI in males at baseline ranged from 6.73 to 9.08 cm^2/m^2 (median, 7.65 cm^2/m^2), while that in females ranged from 4.45 to 7.27 cm^2/m^2 (median, 5.81 cm^2/m^2). At SVR, 36 patients (52.2%) had increased SMI as compared with baseline. In the univariate analysis, age ($p = 0.0392$), hyaluronic acid ($p = 0.0143$), and branched-chain amino acid to tyrosine ratio (BTR) ($p = 0.0024$) were significant pretreatment factors linked to increased SMI at SVR. In the multivariate analysis, only BTR was an independent predictor linked to the increased SMI at SVR ($p = 0.0488$). Conclusion: Pretreatment BTR level can be helpful for predicting increased SMI after SVR in CHC patients undergoing IFN-free DAAs therapy.

Keywords: chronic hepatitis C; direct acting antiviral; sustained virological response; skeletal muscle mass

1. Introduction

The ultimate goal of treatment for chronic hepatitis C (CHC) is to eliminate the hepatitis C virus (HCV) and thereby to suppress the liver disease progression and the liver carcinogenesis [1–3]. In cases with sustained virological response (SVR), the incidence of disease progression or carcinogenesis has been reported to be markedly decreased [1,2,4,5]. CHC therapy has dramatically changed with the recent accessibility of direct acting antivirals (DAAs). Protease inhibitors including telaprevir, simeprevir, or vaniprevir containing pegylated-interferon (Peg-IFN)α2a or Peg-IFNα2b and ribavirin (RBV) combination therapy (IFN-based triple therapy) have demonstrated higher SVR rates [6]. Further, IFN-free DAAs therapies such as daclatasvir (DCV)/asunaprevir (ASV), sofosbuvir (SOF)/RBV, ledipasvir (LDV)/SOF, LDV/SOF/RBV, and SOF/velpatasvir have also demonstrated excellent SVR rates [4,5,7,8]. Recently, almost all CHC patients have been able to eradicate HCV in a comfortable manner [3].

On the other hand, skeletal muscle loss (SML) has been shown to be an adverse predictor in patients with liver diseases and has drawn much caution among clinicians because of its linkage to clinical outcomes [9–11]. Skeletal muscle mass is maintained by a balance between protein synthesis and protein breakdown, and muscle mass loss can occur due to an increment in proteolysis or a reduction in protein synthesis, or both disorders [12–14]. There have been compelling evidences to show that SML is one of the major complications in liver cirrhosis (LC) due to the LC-related double metabolic burdens (i.e., protein metabolic and energy metabolic disorders) [11,12,15–25]. Thus, for CHC patients treated with antiviral therapies, maintaining skeletal muscle mass is crucial. However, to the best of our knowledge, there have been no available data with regard to changes in skeletal muscle mass for CHC patients with SVR who underwent IFN-free DAAs therapy. Further, identifying pretreatment factors linked to the improvement in skeletal muscle mass may be pivotal for creating nutritional strategies in CHC patients after SVR.

The aims of the current study were therefore to examine changes in skeletal muscle mass in CHC patients undergoing IFN-free DAAs therapy who achieved SVR and to identify pretreatment predictors that are associated with the improvement in skeletal muscle mass.

2. Patients and Methods

2.1. Patients and Skeletal Muscle Mass Measurement

This study was a single center retrospective study. All study participants were CHC patients with data for skeletal muscle mass at baseline and SVR. Patients without those data were excluded from the current analysis.

For all analyzed subjects, skeletal muscle mass was assessed using bio-impedance analysis (BIA, Inbody720, Takumi Ltd., Aichi, Japan) in the standing position. BIA is a device which can measure the body fat mass, body water mass, and body muscle mass using differences in frequency [11].

Our current study participants were CHC patients treated with IFN-free DAAs therapy (DCV/ASV, SOF/LDV, SOF/LDV/RBV, SOF/RBV, or others) who were admitted at the Division of Hepatobiliary and Pancreatic disease, Department of Internal Medicine, Hyogo College of Medicine, Hyogo, Japan between August 2013 and August 2015. All patients achieved SVR and had available data for BIA. In this analysis, SVR was defined as the disappearance of serum HCV-RNA at a time point more than 12 weeks after the completion of each DAA therapy. In principal, BIA was routinely performed at baseline and at SVR 24 (24 weeks after the completion of DAAs therapy). All patients had no ascites on radiologic findings. Skeletal muscle index (SMI) was defined as the sum of skeletal muscle mass in the upper and lower extremities divided by height squared (cm^2/m^2), using data from BIA [11]. We compared the changes in SMI at baseline and SMI at SVR. Patients with increased SMI were defined as those with an SMI at SVR that was more than the SMI at baseline. Further, we identified pretreatment parameters contributing to the increased SMI using univariate and multivariate analyses. Included pretreatment parameters (potentially relevant factors with the development of SML in view of current published articles) are listed in Table 1 [9,11–14]. The ethical committee meeting at Hyogo College of Medicine approved our current study protocol and this study strictly followed all provisions of the Declaration of Helsinki.

Table 1. Baseline data (n = 69).

Variables	Number or Median (Range)
Age (years)	63 (25–83)
Gender, male/female	31/38
Body mass index (kg/m^2)	22.1 (15.7–32.8)
Skeletal muscle index (cm^2/m^2), male	7.65 (6.73–9.08)
Skeletal muscle index (cm^2/m^2), female	5.81 (4.45–7.27)
Total bilirubin (mg/dL)	0.8 (0.3–3.0)
Serum albumin (g/dL)	4.1 (2.8–4.9)
Prothrombin time (%)	83.4 (61.1–119.4)
Platelets (×10^4/mm^3)	15.5 (3.3–27.8)
Serum sodium (mmol/L)	140 (129–144)
eGFR (mL/min/1.73 m^2)	84 (33–142)
Total cholesterol (mg/dL)	159 (110–234)
Triglyceride (mg/dL)	88 (33–779)
AST (IU/L)	37 (15–140)
ALT (IU/L)	37 (11–155)
Fasting blood glucose (mg/dL)	94 (74–187)
HbA1c (NSGP)	5.5 (4.1–9.7)
BTR	4.94 (2.13–9.09)
Alpha-fetoprotein (ng/mL)	4.2 (1.3–224.9)
Hyaluronic acid (ng/mL)	103 (9–699)
FIB-4 index	2.46 (0.66–20.04)
HCV genotype, 1/2	55/14
HCV viral load (log IU/L)	6.2 (5.0–7.7)

Data are expressed as number or median (range). eGFR; estimated glomerular filtration rate, AST; aspartate aminotransferase, ALT; alanine aminotransferase, NGSP; National Glycohemoglobin Standardization Program, BTR; branched-chain amino acid to tyrosine ratio, HCV; hepatitis C virus.

2.2. *Statistical Analysis*

First, the distribution of each parameter (normal or not) was assessed by the Shapiro-Wilk test. Categorical variables were compared by Fisher's exact test. Continuous variables were compared by unpaired t-test, paired t-test, or Mann-Whitney U test as applicable. For predicting increased SMI, candidate variables were identified by univariate analysis; variables with $p < 0.10$ were analyzed by a multivariate logistic regression analysis. Data are presented as median value (range) unless otherwise mentioned. Statistical significance was set at $p < 0.05$. Statistical analysis was performed with JMP 11 (SAS Institute Inc., Cary, NC, USA).

3. Results

3.1. *Baseline Characteristics*

Baseline characteristics in the present study are shown in Table 1. Our study cohort (n = 69; 55 in HCV genotype 1 and 14 in genotype 2) included 31 males and 38 females with a median (range) age of 63 (25–83) years. SMI in males at baseline ranged from 6.73 to 9.08 cm^2/m^2 (median, 7.65 cm^2/m^2), while SMI in females at baseline ranged from 4.45 to 7.27 cm^2/m^2 (median, 5.81 cm^2/m^2). According to current guidelines, the proportion of low SMI in males (<7.0 cm^2/m^2) was 22.6% (7/31) and that in females (<5.7 cm^2/m^2) was 44.7% (17/38) [11]. For the entire cohort, SMI had normal distribution.

3.2. *Changes in SMI for the Entire Cohort (n = 69)*

The median SMI for the entire cohort at baseline was 6.62 cm^2/m^2 (range, 4.45–9.08 cm^2/m^2), while the median SMI for the entire cohort at SVR was 6.51 cm^2/m^2 (range, 4.55–9.30 cm^2/m^2). (p = 0.6352, Figure 1A) The proportion of increased SMI at SVR compared with the SMI at baseline was 52.2% (36/69, 19 males and 17 females).

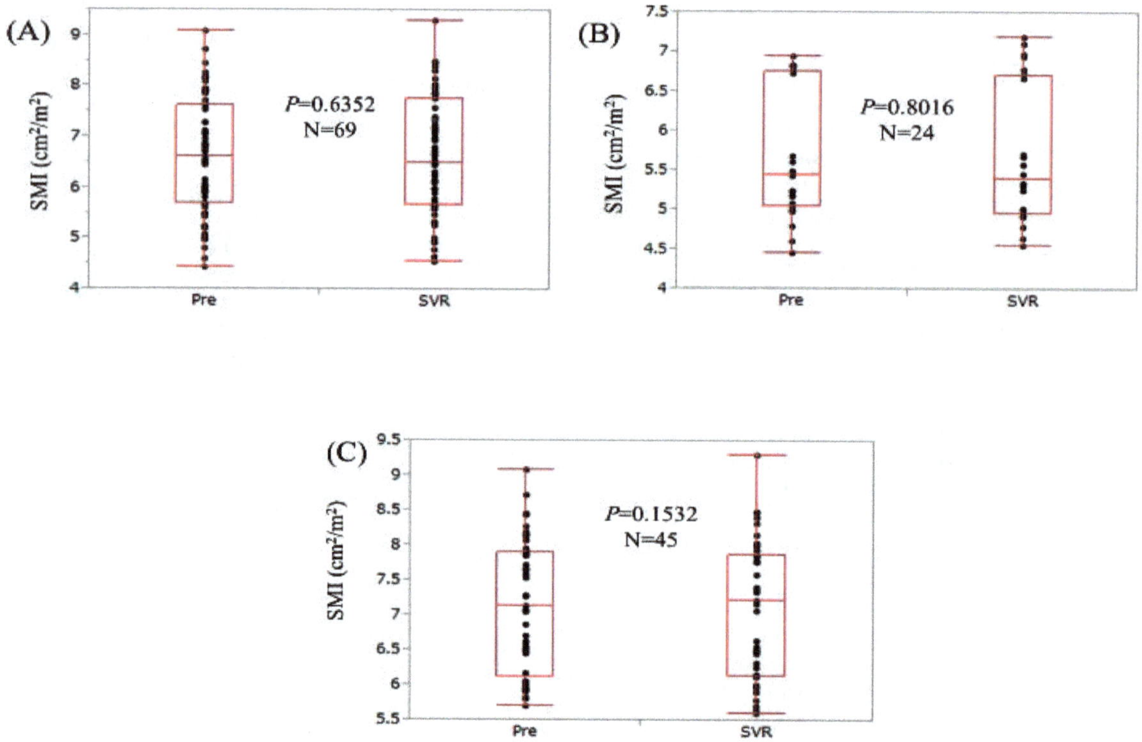

Figure 1. Changes in skeletal muscle index (SMI) during interferon (IFN)-free direct acting antivirals (DAAs) therapy at pretreatment and sustained virological response (SVR). (**A**) For the entire cohort (n = 69); (**B**) For patients with low muscle mass at baseline (n = 24, as defined by current guidelines [11]); (**C**) For patients without low muscle mass at baseline (n = 45, as defined by current guidelines [11]).

3.3. Changes in SMI for Patients with Low Muscle Mass (Low SMI) at Baseline (n = 24)

The median SMI for patients with low muscle mass (low SMI) at baseline was 5.44 cm^2/m^2 (range, 4.45–6.95 cm^2/m^2), while the median SMI for those patients at SVR was 5.40 cm^2/m^2 (range, 4.55–7.20 cm^2/m^2) (p = 0.8016, Figure 1B).

3.4. Changes in SMI for Patients without Low Muscle Mass (Low SMI) at Baseline (n = 45)

The median SMI for patients without low muscle mass (low SMI) at baseline was 7.13 cm^2/m^2 (range, 5.70–9.08 cm^2/m^2), while the median SMI for those patients at SVR was 7.22 cm^2/m^2 (range, 5.59–9.30 cm^2/m^2) (p = 0.1532, Figure 1C).

3.5. Changes in SMI According to Baseline FIB-4 Index

We compared changes in SMI according to FIB-4 index. Patients with baseline FIB-4 index $\geq$2.46 (the median value in our cohort) were defined as the high FIB-4 index group (n = 34), while those with baseline FIB-4 index <2.46 were defined as the low FIB-4 index group (n = 35). In the high FIB-4 index group, SMI at SVR did not significantly increase as compared with baseline levels (p = 0.9812). In the low FIB-4 index group, SMI at SVR tended to significantly increase as compared with baseline levels (p = 0.0879) (Figure 2).

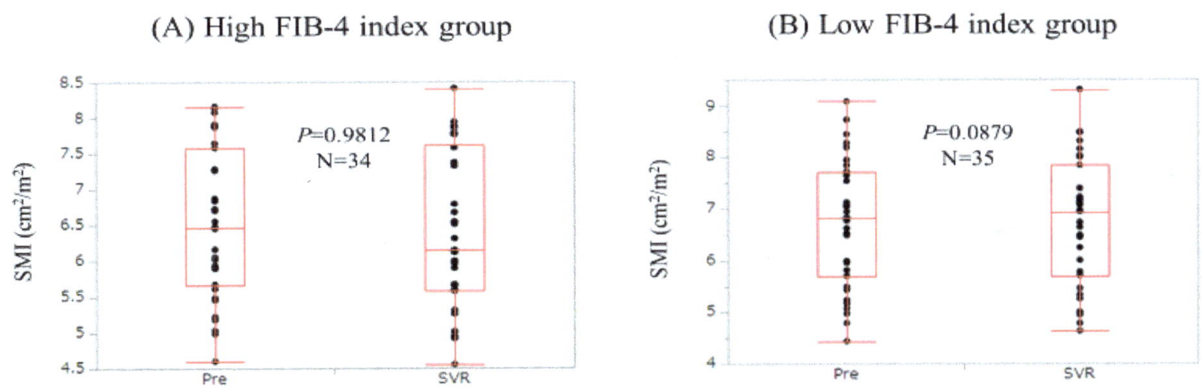

Figure 2. Changes in SMI according to baseline FIB-4 index. (**A**) Patients with baseline FIB-4 index ≥2.46 (the median value in our cohort) were defined as the high FIB-4 index group (n = 34). SMI at SVR did not significantly increase as compared with baseline levels (p = 0.9812); (**B**) Patients with baseline FIB-4 index <2.46 were defined as the low FIB-4 index group (n = 35). SMI at SVR tended to significantly increase as compared with baseline levels (p = 0.0879).

3.6. Changes in SMI According to HCV Serotype

In the HCV serotype 1 group (n = 55), SMI at SVR did not significantly increase as compared with baseline levels (p = 0.5777). In the HCV serotype 2 group (n = 14), SMI at SVR tended to significantly decrease as compared with baseline levels (p = 0.0708) (Figure 3).

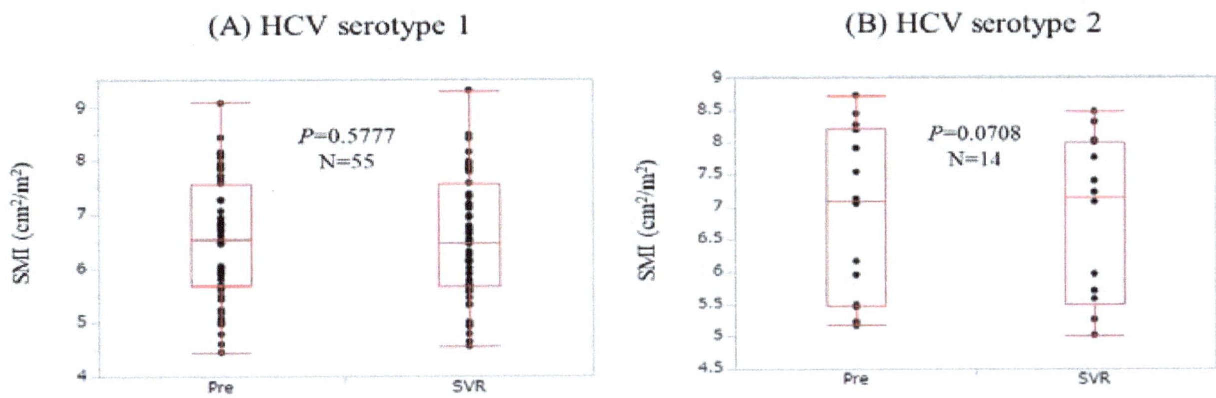

Figure 3. Changes in SMI according to HCV serotype. (**A**) In the HCV serotype 1 group (n = 55), SMI at SVR did not significantly increase as compared with baseline levels (p = 0.5777); (**B**) In the HCV serotype 2 group (n = 14), SMI at SVR tended to significantly decrease as compared with baseline levels (p = 0.0708).

3.7. Changes in SMI According to HCV Viral Load

We compared changes in SMI according to baseline HCV viral load. Patients with baseline HCV viral load >6.2 log IU/mL (the median value in our cohort) were defined as the high HCV viral load group (n = 34), while those with baseline HCV viral load ≤6.2 log IU/mL were defined as the low HCV viral load (n = 35). In the high HCV viral load group, SMI at SVR did not significantly increase as compared with baseline levels (p = 0.3797). In the low HCV viral load group, SMI at SVR did not significantly increase as compared with baseline levels (p = 0.1772) (Figure 4).

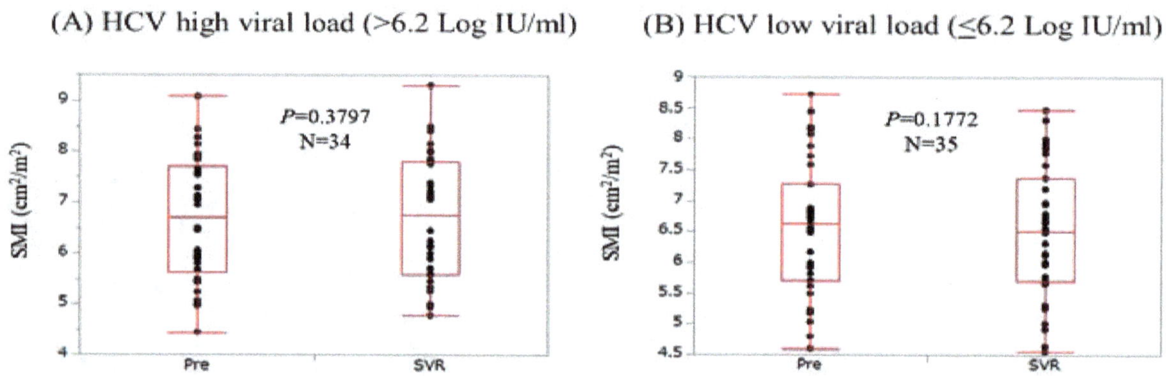

Figure 4. Changes in SMI according to HCV viral load. Patients with baseline HCV viral load >6.2 log IU/mL (the median value in our cohort) were defined as the high HCV viral load group ($n = 34$), while those with baseline HCV viral load ≤6.2 log IU/mL were defined as the low HCV viral load ($n = 35$). (**A**) In the high HCV viral load group, SMI at SVR did not significantly increase as compared with baseline levels ($p = 0.3797$); (**B**) In the low HCV viral load group, SMI at SVR did not significantly increase as compared with baseline levels ($p = 0.1772$).

3.8. Changes in SMI According to Age

We compared changes in SMI according to age. Patients with the age of >63 years (the median value in our cohort) were defined as the elderly group ($n = 34$), while those with the age of ≤63 years were defined as the non-elderly group ($n = 35$). In the elderly group, SMI at SVR did not significantly increase as compared with baseline levels ($p = 0.1662$). In the non-elderly group, SMI at SVR did not significantly increase as compared with baseline levels ($p = 0.5105$) (Figure 5).

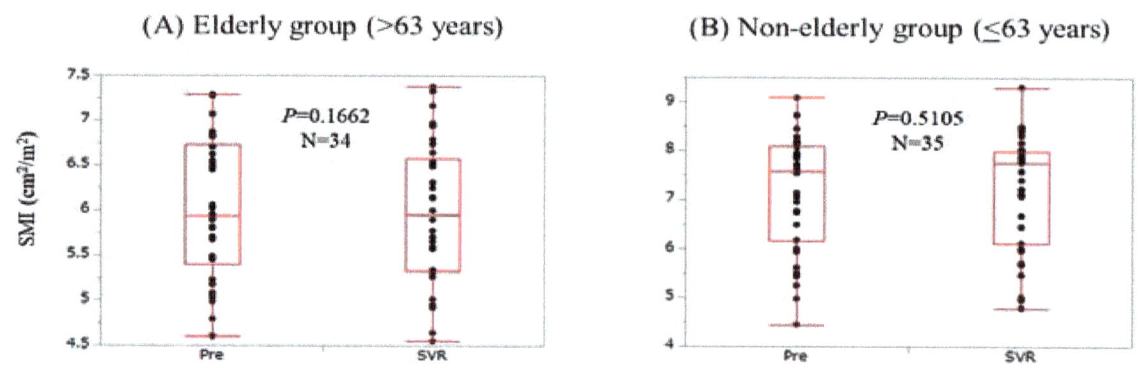

Figure 5. Changes in SMI according age. Patients with the age of >63 years (the median value in our cohort) were defined as the elderly group ($n = 34$), while those with the age of ≤63 years were defined as the non-elderly group ($n = 35$). (**A**) In the elderly group, SMI at SVR did not significantly increase as compared with baseline levels ($p = 0.1662$); (**B**) In the non-elderly group, SMI at SVR did not significantly increase as compared with baseline levels ($p = 0.5105$).

3.9. Comparison of Baseline Characteristics Between Patients with and without Increased SMI

Comparison of baseline characteristics between patients with increased SMI ($n = 36$) and without increased SMI ($n = 33$) is shown in Table 2. Age ($p = 0.0392$) and hyaluronic acid level ($p = 0.0143$) in the increased SMI group were significantly lower than those in the non-increased SMI group. Branched-chain amino acid to tyrosine ratio (BTR) in the increased SMI group was significantly higher than those in the non-increased SMI group ($p = 0.0024$). FIB-4 index in the increased SMI group tended to be significantly lower than that in the non-increased SMI group ($p = 0.0656$).

Table 2. Comparison of baseline characteristics between patients with increased SMI (I-SMI, $n = 36$) and without I-SMI ($n = 33$).

Variables	I-SMI ($n = 36$)	Non-I-SMI ($n = 33$)	p Value
Age (years)	59 (25–78)	65 (39–83)	0.0392
Gender, male/female	18/18	13/20	0.4693
Serum albumin (g/dL)	4.1 (3.3–4.9)	4.1 (2.8–4.6)	0.6883
Total bilirubin (mg/dL)	0.8 (0.3–2.5)	0.7 (0.4–3.0)	0.3416
Prothrombin time (%)	84.05 (67–108.4)	82.8 (61.1–119.4)	0.4161
Platelet count ($\times 10^4/mm^3$)	17.35 (3.6–25.3)	14.2 (3.3–27.8)	0.3433
AST (IU/L)	29.5 (15–140)	45 (19–120)	0.2735
ALT (IU/L)	36.5 (11–155)	39 (13–104)	0.4971
Serum sodium (mmol/L)	140 (129–144)	141 (135–143)	0.7724
Total cholesterol (mg/dL)	158 (110–228)	159 (126–234)	0.5347
Triglyceride (mg/dL)	92 (33–174)	88 (45–779)	0.9091
Fasting blood glucose (mg/dL)	93 (74–187)	96 (85–130)	0.1224
eGFR (mL/min/1.73 m^2)	85 (33–141)	82 (36–142)	0.8803
HbA1c (NSGP)	5.5 (4.7–9.7)	5.5 (4.1–7.0)	0.4911
Body mass index (kg/m^2)	21.95 (15.7–30.8)	22.5 (17.4–32.8)	0.3988
BTR	5.16 (3.01–9.09)	4.19 (2.13–8.36)	0.0024
Hyaluronic acid (ng/mL)	80 (9–437)	156 (17–699)	0.0143
FIB-4 index	1.94 (0.66–20.04)	3.53 (0.96–15.29)	0.0656
Alpha-fetoprotein (ng/mL)	3.1 (1.9–224.9)	7.3 (1.3–183.3)	0.4694
HCV genotype, 1/2	31/5	24/9	0.2331
HCV-RNA (log IU/L)	6.3 (5.1–7.2)	6.2 (5.0–7.7)	0.9380

AST; aspartate aminotransferase, ALT; alanine aminotransferase, eGFR; estimated glomerular filtration rate, NGSP; National Glycohemoglobin Standardization Program, BTR; branched chain amino acid to tyrosine ratio, HCV; hepatitis C virus. Patients with I-SMI indicate those with an SMI at SVR the was more than the SMI at baseline.

3.10. Multivariate Analyses of Factors Linked to the Presence of Increased SMI

Multivariate analysis for the above four factors with $p < 0.10$ (i.e., age, hyaluronic acid, FIB-4 index, and BTR) showed that only BTR was a significant prognostic pretreatment factor linked to the presence of increased SMI ($p = 0.0488$). (Table 3) Odds ratios and 95% confidence intervals are demonstrated in Table 3.

Table 3. Multivariate analysis of factors contributing to the increased SMI.

Variables	Multivariate Analysis	
	OR (95% CI)	p Value
Age (per one year)	1.029 (0.977–1.089)	0.2797
Hyaluronic acid (per one ng/mL)	1.002 (0.998–1.006)	0.3794
BTR (per one)	0.648 (0.398–0.998)	0.0488
FIB-4 index (per one)	0.996 (0.832–1.221)	0.9688

OR; Odds ratio, CI; confidence interval, BTR; branched-chain amino acid to tyrosine ratio.

4. Discussion

Liver disease patients are aging in our country and SML is also associated with aging [11]. In other words, SML in liver disease patients can occur, irrespective of the degree of liver fibrosis stage. CHC therapy has dramatically improved due to the introduction of DAAs [1,4]. As described earlier, SML can be an adverse predictor in patients with liver diseases, although there are limited clinical data showing that skeletal muscle mass improvement can lead to favorable clinical outcomes in CHC patients, and reversing skeletal muscle mass loss is a priority field for therapeutic strategies in these patients [9–13]. In view of these backgrounds, addressing clinical queries to which factors are associated with the improvement of skeletal muscle mass after SVR may be a point of focus, and our current results may therefore be worthy of reporting.

In the multivariate analysis, only pretreatment BTR value was an independent predictor linked to increased SMI. BTR has also been shown to decrease in cirrhotic patients. Furthermore, BTR is widely used in Japan as an easily measurable indicator of amino acid imbalance and it is also closely related to protein synthesis in the muscle [9,26]. In addition, in our previous study, we demonstrated that lower BTR was associated with decreased skeletal muscle mass in patients with chronic liver diseases, which is in agreement with our current data [27]. In a sense, measuring BTR can lead to creating strategies for nutritional intervention from the view point of skeletal muscle mass. In patients with well-preserved protein synthesis ability, as reflected by a higher BTR level, HCV eradication may lead to the acceleration of protein synthesis in the muscle; this is a major finding in the current study. On the contrary, considering our current results, patients with LC status are expected to have poor improvement in skeletal muscle mass even after HCV eradication. Patients with a higher baseline FIB-4 index had poor improvement in skeletal muscle mass at SVR in our results, and this observation can support our hypothesis. In such patients, some interventions including exercise may be recommended [9,12,13]. In compensated LC patients, walking 5000 or more steps per day may be ideal [28]. On the other hand, it is of note that the proportion of low SMI in males was rather lower than that in females (22.6% vs. 44.7%). Significant differences in baseline characteristics between males and females (age; $p < 0.0001$, FIB-4 index; $p = 0.0196$, BTR; $p = 0.0292$, data not shown) may account for our current results.

It is of interest that in the HCV serotype 2 group, SMI at SVR tended to significantly decrease as compared with baseline levels ($p = 0.0708$). One possible reason for these results is that in HCV serotype 2 patients, RBV was used in most cases. RBV-related anemia may cause muscle mass decrease.

Whether SMI increment presents a good prognosis in chronic liver disease patients has yet to be clarified. On the other hand, previous investigators reported that a higher BTR was a favorable predictor for LC patients [29]. In our results, higher BTR was associated with SMI increment. In view of this, SMI increment in CHC patients can result in a good prognosis. However, further studies will be required to confirm these results.

Our study had the drawbacks of a small sample size for analysis, and how these short-term outcomes translate into long-term outcomes has yet to be determined. In addition, several important variables that could influence the outcome were overlooked (diet, exercise, and other pharmacological therapies), as they were not included in the current analysis. The causal relationship between BTR and skeletal muscle mass should also be elucidated. Thus, further well-designed and larger studies with longer observation periods will be needed in the future. However, our results denote that pretreatment BTR level is a useful predictor for improvement in skeletal muscle mass after SVR in CHC patients treated with DAAs.

5. Conclusions

In conclusion, pretreatment BTR levels can be helpful for predicting increased SMI after SVR in CHC patients undergoing IFN-free DAAs therapy.

Acknowledgments: The authors would like to thank all medical staff in our hospital for data collection.

Author Contributions: K.Y., H.N., S.N. and H.E. conceived and designed the experiments; K.Y., H.N. and H.E. performed the experiments; K.Y., H.N. and H.E. analyzed the data; A.I., Y.I., Y.M., N.I., Y.Y., K.H., C.N., T.N., N.A., Y.S., N.I., T.T., R.T. and H.I. contributed reagents/materials/analysis tools; K.Y., H.N. and H.E. wrote the paper.

Abbreviations

CHC	chronic hepatitis C
HCV	hepatitis C virus
SVR	sustained virological response
DAA	direct acting antiviral

SMV	Simeprevir
Peg-IFN	pegylated interferon
RBV	Ribavirin
DCV	Daclatasvir
ASV	Asunaprevir
SOF	Sofosbuvir
LDV	Ledipasvir
SML	skeletal muscle loss
LC	liver cirrhosis
BIA	bio-impedance analysis
SMI	skeletal muscle index
BTR	branched-chain amino acid to tyrosine ratio

References

1. Wang, L.S.; D'Souza, L.S.; Jacobson, I.M. Hepatitis C—A clinical review. *J. Med. Virol.* **2016**, *88*, 1844–1855. [CrossRef] [PubMed]
2. Van der Meer, A.J.; Berenguer, M. Reversion of disease manifestations after HCV eradication. *J. Hepatol.* **2016**, *65*, S95–S108. [CrossRef] [PubMed]
3. Majumdar, A.; Kitson, M.T.; Roberts, S.K. Systematic review: Current concepts and challenges for the direct-acting antiviral era in hepatitis C cirrhosis. *Aliment. Pharmacol. Ther.* **2016**, *43*, 1276–1292. [CrossRef] [PubMed]
4. Gutierrez, J.A.; Lawitz, E.J.; Poordad, F. Interferon-free, direct-acting antiviral therapy for chronic hepatitis C. *J. Viral Hepat.* **2015**, *22*, 861–870. [CrossRef] [PubMed]
5. Jacobson, I.M. The HCV treatment revolution continues: Resistance considerations, pangenotypic efficacy, and advances in challenging populations. *Gastroenterol. Hepatol.* **2016**, *12*, 1–11.
6. Welch, N.M.; Jensen, D.M. Pegylated interferon based therapy with second-wave direct-acting antivirals in genotype 1 chronic hepatitis C. *Liver Int.* **2015**, *35*, 11–17. [CrossRef] [PubMed]
7. Terrault, N.A.; Zeuzem, S.; Di Bisceglie, A.M.; Lim, J.K.; Pockros, P.J.; Frazier, L.M.; Kuo, A.; Lok, A.S.; Shiffman, M.L.; Ben Ari, Z. Effectiveness of ledipasvir-sofosbuvir combination in patients with hepatitis C virus infection and factors associated with sustained virologic response. *Gastroenterology* **2016**, *151*, 1131–1140. [CrossRef] [PubMed]
8. Mir, F.; Kahveci, A.S.; Ibdah, J.A.; Tahan, V. Sofosbuvir/velpatasvir regimen promises an effective pan-genotypic hepatitis C virus cure. *Drug Des. Dev. Ther.* **2017**, *11*, 497–502. [CrossRef] [PubMed]
9. Sinclair, M.; Gow, P.J.; Grossmann, M.; Angus, P.W. Review article: Sarcopenia in cirrhosis-aetiology, implications and potential therapeutic interventions. *Aliment. Pharmacol. Ther.* **2016**, *43*, 765–777. [CrossRef] [PubMed]
10. Petta, S.; Ciminnisi, S.; Di Marco, V.; Cabibi, D.; Cammà, C.; Licata, A.; Marchesini, G.; Craxì, A. Sarcopenia is associated with severe liver fibrosis in patients with non-alcoholic fatty liver disease. *Aliment. Pharmacol. Ther.* **2016**, *45*, 510–518. [CrossRef] [PubMed]
11. Nishikawa, H.; Shiraki, M.; Hiramatsu, A.; Moriya, K.; Hino, K.; Nishiguchi, S. Japan Society of Hepatology guidelines for sarcopenia in liver disease (1st edition): Recommendation from the working group for creation of sarcopenia assessment criteria. *Hepatol. Res.* **2016**, *46*, 951–963. [CrossRef] [PubMed]
12. Dasarathy, S.; Merli, M. Sarcopenia from mechanism to diagnosis and treatment in liver disease. *J. Hepatol.* **2016**, *65*, 1232–1244. [CrossRef] [PubMed]
13. Dasarathy, S. Consilience in sarcopenia of cirrhosis. *J. Cachexia Sarcopenia Muscle* **2012**, *3*, 225–237. [CrossRef] [PubMed]
14. Santilli, V.; Bernetti, A.; Mangone, M.; Paoloni, M. Clinical definition of sarcopenia. *Clin. Cases Miner. Bone Metab.* **2014**, *11*, 177–180. [CrossRef] [PubMed]
15. Cruz-Jentoft, A.J.; Landi, F.; Schneider, S.M.; Zúñiga, C.; Arai, H.; Boirie, Y.; Chen, L.K.; Fielding, R.A.; Martin, F.C.; Michel, J.P. Prevalence of and interventions for sarcopenia in ageing adults: A systematic review. Report of the international sarcopenia initiative (EWGSOP and IWGS). *Age Ageing* **2014**, *43*, 748–759. [CrossRef] [PubMed]

16. Hanai, T.; Shiraki, M.; Nishimura, K.; Ohnishi, S.; Imai, K.; Suetsugu, A.; Takai, K.; Shimizu, M.; Moriwaki, H. Sarcopenia impairs prognosis of patients with liver cirrhosis. *Nutrition* **2015**, *31*, 193–199. [CrossRef] [PubMed]
17. Nardelli, S.; Lattanzi, B.; Torrisi, S.; Greco, F.; Farcomeni, A.; Gioia, S.; Merli, M.; Riggio, O. Sarcopenia is risk factor for development of hepatic encephalopathy after transjugular intrahepatic portosysthemic shunt placement. *Clin. Gastroenterol. Hepatol.* **2017**, *15*, 934–936. [CrossRef] [PubMed]
18. Kalafateli, M.; Mantzoukis, K.; Choi Yau, Y.; Mohammad, A.O.; Arora, S.; Rodrigues, S.; de Vos, M.; Papadimitriou, K.; Thorburn, D.; O'Beirnr, J. Malnutrition and sarcopenia predict post-liver transplantation outcomes independently of the Model for End-stage Liver Disease score. *J. Cachexia Sarcopenia Muscle* **2017**, *8*, 113–121. [CrossRef] [PubMed]
19. Chen, L.K.; Liu, L.K.; Woo, J.; Assantachai, P.; Auyeung, T.W.; Bahyah, K.S.; Chou, M.Y.; Chen, L.Y.; Hsu, P.S.; Krairit, O.; et al. Sarcopenia in Asia: Consensus report of the Asian Working Group for Sarcopenia. *J. Am. Med. Dir. Assoc.* **2014**, *15*, 95–101. [CrossRef] [PubMed]
20. Hiraoka, A.; Michitaka, K.; Ueki, H.; Kaneto, M.; Aibiki, T.; Okudaira, T.; Kawakami, T.; Yamago, H.; Suga, Y.; Tomida, H.; et al. Sarcopenia and two types of presarcopenia in Japanese patients with chronic liver disease. *Eur. J. Gastroenterol. Hepatol.* **2016**, *28*, 940–947. [CrossRef] [PubMed]
21. Dos Santos, L.; Cyrino, E.S.; Antunes, M.; Santos, D.A.; Sardinha, L.B. Sarcopenia and physical independence in older adults: The independent and synergic role of muscle mass and muscle function. *J. Cachexia Sarcopenia Muscle* **2017**, *8*, 245–250. [CrossRef] [PubMed]
22. Kalyani, R.R.; Corriere, M.; Ferrucci, L. Age-related and disease-related muscle loss: The effect of diabetes, obesity, and other diseases. *Lancet Diabetes Endocrinol.* **2014**, *2*, 819–829. [CrossRef]
23. Kaido, T.; Tamai, Y.; Hamaguchi, Y.; Okumura, S.; Kobayashi, A.; Shirai, H.; Yagi, S.; Kamo, N.; Hammad, A.; Inagaki, N.; et al. Effects of pretransplant sarcopenia and sequential changes in sarcopenic parameters after living donor liver transplantation. *Nutrition* **2017**, *33*, 195–198. [CrossRef] [PubMed]
24. Merli, M.; Giusto, M.; Lucidi, C.; Giannelli, V.; Pentassuglio, I.; Di Gregorio, V.; Lattanzi, B.; Riggio, O. Muscle depletion increases the risk of overt and minimal hepatic encephalopathy: Results of a prospective study. *Metab. Brain Dis.* **2013**, *28*, 281–284. [CrossRef] [PubMed]
25. Kalafateli, M.; Konstantakis, C.; Thomopoulos, K.; Triantos, C. Impact of muscle wasting on survival in patients with liver cirrhosis. *World J. Gastroenterol.* **2015**, *21*, 7357–7361. [CrossRef] [PubMed]
26. Suzuki, K.; Suzuki, K.; Koizumi, K.; Ichimura, H.; Oka, S.; Takada, H.; Kuwayama, H. Measurement of serum branched-chain amino acids to tyrosine ratio level is useful in a prediction of a change of serum albumin level in chronic liver disease. *Hepatol. Res.* **2008**, *38*, 267–272. [CrossRef] [PubMed]
27. Nishikawa, H.; Enomoto, H.; Ishii, A.; Iwata, Y.; Miyamoto, Y.; Ishii, N.; Yuri, Y.; Takata, R.; Hasegawa, K.; Nakano, C.; et al. Development of a simple predictive model for decreased skeletal muscle mass in patients with compensated chronic liver disease. *Hepatol. Res.* **2017**. [CrossRef] [PubMed]
28. Hayashi, F.; Matsumoto, Y.; Momoki, C.; Yuikawa, M.; Okada, G.; Hamakawa, E.; Kawamura, E.; Hagihara, A.; Toyama, M.; Fujii, H.; et al. Physical inactivity and insufficient dietary intake are associated with the frequency of sarcopenia in patients with compensated viral liver cirrhosis. *Hepatol. Res.* **2013**, *43*, 1264–1275. [CrossRef] [PubMed]
29. Nishikawa, H.; Osaki, Y. Clinical significance of therapy using branched-chain amino acid granules in patients with liver cirrhosis and hepatocellular carcinoma. *Hepatol. Res.* **2014**, *44*, 149–158. [CrossRef] [PubMed]

13

Sarcopenia Impairs Prognosis of Patients with Hepatocellular Carcinoma: The Role of Liver Functional Reserve and Tumor-Related Factors in Loss of Skeletal Muscle Volume

Kenji Imai *, Koji Takai, Satoshi Watanabe, Tatsunori Hanai, Atsushi Suetsugu, Makoto Shiraki and Masahito Shimizu

Department of Gastroenterology/Internal Medicine, Gifu University Graduate School of Medicine, Gifu 501-1194, Japan; koz@gifu-u.ac.jp (K.T.); ronkalevala777@yahoo.co.jp (S.W.); hanai0606@yahoo.co.jp (T.H.); asue327@yahoo.co.jp (A.S.); mshiraki-gif@umin.ac.jp (M.S.); shimim-gif@umin.ac.jp (M.S.)

* Correspondence: ikenji@gifu-u.ac.jp

Abstract: Sarcopenia impairs survival in patients with hepatocellular carcinoma (HCC). This study aimed to clarify the factors that contribute to decreased skeletal muscle volume in patients with HCC. The third lumbar vertebra skeletal muscle index (L3 SMI) in 351 consecutive patients with HCC was calculated to identify sarcopenia. Sarcopenia was defined as an L3 SMI value $\leq$ 29.0 cm^2/m^2 for women and $\leq$ 36.0 cm^2/m^2 for men. The factors affecting L3 SMI were analyzed by multiple linear regression analysis and tree-based models. Of the 351 HCC patients, 33 were diagnosed as having sarcopenia and showed poor prognosis compared with non-sarcopenia patients ($p = 0.007$). However, this significant difference disappeared after the adjustments for age, sex, Child–Pugh score, maximum tumor size, tumor number, and the degree of portal vein invasion by propensity score matching analysis. Multiple linear regression analysis showed that age ($p = 0.015$) and sex ($p < 0.0001$) were significantly correlated with a decrease in L3 SMI. Tree-based models revealed that sex (female) is the most significant factor that affects L3 SMI. In male patients, L3 SMI was decreased by aging, increased Child–Pugh score ($\geq$56 years), and enlarged tumor size (<56 years). Maintaining liver functional reserve and early diagnosis and therapy for HCC are vital to prevent skeletal muscle depletion and improve the prognosis of patients with HCC.

Keywords: hepatocellular carcinoma; skeletal muscle depletion; sarcopenia; prognostic factor

---

1. Introduction

Hepatocellular carcinoma (HCC) is one of the most common malignancies worldwide. Typically, patients with HCC have a poor clinical course as the prognosis is strongly affected by liver functional reserve and clinical cancer stage [1,2]. The recurrence rate of HCC is extremely high, which is also associated with the poor prognosis [3]. To identify patients with a high mortality risk and to choose the most adequate treatment, a precise prediction of the prognosis of patients with HCC is essential. Thus, several prognostic staging systems, such as Barcelona Clinic Liver Cancer (BCLC) [4], Cancer of the Liver Italian Program (CLIP) [1], and Japan Integrated Staging (JIS) [2], most of which take both clinical cancer stage and liver functional reserve into consideration, have been developed.

Recently, skeletal muscle depletion or sarcopenia, initially defined as the loss of skeletal muscle mass that occurs with aging [5], has garnered attention as a new and promising prognostic factor for various malignancies, including HCC [6–10]. Skeletal muscle volume depletion assessed by computed tomography (CT) predicts poor prognosis of all cancer stages [11], and for sorafenib-treated patients with HCC [12]. Sarcopenia and rapid skeletal muscle depletion are also involved in worse survival in patients with liver cirrhosis [13,14]. These findings strongly suggest that sarcopenia is a significant factor that predicts the prognosis of patients with HCC and liver cirrhosis.

Several pathological conditions, including advanced organ failure, inflammatory disease, malignancy, endocrine disease, sedentary lifestyle, and malnutrition are associated with skeletal muscle depletion [5,15]. In liver disease, the following points can be considered as the main mechanisms of sarcopenia: protein energy malnutrition; imbalance of protein synthesis and breakdown; increased expression of myostatin, a cytokine that strongly suppresses skeletal muscle growth; and increased production of reactive oxygen species and inflammatory cytokines [16]. Therefore, sarcopenia could be a result of various pathological conditions, such as poor liver functional reserve or advanced cancer stages, which in turn affects survival of patients with HCC. However, the precise factors that enhance the progression of sarcopenia and worsen the prognosis of HCC patients have not been evaluated.

The purpose of this study is to identify the factors that contribute to skeletal muscle depletion in HCC patients, especially focusing on liver functional reserve and cancer progression. Based on the results of this study, we will also discuss how to prevent skeletal muscle depletion and improve prognosis in patients with HCC.

2. Materials and Methods

2.1. Patients, Treatment, and Follow-Up Strategy

We evaluated 351 consecutive HCC patients in our hospital between May 2006 and December 2015. HCC nodules were detected using imaging modalities, including dynamic CT, dynamic magnetic resonance imaging (MRI), and abdominal arteriography. HCC was diagnosed based on a typical hypervascular tumor stain on angiography and typical dynamic study findings of enhanced staining in the early phase and attenuation in the delayed phase. The treatment plan in each case was according to the Clinical Practice Guidelines for HCC issued by the Japan Society of Hepatology (JSH) [17]. Patients were thereafter followed on an outpatient basis and had dynamic CT, MRI, or ultrasound every three months after the initial treatment. Recurrent HCC was diagnosed when the typical findings of HCC were observed, and the treatment was still based on the aforementioned guidelines for HCC. Overall survival was defined as the interval from the date of the initial treatment to the date of death or December 2015 for surviving patients. All study participants provided verbal informed consent, which was considered sufficient because this study followed an observational research design that did not require new human biological specimens, and instead relied only on preexisting materials. The study design—including this consent procedure—was approved by the ethics committee of the Gifu University School of Medicine on 7 June 2017 (ethic approval code: 29–26).

2.2. Image Analysis of Skeletal Muscle Volume and Definition of Sarcopenia

Skeletal muscle volume was measured using a CT image that had been taken solely for the purpose of diagnosing HCC prior to the initial treatment. A transverse CT image at the third lumbar vertebra (L3) in the inferior direction was assessed. The muscles in the L3 region—including psoas, erector spinae, quadratus lumborum, transversus abdominis, external and internal obliques, and rectus abdominis—were analyzed using SYNAPSE VINCENT software (version 3.0, Fujifilm Medical, Tokyo, Japan), which enables specific tissue demarcation using Hounsfield unit (HU) thresholds. The muscles were quantified within a range of −29 to +150 HU [18], and tissue boundaries were manually corrected as needed. The cross-sectional areas of the muscle (cm^2) at the L3 level computed from each image were normalized by the square of the height (m^2) to obtain the L3 skeletal muscle index (L3 SMI, cm^2/m^2), which was used as an indicator of skeletal muscle volume in previous reports [11,12,16]. Sarcopenia was defined as an L3 SMI value $\leq$29.0 cm^2/m^2 for women and $\leq$36.0 cm^2/m^2 for men, which is according to a previous study [11].

2.3. Statistical Analysis

Overall survival was estimated using the Kaplan–Meier method, and differences between curves were evaluated using the log-rank test. To exclude the effect of possible confounding factors between sarcopenia and non-sarcopenia groups, we performed rigorous adjustments for the following six factors using a propensity score matching analysis: age, sex, Child–Pugh score (CPS), tumor size, tumor number, and the degree of portal vein invasion, which were considered as prognostic factors for HCC patients by previous studies [1,2,4], and showed significant differences between the two groups. The propensity score matching analysis was performed based on the following algorithm: 1:1 optimal match with calipers of width 0.2 of the standard deviation of the logit of the propensity score and no replacement [19]. To identify which of the six factors contributed to decreased L3 SMI, we conducted a multiple linear regression analysis. A tree-based model analysis, which uses the binary recursive partitioning process of the population, was also performed; thus, L3 SMI is similar in patients within each group but different between groups [20,21]. Statistical significance was defined as $p < 0.05$. All statistical analyses were performed using R version 3.3.1 (The R Project for Statistical Computing, Vienna, Austria; http://www.R-project.org/).

3. Results

3.1. Baseline Characteristics and Laboratory Data of Patients

The baseline characteristics and laboratory data of the 351 patients (242 male and 109 female; average age, 70.4 years) are shown in Table 1. The average L3 SMI for all enrolled patients was 43.7 cm^2/m^2, and 33 patients were classified into the sarcopenia group. The average tumor size was 4.2 cm, and 188 patients received curative treatment.

Table 1. Baseline demographic and clinical characteristics.

Variables	Total (n = 351)
Sex (male/female)	242/109
Age (years)	70.4 ± 10.3
Etiology (HBV/HCV/HBV + HCV/others)	43/204/3/101
BMI (kg/m^2)	23.1 ± 3.4
L3 SMI (cm^2/m^2)	43.7 ± 8.6
Sarcopenia (yes/no)	33/318
Child–Pugh score (5/6/7/8/9/10/11)	179/84/52/20/9/6/1
ALB (g/dL)	3.6 ± 0.6
ALT (IU/L)	46.9 ± 44.3
T-Bil (mg/dL)	1.2 ± 1.0
PLT ($\times 10^4/\mu L$)	13.1 ± 7.8
PT (%)	85.3 ± 16.7
FPG (mg/dL)	110.6 ± 34.2
HbA_{1c} (%)	6.0 ± 1.1
AFP (ng/dL)	11,557 ± 73,374
PIVKA-II (mAU/mL)	21,056 ± 125,773
Tumor size (cm)	4.2 ± 3.7
Tumor number (1/≥2)	193/158
Vp (0/1/2/3/4)	289/15/15/15/17
Stage (I/II/III/IV)	79/126/100/46
Curability of initial treatment (yes/no)	188/163
Oral administration of BCAA (yes/no)	153/198
Co-existing diseases (yes/no)	
Renal disease	22/329
Heart disease	45/306
Respiratory disease	16/335
Neurologic disease	22/329
Malignant disease (except HCC)	27/324

Values are presented as average ± standard deviation. HBV, hepatitis B virus; HCV, hepatitis C virus; BMI, body mass index; L3 SMI, third lumbar vertebra skeletal muscle index; ALT, alanine aminotransferase; T-Bil, total bilirubin; PLT, platelet count; PT, prothrombin time; FPG, fasting plasma glucose; AFP, alpha-fetoprotein; PIVKA-II, protein induced by vitamin K absence or antagonists-II; Vp, the degree of portal vein invasion; BCAA, branched-chain amino acids; HCC, hepatocellular carcinoma.

3.2. Comparison of Overall Survival in Sarcopenia and Non-Sarcopenia Groups before and after Adjustments for Possible Confounding Factors

The one-, three-, and five-year overall survival rates of all enrolled patients were 83.0, 61.8, and 42.2%, respectively (Figure 1a). Table 2 shows the clinical characteristics and laboratory data of the sarcopenia ($n = 33$) and non-sarcopenia ($n = 318$) groups. Significant differences in sex (male/female = 30/3 vs. 212/106, $p = 0.003$), body mass index (BMI; kg/m^2, 20.8 vs. 23.3, $p < 0.0001$), the value of L3 SMI (cm^2/m^2; 30.8 vs. 45.1, $p < 0.0001$), CPS (5/6/7/8/9/10/11 = 15/7/5/2/0/3/1 vs. 164/77/47/18/9/3/0, $p = 0.039$), total bilirubin (mg/dL; 1.6 vs. 1.2, $p = 0.045$), maximum tumor size (cm; 5.6 vs. 4.0, $p = 0.020$), the degree of portal vein invasion (Vp 0/1/2/3/4 = 24/1/2/2/4 vs. 265/14/13/13/13, $p = 0.040$), curability of initial treatment (yes/no, 12/21 vs. 175/142, $p = 0.039$), and prevalence rate of neurologic disease (yes/no, 6/27 vs. 16/302, $p = 0.011$) were found. Sarcopenia patients died significantly earlier than non-sarcopenia patients ($p = 0.007$, Figure 1b).

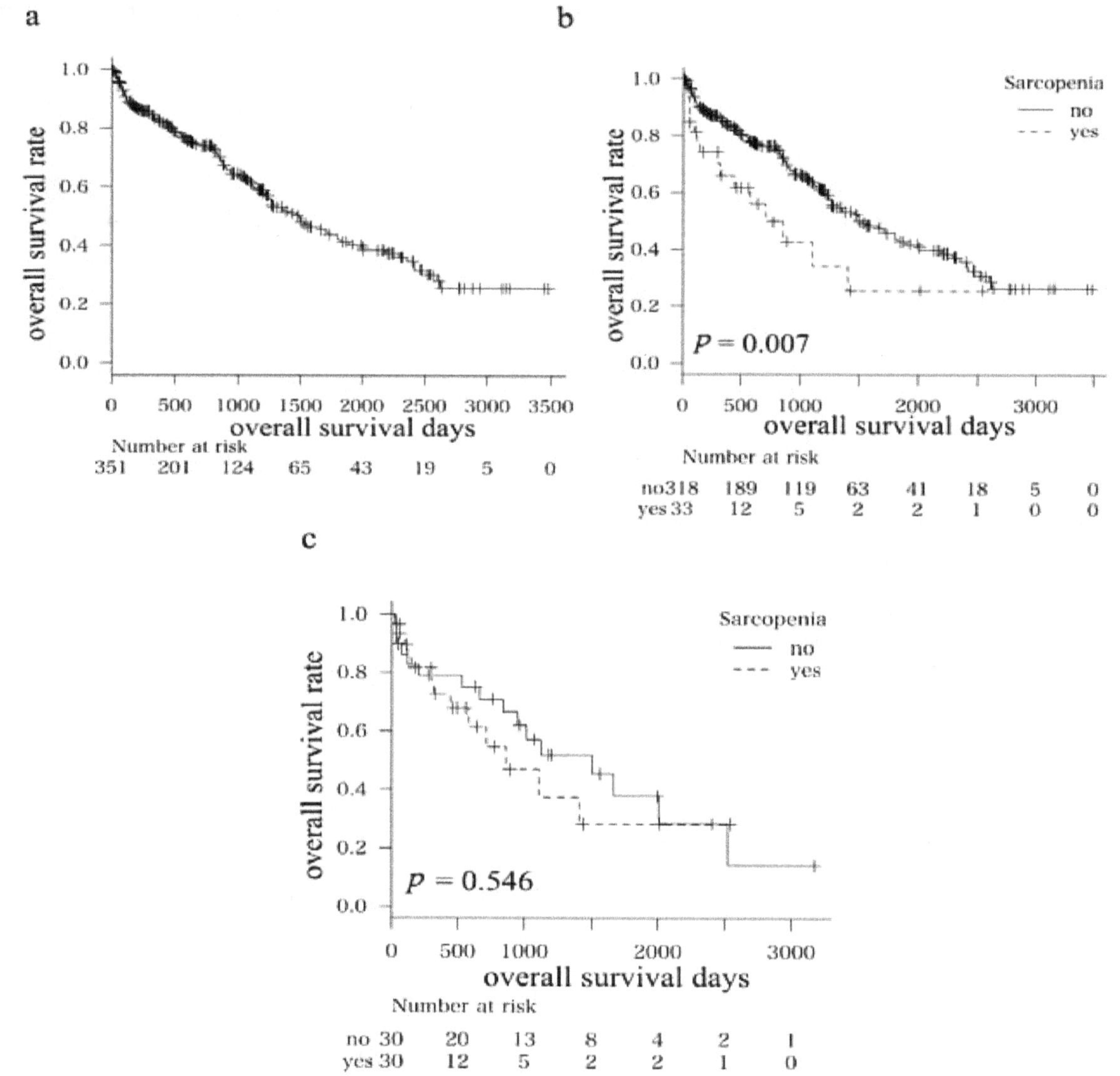

Figure 1. Kaplan–Meier curves for overall survival time in (**a**) all patients; (**b**) subgroups (i.e., sarcopenia and non-sarcopenia groups); and (**c**) subgroups after adjustments for possible confounding factors (age, sex, Child–Pugh score, maximum tumor size, tumor number, and the degree of portal vein invasion) using propensity score matching analysis.

Table 2. Baseline demographic and clinical characteristics of sarcopenia and non-sarcopenia groups.

Variables	Sarcopenia (n = 33)	Non-Sarcopenia (n = 318)	p Value
Sex (male/female)	30/3	212/106	0.003
Age (years)	72.6 ± 1.8	70.2 ± 0.6	0.197
Etiology (HBV/HCV/HBV + HCV/other)	3/22/0/8	40/182/3/93	0.868
BMI (kg/m^2)	20.8 ± 0.6	23.3 ± 0.2	<0.0001
L3 SMI (cm^2/m^2)	30.8 ± 1.3	45.1 ± 0.4	<0.0001
Child–Pugh score (5/6/7/8/9/10/11)	15/7/5/2/0/3/1	164/77/47/18/9/3/0	0.039
ALB (g/dL)	3.5 ± 0.1	3.6 ± 0.03	0.315
ALT (IU/L)	52.2 ± 7.7	46.4 ± 2.5	0.805
T-Bil (mg/dL)	1.6 ± 0.2	1.2 ± 0.06	0.045
PLT (×10^4/μL)	14.5 ± 1.4	13.0 ± 0.4	0.276
PT (%)	89.1 ± 2.9	84.9 ± 0.9	0.176
FPG (mg/dL)	113.3 ± 6.0	110.3 ± 2.0	0.958
HbA$_{1c}$ (%)	6.2 ± 0.2	6.0 ± 0.07	0.356
AFP (ng/dL)	4133 ± 12983	12,319 ± 4158	0.549
PIVKA-II (mAU/mL)	35,910 ± 21,910	19,475 ± 7149	0.476
Tumor size (cm)	5.6 ± 0.6	4.0 ± 0.2	0.020
Tumor number (1/≥2)	20/13	173/145	0.505
Vp (0/1/2/3/4)	24/1/2/2/4	265/14/13/13/13	0.040
Stage (I/II/III/IV)	8/7/12/6	71/117/88/42	0.303
Curability of initial treatment (yes/no)	12/21	176/142	0.039
Oral administration of BCAA (yes/no)	17/16	136/182	0.361
Co-existing diseases (yes/no)			
Renal disease	2/31	20/298	1.000
Heart disease	5/28	40/278	0.593
Respiratory disease	0/33	16/302	0.381
Neurologic disease	6/27	16/302	0.011
Malignant disease (except HCC)	0/33	27/291	0.093

Values are presented as average ± standard deviation. HBV, hepatitis B virus; HCV, hepatitis C virus; BMI, body mass index; L3 SMI, third lumbar vertebra skeletal muscle index; ALT, alanine aminotransferase; T-Bil, total bilirubin; PLT, platelet count; PT, prothrombin time; FPG, fasting plasma glucose; AFP, alpha-fetoprotein; PIVKA-II, protein induced by vitamin K absence or antagonists-II; Vp, the degree of portal vein invasion; BCAA, branched-chain amino acids; HCC, hepatocellular carcinoma.

To clarify the effects of sarcopenia on the prognosis of HCC patients, a propensity score matching analysis was performed after adjusting for liver functional reserve and tumor-related factors. Thirty patients from both sarcopenia and non-sarcopenia groups were chosen (Table 3). No significant differences in all variables except BMI (20.7 vs. 23.2, $p = 0.002$) and L3 SMI (30.5 vs. 46.8, $p < 0.0001$) were found; the adjustments were performed properly. Interestingly, the significant difference in the overall survival between sarcopenia and non-sarcopenia patients observed in the initial analysis (Figure 1b) disappeared after the adjustments for possible confounding factors ($p = 0.546$, Figure 1c).

Table 3. Baseline demographic and clinical characteristics of sarcopenia and non-sarcopenia groups after adjustments for possible confounding factors using propensity score matching analysis.

Variables	Sarcopenia (n = 30)	Non-Sarcopenia (n = 30)	p Value
Sex (male/female)	27/3	28/2	1.000
Age (years)	71.8 ± 9.7	73.0 ± 10.7	0.642
Etiology (HBV/HCV/HBV + HCV/other)	3/21/0/6	3/20/1/6	0.918
BMI (kg/m^2)	20.7 ± 3.0	23.2 ± 2.8	0.002
L3 SMI (cm^2/m^2)	30.5 ± 6.4	46.8 ± 7.4	<0.0001
Child–Pugh score (5/6/7/8/9/10/11)	14/7/5/2/0/1/1	14/9/6/0/1/0/0	0.660
ALB (g/dL)	3.6 ± 0.7	3.6 ± 0.6	0.984
ALT (IU/L)	48.8 ± 57.7	41.8 ± 22.7	0.543
T-Bil (mg/dL)	1.4 ± 1.0	1.0 ± 0.5	0.106
PLT (×10^4/μL)	14.5 ± 13.0	13.4 ± 4.9	0.656
PT (%)	89.8 ± 14.4	87.7 ± 15.5	0.589

Table 3. *Cont.*

Variables	Sarcopenia (n = 30)	Non-Sarcopenia (n = 30)	p Value
FPG (mg/dL)	114.8 ± 40.2	113.6 ± 47.9	0.918
HbA_{1c} (%)	6.3 ± 1.6	5.8 ± 1.2	0.226
AFP (ng/dL)	3531 ± 12,997	1480 ± 4268	0.423
PIVKA-II (mAU/mL)	22,979 ± 89,165	10,893 ± 46,387	0.518
Tumor size (cm)	5.0 ± 3.9	4.4 ± 3.8	0.534
Tumor number (1/≥2)	18/12	18/12	1.000
Vp (0/1/2/3/4)	24/1/2/1/2	22/3/1/2/2	0.852
Stage (I/II/III/IV)	8/7/10/5	7/11/5/7	0.427
Curability of initial treatment (yes/no)	12/18	17/13	0.301

Values are presented as average ± standard deviation. HBV, hepatitis B virus; HCV, hepatitis C virus; BMI, body mass index; L3 SMI, third lumbar vertebra skeletal muscle index; ALT, alanine aminotransferase; T-Bil, total bilirubin; PLT, platelet count; PT, prothrombin time; FPG, fasting plasma glucose; AFP, alpha-fetoprotein; PIVKA-II, protein induced by vitamin K absence or antagonists-II; Vp, the degree of portal vein invasion.

3.3. Significant Factors that Affect L3 SMI Based on Multiple Linear Regression Analysis and Tree-Based Models

Of the six possible confounding factors (age, sex, CPS, tumor size, tumor number, and the degree of portal vein invasion), age (p = 0.015) and sex (p < 0.0001) were significantly correlated with the value of L3 SMI based on multiple linear regression analysis (Table 4). The following regression equation with an intercept of 46.94 (p < 0.0001) was obtained from Equation (1) and (2):

$$\text{L3 SMI (cm}^2/\text{m}^2) = 46.94 - 0.10 \times [\text{Age}] + 5.20 \text{ (for men)} \quad (1)$$

$$\text{L3 SMI (cm}^2/\text{m}^2) = 46.94 - 0.10 \times [\text{Age}] \text{ (for women)} \quad (2)$$

Table 4. Significant factors affecting L3 SMI by multiple linear regression analysis.

Variables	Std. Coefficient	Std. Error	t Value	p Value
Intercept	46.94	3.06	15.33	<0.0001
Age	−0.10	0.04	−2.44	0.015
Sex (vs. man)	5.20	0.95	5.46	<0.0001

Std. coefficient, standard coefficient; Std. error, standard error.

Furthermore, according to the tree-based models, the most significant factor contributing to the value of L3 SMI was sex; the average L3 SMI in men was 46 cm^2/m^2 and that in women was 40 cm^2/m^2. In men, the most significant factor for decreased L3 SMI was aging; the average L3 SMI in men ≥ 56 and < 56 years old was 45 and 50 cm^2/m^2, respectively. In men ≥ 56 years old, a higher CPS was involved in the loss of skeletal muscle mass; the average L3 SMI with CPS ≥ 9 and < 9 was 38 and 45 cm^2/m^2, respectively. In men < 56 years old, an enlarged tumor size was involved in the loss of skeletal muscle mass; the average L3 SMI with tumor size ≥ 5.7 and < 5.7 cm was 45 and 52 cm^2/m^2, respectively. However, these factors observed in men did not affect the L3 SMI in women. The decision tree for this analysis is shown in Figure 2.

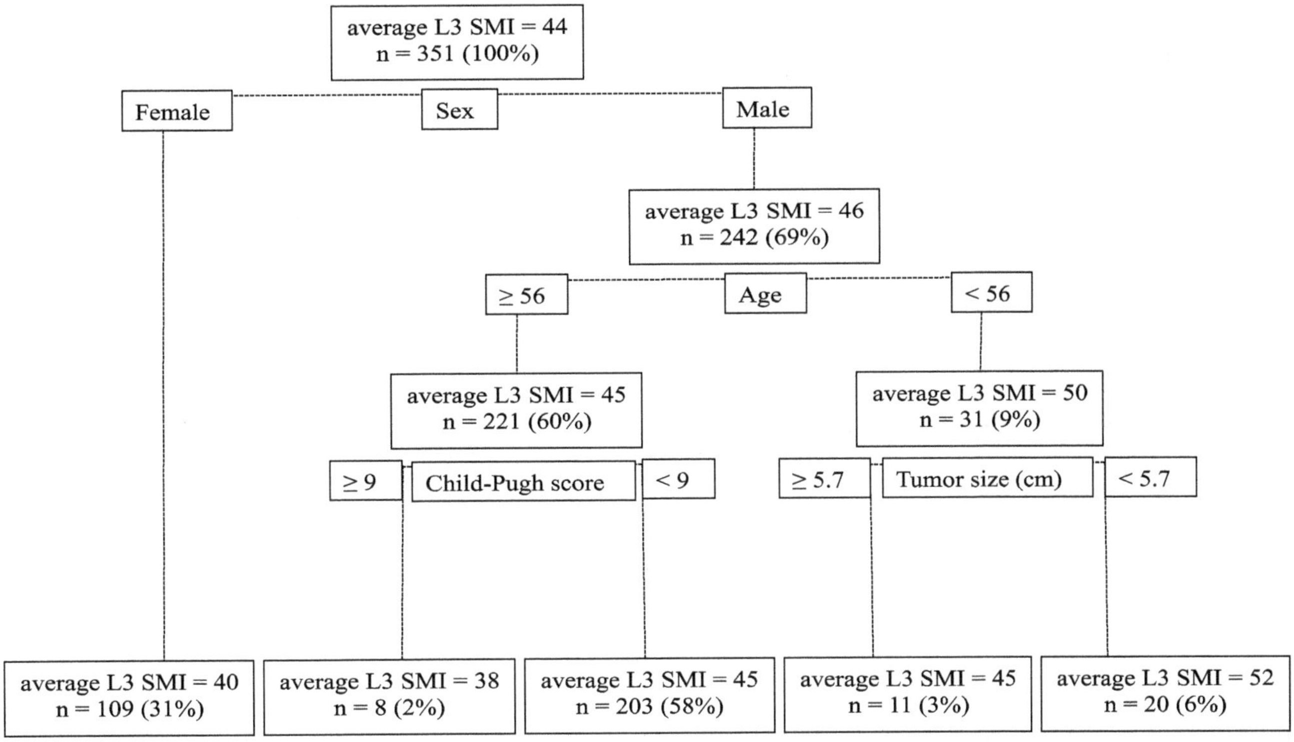

Figure 2. The decision tree for the tree-based models. The differences in L3 SMI between each group become larger with the six factors (age, sex, Child–Pugh score, maximum tumor size, tumor number, and the degree of portal vein invasion).

4. Discussion

The results of this study showed that sarcopenia impairs survival in patients with HCC. These findings are consistent with those of previous studies [6–12]. Thus, skeletal muscle volume measurement using CT, which is commonly used in the clinical setting for HCC, is useful to predict the prognosis of patients with this malignancy.

Here, patients in the sarcopenia group had poorer liver functional reserve, larger tumor size, and more severe portal vein invasion, which significantly contributed to the lower curability of the initial treatment for HCC. Moreover, men, older patients, and those with poorer liver functional reserve and larger tumor size had a lower skeletal muscle volume. Several studies revealed that liver functional reserve and clinical cancer stage are significant prognostic factors for HCC and that, similar to the results in our study, the progression of underlying liver cirrhosis and HCC, in addition to aging, are critically involved in the development of sarcopenia and subsequent poor prognosis of these patients [1,2,4]. The results of the propensity score matching analysis showed that the significant differences in overall survival between the sarcopenia and non-sarcopenia groups disappeared after adjustments for the probable confounding factors associated with the patients' characteristics and tumor factors. This finding may suggest that the sarcopenia group had clinical characteristics—such as old age, poor liver functional reserve, and progressed cancer stage—that affect survival.

Several clinical studies have revealed that sarcopenia might be an independent prognostic factor for HCC [11,12]. In addition, HCC patients with sarcopenia more often have complications with chemotherapy toxicity and this might make the prognosis of the patients more serious [22,23]. On the other hand, skeletal muscle volume in HCC patients was determined, at least in part, by sex, age, CPS, and tumor burden in this study. Based on the findings, it could be said that, at least in men, sarcopenia is a prognostic factor possibly affected by already-known prognostic factors, including liver functional reserve and clinical cancer stage [1,2,4]. Most of the existing prognostic staging systems, such as CLIP and JIS [1,2,4], take liver functional reserve and clinical cancer stage into consideration in predicting prognosis for HCC as accurately as possible. Thus, these findings strongly suggest that maintaining liver functional reserve and early detection and therapy for HCC, which can increase the curability of initial treatment, are effective strategies to improve the prognosis. In addition, reducing the amount of tumor burden and maintaining liver functional reserve, which have been reported repeatedly to improve prognosis for HCC [1,2,4], could be effective measures to prevent skeletal muscle depletion; however, future prospective study is required to evaluate this hypothesis further.

Other possible strategies to prevent skeletal muscle depletion or to increase skeletal muscle mass include nutritional and exercise therapies, both of which have been shown to improve outcomes in patients with liver cirrhosis [24,25]. Oral supplementation with branched chain amino acids is one of the most promising methods [26–28]. Exercise therapy might also be promising in preventing skeletal muscle depletion [29]. Moreover, poor dietary or sedentary lifestyle is considered one of the main causes of sarcopenia [15]; thus, appropriate assessment and modification of lifestyle could be useful to prevent decreased skeletal muscle volume and subsequently to improve the prognosis of patients with HCC and liver cirrhosis. Furthermore, pathological conditions—except liver diseases—that can lead to sarcopenia must also be considered. The aging of HCC patient population is advancing and elderly patients are easily complicated with several diseases which cause sarcopenia. In the present study, the prevalence of patients with neurologic disease, which decreases activities of daily living levels, was significantly high in the sarcopenia group. Therefore, in order to prevent sarcopenia, such patients might especially be recommended to start rehabilitation as early as possible.

In the present study, aging was critically involved in the complication with sarcopenia in men. One of the reasons of this phenomenon might be that decreasing of testosterone caused by aging because this sex hormone is known to promote the growth of skeletal muscle [30]. On the other hand, aging, progression of CPS, and enlargement of tumor size did not have effects on the loss of skeletal muscle volume in women. Because women usually store abundance of fat and generate their energy more preferentially from fat stores than from skeletal muscle stores [31], women might be more resistant to sarcopenia compared to men. In addition to the present study, several clinical trials have defined the optimal cutoff values of skeletal muscle volume which are different between men and women [7,11,32]. These findings may suggest that setting the different cutoff values on every sex is reasonable to evaluate sarcopenia.

This study has some limitations. First, we used our own cutoff values for L3 SMI (i.e., 29.0 cm^2/m^2 for women and 36.0 cm^2/m^2 for men), which are not similar to those of the JSH (i.e., 38.0 cm^2/m^2 for women and 42.0 cm^2/m^2 for men) [16], to determine sarcopenia because the latter could not stratify the risk of mortality for HCC patients. We also did not use the cutoff values reported by the previous reports [7,32], both of which are widely accepted as appropriate values in western countries, because they are not applicable to Japanese HCC patients whose BMIs are small and differ considerably from Western populations. Second, because of the retrospective design of our study, muscle strength such as grip strength and walking speed, which is usually regarded as a diagnostic criterion for sarcopenia [15,16], was not assessed. Future prospective studies that examine the most optimal cutoff values for L3 SMI to diagnose sarcopenia and whether sarcopenia itself worsens the prognosis of patients with HCC should be performed.

5. Conclusions

We demonstrated that L3 SMI, an indicator of skeletal muscle volume, was significantly decreased in female HCC patients. In male patients, L3 SMI was significantly affected by aging, liver functional reserve ($\geq$56 years), and tumor size (<56 years). These findings strongly suggest that more emphasis should be put on maintaining liver functional reserve and reducing tumor burden, both of which are well-reported prognostic factors for HCC [1,2,4], especially in patients with sarcopenia. In conclusion, in addition to the measure for sarcopenia, maintaining liver functional reserve and early detection and curative therapy for HCC are effective ways to improve the prognosis of chronic liver disease patients, especially those with HCC.

Acknowledgments: No funding sources support the preparation of this manuscript.

Author Contributions: Kenji Imai designed the study, analyzed the data, and wrote the manuscript. Koji Takai supervised the treatment for the participants. Satoshi Watanabe, Tatsunori Hanai, Atsushi Suetsugu, and Makoto Shiraki contributed to select the participants and collect the data. Masahito Shimizu mainly reviewed and amended the manuscript. All authors read and approved the final manuscript.

References

1. A new prognostic system for hepatocellular carcinoma: A retrospective study of 435 patients: The cancer of the liver italian program (clip) investigators. *Hepatology* **1998**, *28*, 751–755.
2. Kudo, M.; Chung, H.; Osaki, Y. Prognostic staging system for hepatocellular carcinoma (clip score): Its value and limitations, and a proposal for a new staging system, the japan integrated staging score (jis score). *J. Gastroenterol.* **2003**, *38*, 207–215. [CrossRef] [PubMed]
3. Poon, R.T. Prevention of recurrence after resection of hepatocellular carcinoma: A daunting challenge. *Hepatology* **2011**, *54*, 757–759. [CrossRef] [PubMed]
4. Llovet, J.M.; Bru, C.; Bruix, J. Prognosis of hepatocellular carcinoma: The bclc staging classification. *Semin. Liver Dis.* **1999**, *19*, 329–338. [CrossRef] [PubMed]
5. Rosenberg, I.H. Sarcopenia: Origins and clinical relevance. *J. Nutr.* **1997**, *127*, 990S–991S. [CrossRef] [PubMed]
6. Fujiwara, N.; Nakagawa, H.; Kudo, Y.; Tateishi, R.; Taguri, M.; Watadani, T.; Nakagomi, R.; Kondo, M.; Nakatsuka, T.; Minami, T.; et al. Sarcopenia, intramuscular fat deposition, and visceral adiposity independently predict the outcomes of hepatocellular carcinoma. *J. Hepatol.* **2015**, *63*, 131–140. [CrossRef] [PubMed]
7. Prado, C.M.; Lieffers, J.R.; McCargar, L.J.; Reiman, T.; Sawyer, M.B.; Martin, L.; Baracos, V.E. Prevalence and clinical implications of sarcopenic obesity in patients with solid tumours of the respiratory and gastrointestinal tracts: A population-based study. *Lancet Oncol.* **2008**, *9*, 629–635. [CrossRef]
8. Sabel, M.S.; Lee, J.; Cai, S.; Englesbe, M.J.; Holcombe, S.; Wang, S. Sarcopenia as a prognostic factor among patients with stage iii melanoma. *Ann. Surg. Oncol.* **2011**, *18*, 3579–3585. [CrossRef] [PubMed]
9. Tan, B.H.; Birdsell, L.A.; Martin, L.; Baracos, V.E.; Fearon, K.C. Sarcopenia in an overweight or obese patient is an adverse prognostic factor in pancreatic cancer. *Clin. Cancer Res. Off. J. Am. Assoc. Cancer Res.* **2009**, *15*, 6973–6979. [CrossRef] [PubMed]
10. Van Vledder, M.G.; Levolger, S.; Ayez, N.; Verhoef, C.; Tran, T.C.; Ijzermans, J.N. Body composition and outcome in patients undergoing resection of colorectal liver metastases. *Br. J. Surg.* **2012**, *99*, 550–557. [CrossRef] [PubMed]
11. Iritani, S.; Imai, K.; Takai, K.; Hanai, T.; Ideta, T.; Miyazaki, T.; Suetsugu, A.; Shiraki, M.; Shimizu, M.; Moriwaki, H. Skeletal muscle depletion is an independent prognostic factor for hepatocellular carcinoma. *J. Gastroenterol.* **2015**, *50*, 323–332. [CrossRef] [PubMed]
12. Imai, K.; Takai, K.; Hanai, T.; Ideta, T.; Miyazaki, T.; Kochi, T.; Suetsugu, A.; Shiraki, M.; Shimizu, M. Skeletal muscle depletion predicts the prognosis of patients with hepatocellular carcinoma treated with sorafenib. *Int. J. Mol. Sci.* **2015**, *16*, 9612–9624. [CrossRef] [PubMed]
13. Hanai, T.; Shiraki, M.; Nishimura, K.; Ohnishi, S.; Imai, K.; Suetsugu, A.; Takai, K.; Shimizu, M.; Moriwaki, H. Sarcopenia impairs prognosis of patients with liver cirrhosis. *Nutrition* **2015**, *31*, 193–199. [CrossRef] [PubMed]
14. Hanai, T.; Shiraki, M.; Ohnishi, S.; Miyazaki, T.; Ideta, T.; Kochi, T.; Imai, K.; Suetsugu, A.; Takai, K.; Moriwaki, H.; et al. Rapid skeletal muscle wasting predicts worse survival in patients with liver cirrhosis. *Hepatol. Res.* **2016**, *46*, 743–751. [CrossRef] [PubMed]
15. Cruz-Jentoft, A.J.; Baeyens, J.P.; Bauer, J.M.; Boirie, Y.; Cederholm, T.; Landi, F.; Martin, F.C.; Michel, J.P.; Rolland, Y.; Schneider, S.M.; et al. Sarcopenia: European consensus on definition and diagnosis: Report of the european working group on sarcopenia in older people. *Age Ageing* **2010**, *39*, 412–423. [CrossRef] [PubMed]
16. Nishikawa, H.; Shiraki, M.; Hiramatsu, A.; Moriya, K.; Hino, K.; Nishiguchi, S. Japan society of hepatology guidelines for sarcopenia in liver disease (1st edition): Recommendation from the working group for creation of sarcopenia assessment criteria. *Hepatol. Res.* **2016**, *46*, 951–963. [CrossRef] [PubMed]

17. Clinical practice guidelines for hepatocellular carcinoma—The Japan society of hepatology 2009 update. *Hepatol. Res. Off. J. Jpn. Soc. Hepatol.* **2010**, *40*, 2–144.
18. Mitsiopoulos, N.; Baumgartner, R.N.; Heymsfield, S.B.; Lyons, W.; Gallagher, D.; Ross, R. Cadaver validation of skeletal muscle measurement by magnetic resonance imaging and computerized tomography. *J. Appl. Physiol.* **1998**, *85*, 115–122. [PubMed]
19. Austin, P.C. Propensity-score matching in the cardiovascular surgery literature from 2004 to 2006: A systematic review and suggestions for improvement. *J. Thorac. Cardiovasc. Surg.* **2007**, *134*, 1128–1135. [CrossRef] [PubMed]
20. Pociot, F.; Karlsen, A.E.; Pedersen, C.B.; Aalund, M.; Nerup, J.; European Consortium for I.G.S. Novel analytical methods applied to type 1 diabetes genome-scan data. *Am. J. Hum. Genet.* **2004**, *74*, 647–660. [CrossRef] [PubMed]
21. Banerjee, M.; Muenz, D.G.; Chang, J.T.; Papaleontiou, M.; Haymart, M.R. Tree-based model for thyroid cancer prognostication. *J. Clin. Endocrinol. Metab.* **2014**, *99*, 3737–3745. [CrossRef] [PubMed]
22. Mir, O.; Coriat, R.; Blanchet, B.; Durand, J.P.; Boudou-Rouquette, P.; Michels, J.; Ropert, S.; Vidal, M.; Pol, S.; Chaussade, S.; et al. Sarcopenia predicts early dose-limiting toxicities and pharmacokinetics of sorafenib in patients with hepatocellular carcinoma. *PLoS ONE* **2012**, *7*, e37563. [CrossRef] [PubMed]
23. Prado, C.M.; Antoun, S.; Sawyer, M.B.; Baracos, V.E. Two faces of drug therapy in cancer: Drug-related lean tissue loss and its adverse consequences to survival and toxicity. *Curr. Opin. Clin. Nutr. Metab. Care* **2011**, *14*, 250–254. [CrossRef] [PubMed]
24. Jones, J.C.; Coombes, J.S.; Macdonald, G.A. Exercise capacity and muscle strength in patients with cirrhosis. *Liver Transplant.* **2012**, *18*, 146–151. [CrossRef] [PubMed]
25. Plauth, M.; Cabre, E.; Riggio, O.; Assis-Camilo, M.; Pirlich, M.; Kondrup, J.; Ferenci, P.; Holm, E.; Vom Dahl, S.; Muller, M.J.; et al. Espen guidelines on enteral nutrition: Liver disease. *Clin. Nutr.* **2006**, *25*, 285–294. [CrossRef] [PubMed]
26. Marchesini, G.; Bianchi, G.; Merli, M.; Amodio, P.; Panella, C.; Loguercio, C.; Rossi Fanelli, F.; Abbiati, R. Nutritional supplementation with branched-chain amino acids in advanced cirrhosis: A double-blind, randomized trial. *Gastroenterology* **2003**, *124*, 1792–1801. [CrossRef]
27. Moriwaki, H.; Shiraki, M.; Fukushima, H.; Shimizu, M.; Iwasa, J.; Naiki, T.; Nagaki, M. Long-term outcome of branched-chain amino acid treatment in patients with liver cirrhosis. *Hepatol. Res.* **2008**, *38*, S102–S106. [CrossRef] [PubMed]
28. Muto, Y.; Sato, S.; Watanabe, A.; Moriwaki, H.; Suzuki, K.; Kato, A.; Kato, M.; Nakamura, T.; Higuchi, K.; Nishiguchi, S.; et al. Effects of oral branched-chain amino acid granules on event-free survival in patients with liver cirrhosis. *Clin. Gastroenterol. Hepatol.* **2005**, *3*, 705–713. [CrossRef]
29. Vincent, H.K.; Raiser, S.N.; Vincent, K.R. The aging musculoskeletal system and obesity-related considerations with exercise. *Ageing Res. Rev.* **2012**, *11*, 361–373. [CrossRef] [PubMed]
30. Grossmann, M.; Hoermann, R.; Gani, L.; Chan, I.; Cheung, A.; Gow, P.J.; Li, A.; Zajac, J.D.; Angus, P. Low testosterone levels as an independent predictor of mortality in men with chronic liver disease. *Clin. Endocrinol.* **2012**, *77*, 323–328. [CrossRef] [PubMed]
31. Riggio, O.; Angeloni, S.; Ciuffa, L.; Nicolini, G.; Attili, A.F.; Albanese, C.; Merli, M. Malnutrition is not related to alterations in energy balance in patients with stable liver cirrhosis. *Clin. Nutr.* **2003**, *22*, 553–559. [CrossRef]
32. Montano-Loza, A.J.; Meza-Junco, J.; Prado, C.M.; Lieffers, J.R.; Baracos, V.E.; Bain, V.G.; Sawyer, M.B. Muscle wasting is associated with mortality in patients with cirrhosis. *Clin. Gastroenterol. Hepatol.* **2012**, *10*, 166–173, 173.e1. [CrossRef] [PubMed]

Gut Permeability Might be Improved by Dietary Fiber in Individuals with Nonalcoholic Fatty Liver Disease (NAFLD) Undergoing Weight Reduction

Marcin Krawczyk [1,2], Dominika Maciejewska [3], Karina Ryterska [3], Maja Czerwińka-Rogowska [3], Dominika Jamioł-Milc [3], Karolina Skonieczna-Żydecka [3], Piotr Milkiewicz [4,5], Joanna Raszeja-Wyszomirska [4] and Ewa Stachowska [3,*]

1 Department of Medicine II, Saarland University Medical Center, Saarland University, 66421 Homburg, Germany; marcin.krawczyk@uks.eu
2 Laboratory of Metabolic Liver Diseases, Centre for Preclinical Research, Department of General, Transplant and Liver Surgery, Medical University of Warsaw, 02-097 Warsaw, Poland
3 Department of Biochemistry and Human Nutrition, Pomeranian Medical University, 71-210 Szczecin, Poland; domi.maciejka@wp.pl (D.M.); ryterska.karina@gmail.com (K.R.); majaczerwinska89@gmail.com (M.C.-R.); dominikajamiol@interia.pl (D.J.-M.); karzyd@pum.edu.pl (K.S.-Ż.)
4 Liver and Internal Medicine Unit, Department of General, Transplant and Liver Surgery of the Medical University of Warsaw, 02-097 Warsaw, Poland; p.milkiewicz@wp.pl (P.M.); jorasz@gmail.com (J.R.-W.)
5 Translational Medicine Group, Pomeranian Medical University, 71-210 Szczecin, Poland
* Correspondence: ewa.stachowska@pum.edu.pl or ewast@pum.edu.pl

Abstract: (1) Introduction: Zonulin (ZO) has been proposed as a marker of intestinal permeability. Only a few studies have analyzed to date how diet influences the serum concentration of ZO among patients with non-alcoholic fatty liver disease (NAFLD). We performed a six-month dietetic intervention to evaluate the association between fiber intake and ZO concentration in 32 individuals with NAFLD. (2) Methods: Fiber content in the diet was estimated by Food Frequency Questionnaire (FFQ) and by analyzing 72-h nutritional diaries. ZO concentrations in serum were measured before and after the intervention by immunoenzymatic assay (ELISA). Fatty liver was quantified using the Hamaguchi score before and after the dietetic intervention. (3) Results: During the intervention, the dietary fiber intake increased from 19 g/day to the 29 g/day concomitant with an increase in the frequency of fiber consumption. All patients experienced significant (all $p < 0.05$) improvements in serum aspartate aminotransferase (AST), alanine aminotransferase (ALT) and gamma-glutamyltransferase (GGTP) activities. We also detected decreased serum triglycerides ($p = 0.036$), homeostatic model assessment insulin resistance (HOMA-IR ($p = 0.041$) and insulin content ($p = 0.34$), and improvement of fatty liver status according to the Hamaguchi score ($p = 0.009$). ZO concentration in serum decreased by nearly 90% (7.335 ± 13.492 vs. 0.507 ± 0.762 ng/mL, $p = 0.001$) and correlated with the amount of dietary fiber intake ($p = 0.043$) as well as the degree of fatty liver ($p = 0.037$). (4) Conclusion: Increasing nutritional fiber results in reduced serum ZO levels, reduced liver enzymes and improved hepatic steatosis in patients with NAFLD, possibly by altering intestinal permeability. Increased dietary fiber intake should be recommended in patients with NAFLD.

Keywords: NAFLD; zonulin; fiber; diet

1. Introduction

The gut epithelium represents a key protective barrier separating internal organs from the adverse environment of the gut lumen [1]. Its permeability is controlled by several multiprotein adhesive complexes including tight junctions (TJ), subjacent adherens junctions (AJ), and desmosomes [1]. The intestinal barrier is a highly dynamic structure shaped by interactions with internal and external stimuli, such as cytokines, growth factors, and bacteria [1–3]. Diet-derived substances also interact with the barrier and modulate its permeability. For instance, glutamine [4,5] and tryptophan [6], peptides derived from cheese and milk [7,8], and polyphenols [9] act as positive regulators of epithelial permeability, whereas other compounds such as gliadin [10] or medium-chain fatty acids [11,12] negatively regulate intestinal barrier permeability. Zonulin (ZO) is a 47-kDa protein that regulates intestinal permeability by modulating intracellular TJ structure and function [13]. The secretion of ZO into serum is believed to be regulated by several factors, including components of the diet [14,15].

Nonalcoholic fatty liver disease (NAFLD) is now the most common cause of chronic liver disease. It is currently detected in over 20% of Europeans, and its prevalence is predicted to increase over the years [16,17]. NAFLD is considered the hepatic manifestation of the metabolic syndrome, and the steatotic phenotype appears to be worsened by disruptions in the host gut microbiota [18,19]. An increasing body of evidence demonstrates that NAFLD correlates positively with the phenomenon of "leaky gut", the mechanism encompassing TJ damage [20] in both young patients [13] and adults [21,22]. The disturbances of the gut-liver axis might explain, at least to a certain extent, the phenotype of fatty liver [23]. For example, gut dysbiosis and skewed production of inflammatory markers, among others lipopolysachcaride, might modulate the progression of NAFLD. This is underscored by the association between endotoxemia and severe forms of fatty liver [24]. Moreover, a dysbiotic gut ecosystem might result in increased production of endogenous ethanol, which could disrupt the integrity of the intestinal barrier and further increase liver injury in the setting of increased hepatic fat accumulation [25]. Several studies have reported that ZO concentrations increase significantly with the severity of steatosis [13,20,21] and positively correlate with body mass index (BMI), liver histopathology, fasting insulin, and HOMA-IR as well as concentrations of inflammatory markers (e.g., serum IL-6) [21]. To the best of our knowledge, there is only one study that has described how a reduction diet among NAFLD patients might influence the serum concentration of ZO [13]. Here we present the impact of a six-month dietetic intervention, comprising an increased intake of fiber and a decreased intake of fat and simple sugars, on the liver status and ZO serum concentrations in a cohort of 32 patients with NAFLD.

2. Materials and Methods

2.1. Study Design

In the present study we included subjects selected from the Nutrient-Induced Insulin Output Ratio (NIOR) study, which was intended to investigate nutritional strategies for the individualized treatment of NAFLD [22]. In brief, this study was designed as a randomized controlled intervention trial to compare the influence of three nutrigenetic dietary strategies on fatty liver during a six-month intervention [26]. The exclusion criteria were: Diabetes mellitus (DMII); chronic and acute liver diseases other than NAFLD; high levels of physical activity (>3000 kcal/week in leisure-time physical activity); changes in physical activity during the dietary intervention; use of statins; any condition that could limit the mobility of the participant; not being able to attend control visits; vegetarianism or a need for other special diets; excessive consumption of alcohol (more than 20 g in women and more than 30 g in men, per day); and other drug addiction. Compliance with the diet was evaluated at 3 control points (at 1, 2, and 6 months after commencement of the diet) (Figure 1). All subjects were instructed to maintain their usual physical activity (metabolic equivalent of the task; MET), which was controlled by a 2-h physical activity questionnaire. Initially, 171 Caucasian adults were enrolled in the NIOR study; however, 5 subjects did not meet the inclusion criteria. After the first month of the study further 29 individuals were excluded from the study: Either they did not comply with the prescribed diet, engaged in too much physical activity or they failed to complete the dietary intake questionnaire.

At the second control meeting (i.e., 2 months after the beginning of the diet), 14 participants were excluded from the study for similar reasons. During the final visit (after 6 months), a further 13 participants were excluded. As a result, a total of 110 participants were adherent to the intervention protocol and remained in the study (Figure 1). We used an online randomization tool [26] to select patients for biochemical analyses. Serum samples from 32 participants (22 males and 10 females) were available for the current analysis. The fiber consumption was analyzed (soluble fiber as well as insoluble fiber) with the help of the Fineli base (https://fineli.fi/fineli/en/index) and the Diet program (IZZ Poland). The study protocol was approved by the ethics committee of the Pomeranian Medical University and conformed to the ethical guidelines of the 1975 Declaration of Helsinki (Szczecin, Poland, 25 01 2010 KB-0012/09/10). Participants provided written informed consent before the study.

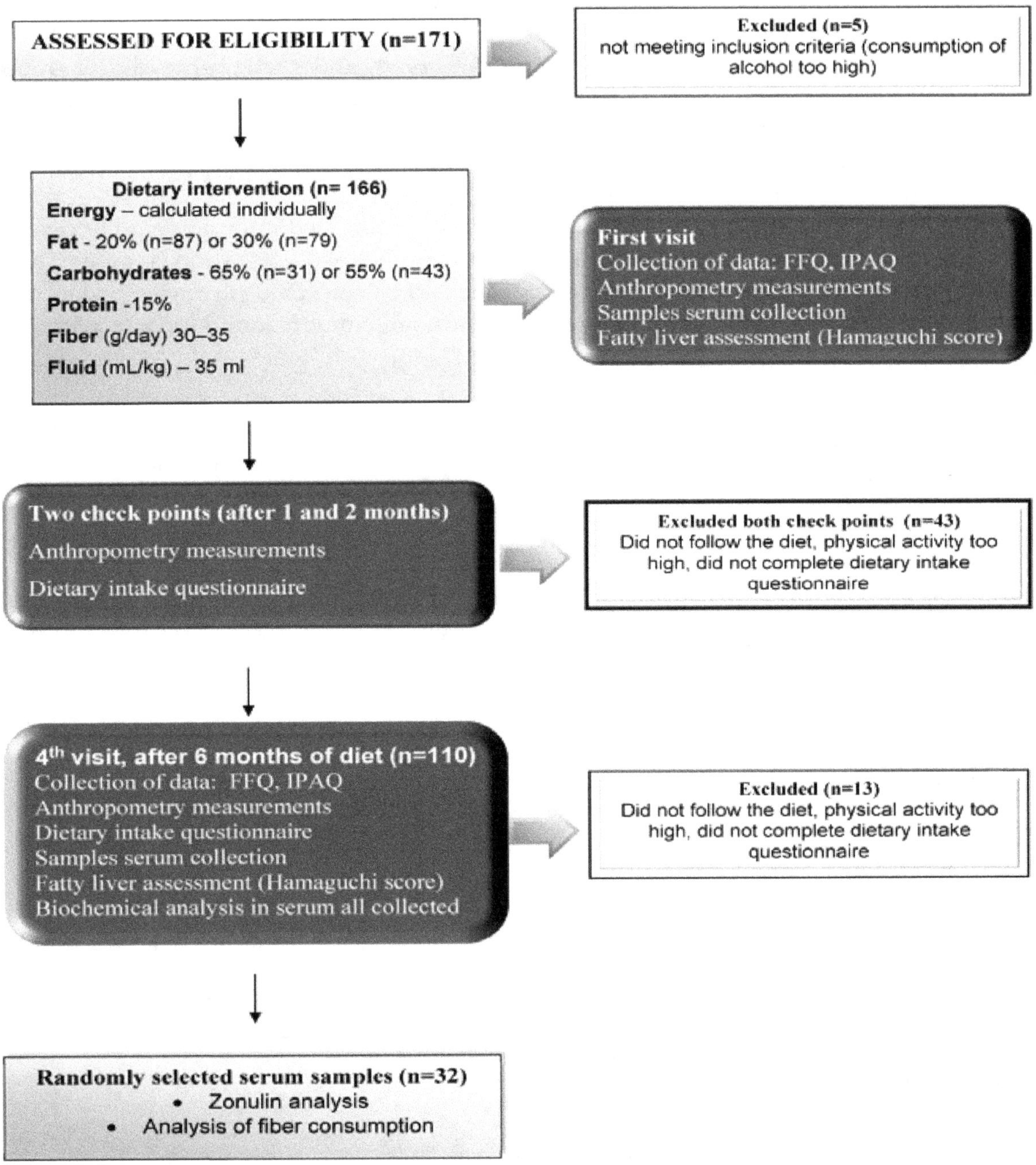

Figure 1. Flowchart for the inclusion of individuals in the study.

2.2. *The Nutritional Intervention and Control*

The NIOR diet was modified on the basis of the of the American Heart Association (AHA) guidelines, including 3–5 meals/day, modified by the genetic result of NIOR as described in detail [27]. Menus were prepared as a daily plan for the 7 days of the week and included guidance on the daily timing of the five meals.

Nutrition patterns were analyzed with a Food Frequency Questionnaire (FFQ) and a 72-h food diary (including 2 working days and one day free of work) [27]. Fiber content (soluble and insoluble) was estimated by means of two methods: frequency of consumption by means of the FFQ and by analyzing the 72 nutritional diaries (from the three control points) via the Diet 5 program (IZZ Poland) and Fineli (the Finnish database). Dietary content, nutritional sources and the products used are presented in Table 1. Three portions of vegetables and two portions of fruit were introduced to the patients' diet. The recommended sources of insoluble fiber were as follows: Whole wheat bread, whole-wheat pasta, cereal and brown rice, whole rye bread, and graham bread. Recommended vegetables were: Tomatoes, savoy cabbages (fresh and pickled), napa cabbages, green beans, paprika, fresh and pickled cucumbers, onions, chives, red beans, lentils, spinach, carrots, leeks, celery, broccoli, lettuce, and dill. Recommended fruits were: apples, plums, and apricots (including dried). Finally, recommended seeds and nuts were: pumpkin seeds and walnuts. The level of physical activity was assessed using the questionnaire technique with validated International Physical Activity Questionnaire (IPAQ). Physical exercise was estimated with MET units (min/week). During the first and final visit, the degree of fatty liver was evaluated by a trained physician according to the Hamaguchi score [28], using a high-resolution B-mode abdominal ultrasound scanner (Acuson X300). Hamaguchi score ≥ 2.0 was set as the cut-off for NAFLD [28].

Table 1. The nutritional products used in the diet.

Variable	Recommendation	Recommended Sources
Energy	**Calculated Individually**	
Fiber (g/day)	30–35	3 portions of vegetables a day; 2 portions of fruit as: fresh, fermented or boiled, wheat bread, whole-wheat pasta, cereal and brown rice
Fat as percentage of total calories (%)	20–30	Vegetable fats with a predominance of rapeseed oil and olive oil.
Carbohydrates (low and medium IG), percentage of total calories (%)	55–65	Low and medium glycemic index as: wheat and mix rye/wheat bread, whole-pasta, cereal and brown rice, fruit and vegetables.
Simple carbohydrate, percentage of total calories (%)	5–10	Dry fruits
Protein (%)	15	Poultry (chicken and turkey), fish (oily fish 3 times a week), fermented dairy products (2 times a day), eggs (4–5 a week), lean cottage cheese, cheese with reduced fat content.
Fluid (mL/kg)	35	Water, coffee (1–2 cup a day) tea (black, green).
Vitamins and minerals	Consistent with recommended daily allowance	Natural sources from vegetables and fruit

2.3. *Laboratory Analyses*

Venous fasted blood samples were collected into tubes containing anticoagulant Ethylenediaminetetraacetic acid (EDTA). Blood samples were centrifuged at 3500 rpm for 10 min at 4 °C within 2 h of collection. Standard blood biochemical analyses were carried out at the University Hospital Laboratory (Szczecin, Poland). Plasma ZO concentrations were measured by ELISA (Immundiagnostik AG, Bensheim, Germany) according to manufacturer's instructions.

2.4. Statistics

For statistical analyses, R software 3.0.2 was used and all results were expressed as mean and standard deviation. Since the distribution in most cases deviated from normality (Shapiro-Wilk test), non-parametric paired tests were used (Wilcoxon signed-rank test) and $p < 0.05$ was considered as statistically significant. The correlations between quantitative variables were calculated using the Spearman's correlation test.

3. Results

3.1. The Amount of Zonulin in Serum Decreases with the Improvement of Fatty Liver

As shown in Figure 2, the six-month dietetic intervention resulted in a significant improvement of liver injury markers in the studied group of 32 individuals as reflected by decreases of serum AST ($p = 0.001$), ALT ($p = 0.001$) and GGTP ($p = 0.03$). As shown in Table 2, it also led to a reduction of the Hamaguchi score (2.87 $\pm$ 0.59 vs. 1.40 $\pm$ 0.93; $p = 0.009$). Furthermore, serum triglyceride concentrations ($p = 0.036$), HOMA-IR ($p = 0.041$) index as well serum insulin ($p = 0.34$) decreased as a result of the dietetic intervention. Notably, we also detected a significant ($p = 0.001$), almost 90% reduction of serum ZO concentration as shown in Figure 2A. Table 3 demonstrates that serum ZO correlated with the degree of fatty liver (i.e., with Hamaguchi score ($p = 0.037$) serum AST ($p = 0.041$) and ALT ($p = 0.043$)), total lipids ($p = 0.041$), as well as low-density lipoprotein ($p = 0.029$). Interestingly, we detected a negative correlation between high-density lipoprotein and serum ZO contents (Table 3) but no significant link between ZO concentration and BMI or glucose metabolism parameters (all $p > 0.05$).

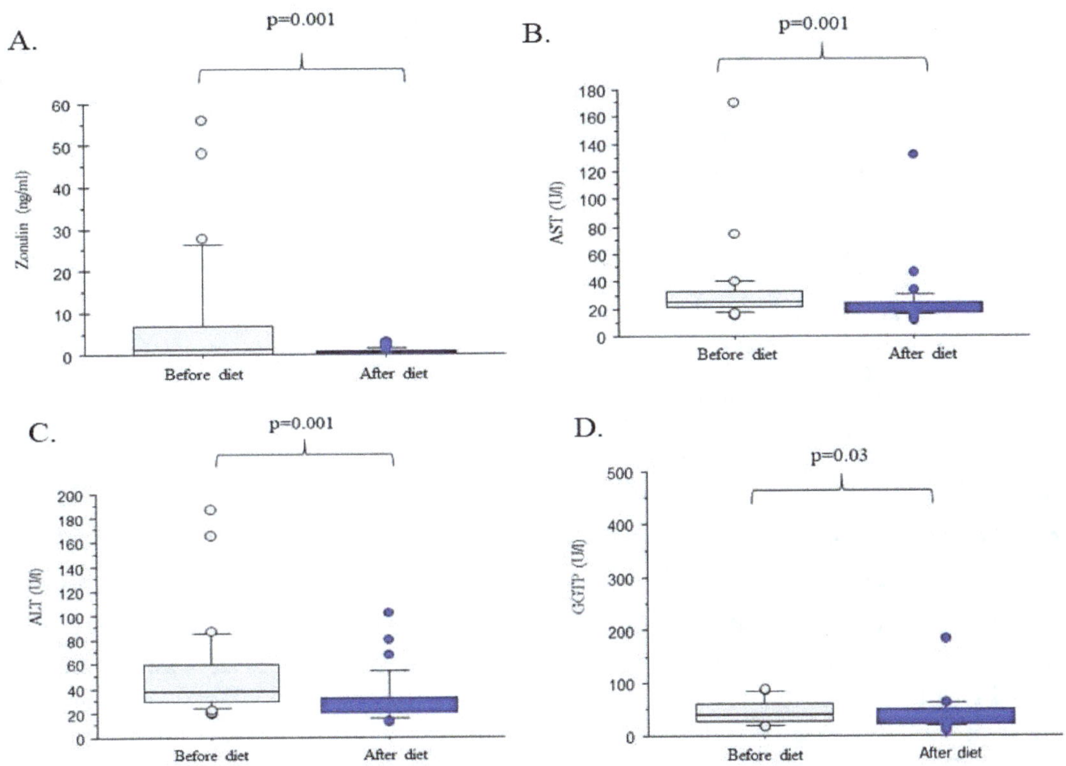

Figure 2. Zonulin concentration and liver function tests before and after the dietetic intervention. (**A**) Zonulin concentration. (**B**) Aspartate aminotransferase (AST) activity. (**C**) Alanine aminotransferase (ALT) activity. (**D**) Gamma-glutamyltransferase (GGTP) activity.

Table 2. Baseline characteristics of the study cohort ($n = 32$), as well as effects of the dietetic intervention.

Parameters	Before Diet	After Diet	p Value
Age (year)	48.03 ±13.13	-	-
Body Mass (kg)	98.76 ± 19.80	91.64 ± 16.60	NS
BMI (kg/m^2)	33.19 ±5.71	30.91 ± 5.45	NS
Fat mass (kg)	38.08 ± 6.06	32.84 ± 9.41	NS
Lean body mass (kg)	60.93 ± 12.90	58.48 ± 12.04	NS
Water content (kg)	45.25 ± 9.16	43.81 ± 8.07	NS
Fatty liver (Hamaguchi score)	2.87 ± 0.60	1.40 ± 0.93	0.009
Triacylglycerols (mg/dL)	219.09 ± 326.01	166.31 ± 219.71	0.036
Total cholesterol (mg/dL)	206.06 ± 52.54	200.56 ± 45.44	NS
High density lipoprotein (mg/dL)	44.84 ± 10.09	49.47 ± 14.47	NS
Low density lipoprotein (mg/dL)	121.15 ± 33.43	122. ± 60.32	NS
Total lipids (mg/dL)	731.06 ± 414.63	706.44 ± 300.43	NS
Glucose (mg/mL)	104.50 ± 20.01	100.78 ± 10.72	NS
Insulin (U/mL)	17.90 ± 11.44	7.47 ± 5.34	0.034
HOMA-IR	4.85 ± 3.14	1.89 ± 1.36	0.041

Abbreviation: BMI, body mass index; HOMA-IR, homeostasis model assessment of insulin resistance; NS, not significant.

Table 3. Correlations between serum zonulin content and patient characteristics.

Parameters	RHO	p Value
Age (years)	0.05	NS
Body Mass (kg)	<0.01	NS
BMI (kg/m^2)	(−) 0.18	NS
Fat mass (kg)	(−) 0.13	NS
Fat content (%)	(−) 0.17	NS
Lean body mass (kg)	0.09	NS
Water content (kg)	0.13	NS
Aspartate transaminase (U/L)	0.35	0.041
Alanine transaminase (U/L)	0.36	0.043
Gamma-glutamyltransferase (U/L)	0.19	NS
Triacylglycerols (mg/dL)	0.17	NS
Total cholesterol (mg/dL)	0.22	NS
High density lipoprotein (mg/dL)	(−) 0.30	0.029
Low density lipoprotein (mg/dL)	0.37	0.032
Total Lipids (mg/dL)	0.31	0.041
Glucose (mg/mL)	(−) 0.07	NS
Insulin (U/mL)	(−) 0.10	NS
Fatty liver (Hamaguchi score)	0.33	0.037

3.2. The Content of Zonulin in the Serum May be Related to the Increase in Fiber Consumption

The analysis of nutritional diaries showed that all patients included in the analysis followed the suggested nutritional recommendations. No significant deviations from the proposed energy supply or key nutrients intake (proteins, carbohydrates and fats) were observed. Recruited patients consumed on average 29.24 ± 10.97 g fiber per day, which is higher than the fiber intake as estimated for the Polish population i.e., 19 g per day [29]. This included: soluble fiber (6.69 ± 3.21 g per day) and insoluble fiber (17.44 ± 7.11 g per day). These calculations were done based on a 72-h recall diary subjected to the Fineli base. According to the database of the Institute of Nutrition in Poland (IZZ), the calculated fiber content was slightly lower: 28.18 g per day. We estimated that the frequency of consumption of fruits and vegetables rose among study participants from a few portions per week to a few portions per day (Table 4). The Spearman's rank analysis indicated the existence of a correlation between the amount of fiber in the diet and the concentration of ZO in blood ($p = 0.043$) (Table 5). No other analyzed food constituent proved to correlate with serum ZO ($p > 0.05$).

Table 4. Changes in patients dietary patterns during the intervention.

Frequency of Consumption According FFQ	Before Intervention	During the Diet	Change in Frequency
Dairy products	Every day	Every day	No change
Cereal products	A few times a day	A few times a day	No change
Fats	Every day	Every day	No change
Fruits	A few times a week	A few times a day	Increased
Vegetables and grains	A few times a week	A few times a day	Increased
Poultry, meet and fish	Every day	Every day	No change

Abbreviation: FFQ, food frequency questionnaire.

Table 5. Correlations between diet compounds and the concentration of serum zonulin.

Parameters	RHO	*p* Value
Energy of diet (kcal)	0.01	NS
Protein (%)	(−) 0.01	NS
Fat (%)	(−) 0.07	NS
Saturated fatty acids (%)	(−) 0.02	NS
Monounsaturated fatty acids (%)	(−) 0.03	NS
Polyunsaturated fatty acids (%)	(−) 0.20	NS
Carbohydrates (%)	0.07	NS
Fiber (%)	(−) 0.30	0.043

4. Discussion

NAFLD is turning into the most frequent liver condition worldwide, and diet is regarded as one of the major drivers of the steatotic phenotype. In our study we reconstructed the amount and frequency of dietary fiber consumption in patients with NAFLD and detected a correlation between ZO concentrations and fiber intake. Previously Pacifico et al. [13] demonstrated that serum ZO is elevated in the blood of obese children with NAFLD: ZO values correlated with steatosis, but not with fibrosis score, or the presence of nonalcoholic steatohepatitis (NASH). The results presented in the study by Hendy et al. [21] suggest that ZO levels could be used for a quick and noninvasive diagnosis of liver inflammation. It was observed that once ZO serum concentration in a patient with NAFLD exceeds 8.3 ng/mL, the risk of developing NASH rises considerably. This might be significant for the development of non-invasive biomarker panels that could substitute liver biopsy [21].

In our study, we examined whether ZO concentrations decreased during the introduction of calorie restriction. Damms-Machado et al. [30] evaluated ZO contents in the stool of patients who underwent a 12-month dietary intervention and showed that ZO concentrations in stool are not influenced by weight reduction therapy and do not correlate with anthropometric variables. In our study we did not detect any significant correlations between serum ZO concentrations and the reduction of body mass parameters either. Similarly to Damms-Machado et al. [30], we observed a correlation between ZO and lipid parameters, enzymatic markers of liver injury and the degree of steatosis. Damms-Machado et al. observed that ZO concentrations among patients did not change significantly with steatosis over the course of the study [30]. They concluded that the lack of fecal ZO alterations after the intervention was a result of ZO-independent regulation of TJ occurring during the course of weight reduction, which leads to the differences in gut permeability. We previously described a similar phenomenon (ZO-independent regulation) in a study in which we analyzed the permeability of the barrier after the use of colostrum [15].

We speculate that changes in fiber intake were responsible for the reduction of ZO in the blood of our patients. Indeed, the level of dietary fiber rose in the diet of our patients regardless of the supply of other nutrients (i.e., fat or carbohydrates). Our patients were subjected to control visits four times during the 6-month dietary intervention, and only those patients who significantly increased their frequency of consumption and supply of soluble and insoluble fiber completed the study. A recently published study found that fruit fiber consumption was associated with improved liver health [31]. According to these results it was postulated that higher insoluble fiber consumption ($\geq$7.5 g/day) leads to improvements in fatty liver parameters. Notably, a regression model proved a relationship between liver status and fruit derived fiber [31]. Our study has some limitations that should be kept in mind when interpreting the data. First of all, included patients were not biopsied, hence we did not have data on the presence of NASH. For the same reason, we did not have data on the degree of liver fibrosis in our patients. We focused on the measurements of zonulin, however other markers of intestinal permeability such as bacterial endotoxin levels, LBP protein concentration or serum citrulin might also provide additional insights into observed changes during diet. Finally, the studied cohort was relatively small and the Hamaguchi score [28], which we applied to quantify NAFLD, has not been thoroughly validated in Caucasians.

Why might the above results be of significance? Fibers fermenting in the intestine provide short-chain fatty acids that fulfill a protective and nourishing role for colonocytes, ensuring the preservation of the intestinal barrier [32]. Plant fiber provides nourishment for intestinal microbiota, which are of prime importance to the preservation of the intestinal barrier integrity [31]. The results of our study imply that appropriate fiber intake helps to maintain the proper structure and function of the intestinal barrier. The lifestyle recommendations for successful management of NAFLD promote fruit and vegetables in the diet of NAFLD patients. As our results show, the increased supply of fiber positively influences the NAFLD-associated parameters and it should be promoted among the specialists designing the diets for patients with fatty liver.

Author Contributions: Conceptualization, E.S., P.M. and M.K.; Methodology E.S., J.R.W.; Software, D.M.; Validation, K.R.; Formal Analysis, M.K., E.S., P.M.; Investigation D.J.M., M.C.R., J.R.; Resources, K.R., E.S.; Data Curation, K.R.; Writing-Original Draft Preparation, E.S., Writing-Review & Editing, M.K.; Visualization, D.M.; Supervision, P.M.; Project Administration, K.R.; Funding Acquisition, E.S.

Acknowledgments: We are grateful to Małgorzta Standowicz, Anna Sabinicz, Małgorzata Napierała for their dietary supervision as well as to Roman Liebe for the proofreading of the manuscript.

References

1. Lechuga, S.; Ivanov, A.I. Disruption of the epithelial barrier during intestinal inflammation: Quest for new molecules and mechanisms. *Biochim. Biophys. Acta* **2017**, *7*, 1183–1194. [CrossRef] [PubMed]
2. Choi, W.; Yeruva, S.; Turner, J.R. Contributions of intestinal epithelial barriers to health and disease. *Exp. Cell Res.* **2017**, *358*, 71–77. [CrossRef] [PubMed]
3. Shimizu, M. Interaction between food substances and the intestinal epithelium. *Biosci. Biotechnol. Biochem.* **2010**, *74*, 232–241. [CrossRef] [PubMed]
4. Peng, X.; Yan, H.; You, Z.; Wang, P.; Wang, S. Effects of enteral supplementation with glutamine granules on intestinal mucosal barrier function in severe burned patients. *Burns* **2004**, *30*, 135–139. [CrossRef] [PubMed]
5. Ding, L.A.; Li, J.S. Effects of glutamine on intestinal permeability and bacterial translocation in TPN-rats with endotoxemia. *World J. Gastroenterol.* **2003**, *9*, 1327–1332. [CrossRef] [PubMed]
6. Watanabe, J.; Fukumoto, K.; Fukushi, E.; Sonoyama, K.; Kawabata, J. Isolation of tryptophan as an inhibitor of ovalbumin permeation and analysis of its suppressive effect on oral sensitization. *Biosci. Biotechnol. Biochem.* **2004**, *68*, 59–65. [CrossRef] [PubMed]
7. Yasumatsu, H.; Tanabe, S. The casein peptide Asn-Pro-Trp-Asp-Gln enforces the intestinal tight junction partly by increasing occludin expression in Caco-2 cells. *Br. J. Nutr.* **2010**, *104*, 951–956. [CrossRef] [PubMed]
8. Hashimoto, K.; Nakayama, T.; Shimizu, M. Effects of beta-lactoglobulin on the tight-junctional stability of Caco-2-SF monolayer. *Biosci. Biotechnol. Biochem.* **1998**, *62*, 1819–1821. [CrossRef] [PubMed]
9. Suzuki, T. Regulation of intestinal epithelial permeability by tight junctions. *Cell. Mol. Life Sci.* **2013**, *70*, 631–659. [CrossRef] [PubMed]
10. Hollon, J.; Puppa, E.L.; Greenwald, B.; Goldberg, E.; Guerrerio, A.; Fasano, A. Effect of gliadin on permeability of intestinal biopsy explants from celiac disease patients and patients with non-celiac gluten sensitivity. *Nutrients* **2015**, *7*, 1565–1576. [CrossRef] [PubMed]

11. Usami, M.; Muraki, K.; Iwamoto, M.; Ohata, A.; Matsushita, E.; Miki, A. Effect of eicosapentaenoic acid (EPA) on tight junction permeability in intestinal monolayer cells. *Clin. Nutr.* **2001**, *20*, 351–359. [CrossRef] [PubMed]
12. Usami, M.L.; Komurasaki, T.; Hanada, A.; Ohata, A.; Matsushita, E.; Miki, A. Effect of gamma-linolenic acid or docosahexaenoic acid on tight junction permeability in intestinal monolayer cells and their mechanism by protein kinase C activation and/or eicosanoid formation. *Nutrition* **2003**, *19*, 150–166. [CrossRef]
13. Pacifico, L.; Bonci, E.; Marandola, L.; Romaggioli, S.; Bascetta, S.; Chiesa, C. Increased circulating zonulin in children with biopsy-proven nonalcoholic fatty liver disease. *World J. Gastroenterol.* **2014**, *20*, 17107–17114. [CrossRef] [PubMed]
14. Fasano, A. Zonulin, regulation of tight junctions, and autoimmune diseases. *Ann. N. Y. Acad. Sci.* **2012**, *1258*, 25–33. [CrossRef] [PubMed]
15. Hałasa, M.; Maciejewska, D.; Baśkiewicz-Hałasa, M.; Machaliński, B.; Safranow, K.; Stachowska, E. Oral Supplementation with Bovine Colostrum Decreases Intestinal Permeability and Stool Concentrations of Zonulin in Athletes. *Nutrients* **2017**, *9*, e370. [CrossRef] [PubMed]
16. European Association for the Study of the Liver (EASL); European Association for the Study of Diabetes (EASD); European Association for the Study of Obesity (EASO). EASL-EASD-EASO Clinical Practice Guidelines for the management of non-alcoholic fatty liver disease. *J. Hepatol.* **2016**, *64*, 1388–1402. [CrossRef] [PubMed]
17. Estes, C.; Anstee, Q.M.; Arias-Loste, M.T.; Bantel, H.; Bellentani, S.; Caballeria, J.; Colombo, M.; Craxi, A.; Crespo, J.; Day, C.P.; et al. Modeling NAFLD Disease Burden in China, France, Germany, Italy, Japan, Spain, United Kingdom, and United States for the period 2016–2030. *J. Hepatol* **2018**, in press. [CrossRef] [PubMed]
18. Henao-Mejia, J.; Elinav, E.; Jin, C.; Hao, L.; Mehal, W.Z.; Strowig, T.; Thaiss, C.A.; Kau, A.L.; Eisenbarth, S.C.; Jurczak, M.J.; et al. Inflammasome-mediated dysbiosis regulates progression of NAFLD and obesity. *Nature* **2012**, *482*, 179–185. [CrossRef] [PubMed]
19. Shen, F.; Zheng, R.D.; Sun, X.Q.; Ding, W.J.; Wang, X.Y.; Fan, J.G. Gut microbiota dysbiosis in patients with non-alcoholic fatty liver disease. *Hepatobiliary Pancreat. Dis. Int.* **2017**, *16*, 375–381. [CrossRef]
20. Miele, L.; Marrone, G.; Lauritano, C.; Cefalo, C.; Gasbarrini, A.; Day, C.; Grieco, A. Gut-liver axis and microbiota in NAFLD: Insight pathophysiology for novel therapeutic target. *Curr. Pharm. Des.* **2013**, *19*, 5314–5324. [CrossRef] [PubMed]
21. Hendy, O.M.; Elsabaawy, M.M.; Aref, M.M.; Khalaf, F.M.; Oda, A.M.A.; El Shazly, H.M. Evaluation of circulating zonulin as a potential marker in the pathogenesis of nonalcoholic fatty liver disease. *Metabolism* **2017**, *69*, 43–50. [CrossRef] [PubMed]
22. Wybranska, I.; Malczewska-Malec, M.; Partyka, L.; Kiec-Wilk, B.; Kosno, K.; Leszczynska-Golabek, I.; Zdzienicka, A.; Gruca, A.; Kwasniak, M.; Dembinska-Kiec, A. Evaluation of genetic predisposition to insulin resistance by nutrient-induced insulin output ratio (NIOR). *Clin. Chem. Lab. Med.* **2007**, *45*, 1124–1132. [CrossRef] [PubMed]
23. Poeta, M.; Pierri, L.; Vajro, P. Gut-Liver Axis Derangement in Non-Alcoholic Fatty Liver Disease. *Children* **2017**, *4*, 66. [CrossRef] [PubMed]
24. Pang, J.; Xu, W.; Zhang, X.; Wong, G.H.; Chan, A.H.; Chan, H.Y.; Tse, C.H.; Shu, S.T.; Choi, P.L.; Chan, H.Y.; et al. Significant positive association of endotoxemia with histological severity in 237 patients with non-alcoholic fatty liver disease. *Aliment. Pharmacol. Ther.* **2017**, *46*, 175–182. [CrossRef] [PubMed]
25. Engstler, A.J.; Aumiller, T.; Degen, C.; Dürr, M.; Weiss, E.; Maier, I.B.; Schattenberg, J.M.; Jin, C.J.; Sellmann, C.; Bergheim, I. Insulin resistance alters hepatic ethanol metabolism: Studies in mice and children with non-alcoholic fatty liver disease. *Gut* **2016**, *65*, 1564–1571. [CrossRef] [PubMed]
26. QuickCalcs. Available online: https://www.graphpad.com/quickcalcs/randomselect2 (accessed on 2 November 2016).
27. Stachowska, E.; Ryterska, K.; Maciejewska, D.; Banaszczak, M.; Milkiewicz, P.; Milkiewicz, M.; Gutowska, I.; Ossowski, P.; Kaczorowska, M.; Jamioł-Milc, D.; et al. Nutritional Strategies for the Individualized Treatment of Non-Alcoholic Fatty Liver Disease (NAFLD) Based on the Nutrient-Induced Insulin Output Ratio (NIOR). *Int. J. Mol. Sci.* **2016**, *17*, 1172. [CrossRef] [PubMed]
28. Hamaguchi, M.; Kojima, T.; Itoh, Y.; Harano, Y.; Fujii, K.; Nakajima, T.; Kato, T.; Takeda, N.; Okuda, J.; Ida, K.; et al. The severity of ultrasonographic findings in nonalcoholic fatty liver disease reflects the

metabolic syndrome and visceral fat accumulation. *Am. J. Gastroenterol.* **2007**, *102*, 2708–2715. [CrossRef] [PubMed]

29. Laskowski, W. *Wartość Odżywcza Diety Polaków Oraz jej Zmiany*; Współczesne Kierunki Działań Prozdrowotnych, red. A.; Wolska-Adamczyk, WSIiZ: Warszawa, Poland, 2015.
30. Damms-Machado, A.; Louis, S.; Schnitzerm, A.; Volynets, V.; Rings, A.; Basrai, M. Gut permeability is related to body weight, fatty liver disease, and insulin resistance in obese individuals undergoing weight reduction. *Am. J. Clin. Nutr.* **2017**, *105*, 127–135. [CrossRef] [PubMed]
31. Cantero, I.; Abete, I.; Monreal, J.I.; Martinez, J.A.; Zulet, M.A. Fruit Fiber Consumption Specifically Improves Liver Health Status in Obese Subjects under Energy Restriction. *Nutrients* **2017**, *9*, e667. [CrossRef] [PubMed]
32. Rinella, M.E.; Sanyal, A.J. Management of NAFLD: A stage-based approach. *Nat. Rev. Gastroenterol. Hepatol.* **2016**, *13*, 196–205. [CrossRef] [PubMed]

15

Dissociation of Fatty Liver and Insulin Resistance in I148M PNPLA3 Carriers: Differences in Diacylglycerol (DAG) FA18:1 Lipid Species as a Possible Explanation

Andras Franko [1,2,3,*], Dietrich Merkel [4], Marketa Kovarova [1,2,3], Miriam Hoene [1], Benjamin A. Jaghutriz [1,2,3], Martin Heni [1,2,3], Alfred Königsrainer [5], Cyrus Papan [4], Stefan Lehr [3,6], Hans-Ulrich Häring [1,2,3] and Andreas Peter [1,2,3]

1 Department of Internal Medicine IV, Division of Endocrinology, Diabetology, Angiology, Nephrology and Clinical Chemistry, University Hospital Tübingen, 72076 Tübingen, Germany; kovarova-marketa@seznam.cz (M.K.); miriam.hoene@med.uni-tuebingen.de (M.H.); benjamin.jaghutriz@med.uni-tuebingen.de (B.A.J.); martin.heni@med.uni-tuebingen.de (M.H.); hans-ulrich.haering@med.uni-tuebingen.de (H.-U.H.); andreas.peter@med.uni-tuebingen.de (A.P.)

2 Institute for Diabetes Research and Metabolic Diseases of the Helmholtz Center Munich, University of Tübingen, 72076 Tübingen, Germany

3 German Center for Diabetes Research (DZD e.V.), 85764 Neuherberg, Germany; stefan.lehr@ddz.uni-duesseldorf.de

4 Sciex Germany GmbH, 64293 Darmstadt, Germany; dietrich.merkel@sciex.com (D.M.); cyrus.papan@sciex.com (C.P.)

5 Department of General, Visceral and Transplant Surgery, University Hospital Tübingen, 72076 Tübingen, Germany; alfred.koenigsrainer@med.uni-tuebingen.de

6 Institute for Clinical Biochemistry and Pathobiochemistry of DDZ, University of Düsseldorf, 40225 Düsseldorf, Germany

* Correspondence: andras.franko@med.uni-tuebingen.de

Abstract: Fatty liver is tightly associated with insulin resistance and the development of type 2 diabetes. I148M variant in patatin-like phospholipase domain-containing protein 3 (PNPLA3) gene is associated with high liver fat but normal insulin sensitivity. The underlying mechanism of the disassociation between high liver fat but normal insulin sensitivity remains obscure. We investigated the effect of I148M variant on hepatic lipidome of subjects with or without fatty liver, using the Lipidyzer method. Liver samples of four groups of subjects consisting of normal liver fat with wild-type PNPLA3 allele (group 1); normal liver fat with variant PNPLA3 allele (group 2); high liver fat with wild-type PNPLA3 allele (group 3); high liver fat with variant PNPLA3 allele (group 4); were analyzed. When high liver fat to normal liver fat groups were compared, wild-type carriers (group 3 vs. group 1) showed similar lipid changes compared to I148M PNPLA3 carriers (group 4 vs. group 2). On the other hand, in wild-type carriers, increased liver fat significantly elevated the proportion of specific DAGs (diacylglycerols), mostly DAG (FA18:1) which, however, remained unchanged in I148M PNPLA3 carriers. Since DAG (FA18:1) has been implicated in hepatic insulin resistance, the unaltered proportion of DAG (FA18:1) in I148M PNPLA3 carriers with fatty liver may explain the normal insulin sensitivity in these subjects.

Keywords: NAFLD; liver; PNPLA3; diacylglycerol; lipidomics

1. Introduction

Nonalcoholic fatty liver disease (NAFLD) is characterized by elevated hepatic lipid content [1]. NAFLD is claimed to be a benign illness, however, it can further develop to nonalcoholic steatohepatitis (NASH), liver fibrosis, cirrhosis and hepatocellular carcinoma [2]. The prevalence of NAFLD is continuously increasing, and currently it is estimated to be higher than 20% in industrialized countries [3]. Despite this high prevalence of NAFLD and its complication NASH, there is no established effective drug therapy, which is generally approved for these illnesses [4]. NAFLD/NASH patients are advised to lose weight with lifestyle intervention (mostly consisting of healthy diet and exercise [4]), however, not all patients benefit from these interventions [5]. To treat NAFLD/NASH, several drugs have been shown to be beneficial in animal models [6,7], and novel activators for peroxisome proliferator-activated receptor (PPAR) (elafibranor) and farnesoid X receptor (FXR) (obeticholic acid) are currently under phase 3 studies in human cohorts with promising results [4]. NAFLD is a strong determinant of insulin sensitivity and the development of type 2 diabetes, however, some distinct genetic causes for the dissociation of liver fat content and insulin sensitivity have been identified [1].

The rs738409 C>G single nucleotide polymorphism (SNP) in the patatin-like phospholipase domain-containing protein 3 (PNPLA3) gene is a common inherited trait, which results in an amino acid exchange I148M leading to a functional mutation of PNPLA3 [8]. At this position, both hetero- (I148M) and homozygous (M148M) variants are described. The prevalence of PNPLA3 variants vary due to ethnicity of the population [9] and 34–37% (I148M) and 4–9% (M148M) are described in studies analyzing German or European-American populations, respectively [8,10]. Several studies demonstrated that I148M PNPLA3 carriers showed an altered metabolic phenotype on nutritional challenges compared to wild-type subjects. Dietary intake of carbohydrates was shown to modify the association between PNPLA3 genotype and circulating triglyceride levels [11]. Carbohydrate overfeeding led to an increased de-novo lipogenesis in proportion to the increase in liver fat and serum triglycerides in subjects with I148I carriers, which however, was not observed in M148M carriers [12]. Furthermore, the M148M PNPLA3 variant influenced the changes in liver fat and docosahexaenoic acid tissue enrichment during a 15–18 months addition of omega 3 fatty acids [13]. The presence of rs738409 SNP was positively associated with elevated liver fat, however, carriers do not show insulin resistance [8,10,14]. On the other hand, some subjects carrying the I148M variant show normal liver fat content, and the function of PNPLA3 in these subjects is not studied yet. PNPLA3 has several enzyme activities, it was reported to be involved in lipid hydrolysis (as a triacylglycerol lipase) and synthesis (as a lysophosphatidic acyltransferase) [15]. The I148M variant is claimed to show lower lipolysis of hepatic triacylglycerols (TAGs) [16] and elevated hepatic TAG synthesis [17]. However, for subjects carrying I148M PNPLA3 variant a lower de novo lipogenesis is also reported [18]. The discrepancy between high liver TAG level and normal insulin sensitivity in I148M carriers is not resolved yet [19], but altered hepatic TAG pattern, especially long-chain polyunsaturated fatty acid content, is reported in rodent and human studies analyzing I148M PNPLA3 carriers [14,15,20]. Several lipid species are implicated in the state of insulin resistance in patients with NAFLD [21]. Elevated ceramide [15] or high diacylglycerol (DAG) content [22,23] have been found in the liver of rodents and human subjects with insulin resistance. Furthermore, quantitative measurements of unique lipid species have been previously shown to broaden our knowledge to understand complex diseases, such as cystic fibrosis, NAFLD and type 1 diabetes and pave the way for identifying new lipid biomarkers [24–27].

In order (i) to study the function of I148M PNPLA3 variant in subjects with normal and high liver fat and, (ii) to analyze the key metabolic lipids (also including detailed measurements of individual ceramide and diacylglycerol lipid species) possibly evoking insulin resistance in wild-type but not in I148M PNPLA3 carriers, we studied the liver of subjects with normal and high hepatic TAG content with wild-type or I148M (heterozygous), as well as M148M (homozygous) PNPLA3 variants. To examine the lipid profiles, we decided to perform an unbiased lipidomic analysis using the Lipidyzer platform, which was originally established for plasma samples [28], therefore, we applied it with an adapted protocol for solid tissue lysates.

2. Materials and Methods

2.1. Human Liver Samples, Total Liver TAG Measurement, and PNPLA3 Genotyping

For the analysis of liver tissue samples, a cohort of European descendent men and women undergoing liver surgery at the Department of General, Visceral, and Transplant Surgery at the University Hospital of Tübingen was included in the present study. None of the patients were diagnosed with an abuse of alcohol, however, no detailed data on alcohol consumption was consistently collected. The liver tissue was collected during hepatic surgery that was performed for different reasons, e.g., hepatic hemangioma, curative resection of hepatic metastases of colorectal malignancies or hepatocellular carcinoma. Patients fasted overnight before collection of liver samples. Exclusion criteria were viral hepatitis infection and liver cirrhosis. Informed, written consent was obtained from all participants, and the Ethics Committee of the University of Tübingen approved the protocol (239/2013BO1) according to the Declaration of Helsinki. Liver samples taken from normal, non-diseased tissue, were quickly frozen in liquid nitrogen and stored at −80 °C. To measure total TAG content, liver tissue samples were homogenized in phosphate buffered saline containing 1% Triton X-100 with a TissueLyser (Qiagen, Hilden, Germany) and determined as described previously [29,30]. In order to match subjects for similar body weight, BMI (body mass index) and age as well as for different liver TAG content, subjects showing less than 3.0% liver TAG content were classified as normal TAG group and subjects showing more than 4.3% liver TAG were classified as high TAG group. For PNPLA3 genotyping, total DNA was isolated from whole blood using a DNA isolation kit (NucleoSpin, Macherey and Nagel, Düren, Germany). The I148M PNPLA3 variations were genotyped using Sequenom's massARRAY System with iPLEX software (Sequenom, Hamburg, Germany) as described previously [14]. Plasma ALT levels were measured with routine clinical chemistry [10].

2.2. Lipidyzer Platform

The Lipidyzer™ platform (SCIEX, Darmstadt, Germany) was used for the whole lipid analysis work flow. Briefly, 10 mg liver was solubilized in 100 μL internal standards (IS, Avanti Polar Lipids, Inc., AL, USA) and 200 μL of 75% methanol was added and hepatic lipids were extracted using methyl tert-butyl ether (MTBE) as described previously [31]. The following isotopes labeled internal standards were used dCER(d16:0), dCE(16:0), dCE(16:1), dCE(18:1), dCE(18:2), dCE(20:3), dCE(20:4), dCE(20:5), dCE(22:6), dDAG(16:0/16:0), dDAG(16:0/18:0), dDAG(16:0/18:1), dDAG(16:0/18:2), dDAG(16:0/18:3), dDAG(16:0/20:4), dDAG(16:0/20:5), dDAG(16:0/22:6), dFFA(16:0), dFFA(17:1), dLPC(16:0), dLPE(18:0), dPC(16:0/16:1), dPC(16:0/18:1), dPC(16:0/18:2), dPC(16:0/18:3), dPC(16:0/20:3), dPC(16:0/20:4), dPC(16:0/20:5), dPC(16:0/22:4), dPC(16:0/22:5), dPC(16:0/22:6), dPE(18:0/18:1), dPE(18:0/18:2), dPE(18:0/18:3), dPE(18:0/20:3), dPE(18:0/20:4), dPE(18:0/20:5), dPE(18:0/22:5), dPE(18:0/22:6), dSM(16:0), dSM(18:1), dSM(24:0), dSM(24:1), dTAG50:1-FA16:0, dTAG52:1-FA18:0, dTAG52:2-FA18:1, dTAG52:3-FA18:2, dTAG52:4-FA18:3, dTAG54:4-FA20:3, dTAG54:5-FA20:4, dTAG56:7-FA22:6, dDCER(16:0), dHCER(16:0), and dLCER(16:0). For each injection, 50 μL of extracted lipid sample was introduced by flow injection (FIA) using a Nexera X2 system (Shimadzu Germany GmbH, Duisburg, Germany), equipped with a 50 μL-sample loop. A Lipidyzer™ included 750 × 0.05 mm PEEKsil™ (Trajan Scientific Europe Ltd., Milton Keynes, UK) sample tubing was used to connect the autosampler valve with the grounding union on the electrospray ionization (ESI) source, and a 350 × 0.05 mm PEEKsil™ (Trajan Scientific Europe Ltd, Milton Keynes, UK) sample tubing was used to connect the grounding union with the ESI electrode having 65 μm inner diameter. The flow profile for the flow injection was determined by the Lipidyzer™ acquisition method with a flow rate during the data acquisition period being 7 μL/min. The mass spectrometry analysis was performed on a Lipidyzer™ Platform, including the Sciex QTRAP® (SCIEX, Darmstadt, Germany) 5500 system equipped with SelexION® (SCIEX, Darmstadt, Germany) Technology (differential mobility separation, DMS). Multiple reaction monitoring (MRM) was used to target and quantitate several hundreds of lipid molecular species from 13 different lipid classes. All samples were first measured in positive and negative polarity with SelexION separation, followed by measurement without SelexION separation. The acquisition time per sample took approximately 25 min for the complete acquisition. All data was acquired and processed automatically using the Lipid Manager Workflow software (SCIEX, Darmstadt, Germany). This provides the following data tables: (i) quantitative results for each lipid class as a sum of individual species; (ii) mole percent composition obtained computationally from lipid molecular species data; and (iii) accurate lipid species compositions.

2.3. Data Evaluation

Missing values, which were not possible to measure and showed zero values, were handled as follows: From the complete data set, lipids, which showed higher values than zero at least in 50% of any group were kept, otherwise they were discarded. To determine whether the groups separate from each other according to PNPLA3 genotype or hepatic TAG content, multivariate partial least squares discriminant analysis (PLS-DA) were performed using soft independent modeling of class analogy (SIMCA, Umetrics, Umea, Sweden). The 761 individual lipid species and the 84 sum of lipid classes were summed up and these 845 lipid values were logarithmic transformed and were statistically evaluated, as written below.

2.4. Statistics

To determine statistical different lipid species caused by increased liver fat, group 3 (high liver fat, wild-type PNPLA3 allele) was compared to group 1 (normal liver fat, wild-type PNPLA3 allele) as well as group 4 (high liver fat, variant PNPLA3 allele) was compared to group 2 (normal liver fat, variant PNPLA3 allele) using GraphPad Prism (7.03). Multiple t-tests were applied with Benjamini-Hochberg correction and false discovery rate (FDR) was set <5%. Furthermore, analysis of variance (ANOVA) with Holm-Sidak´s post hoc test were applied as it is indicated.

3. Results

3.1. Characteristics of Study Groups

To distinguish between the effect of increased liver TAG content and PNPLA3 genotype, subjects were matched for body weight, BMI and age and divided into the following four groups: subjects showing normal liver fat with wild-type PNPLA3 (group 1); normal liver fat with I148M PNPLA3 variant (group 2); high liver fat with wild-type PNPLA3 (group 3) and high liver fat with I148M PNPLA3 variant (group 4) (Table 1).

Our study groups consisted of overweight subjects with similar age, weight, BMI and ALT levels (Table 1). Liver fat was significantly higher in high TAG groups compared to normal groups (group 3 vs. 1 and group 4 vs. 2), but was not different in I148M PNPLA3 carriers compared to wild-type carriers (Table 1). Both variant PNPLA3 groups (groups 2 and 4) consisted of one homozygous M148M (MM) carrier and the rest of the subjects were heterozygous I148M (IM) carriers (Table 1).

In order to study the effect of I148M PNPLA3 variant on hepatic lipid species in subjects with normal and high liver fat, a complete lipid profile was measured using a novel Lipidyzer approach. The following 13 lipid classes were analyzed: triacylglycerols (TAG), diacylglycerols (DAG), free fatty acids (FFA), ceramides (CER), dihydroceramides (DCER), hexosylceramides (HCER), lactosylceramides (LCER), phosphatidylcholines (PC), lysophosphatidylcholines (LPC), phosphatidylethanolamines (PE), lysophosphatidylethanolamines (LPE), cholesterol esters (CE), and sphingomyelins (SM). Among these lipid classes, 761 individual lipid species were measured and 84 sums of individual classes were calculated. In order to investigate whether the hepatic lipid profile of groups with different PNPLA3 genotype or various liver TAG content was different from each other, we first analyzed the data with multivariate partial least squares discriminant analysis (PLS-DA). PLS-DA showed that normal TAG, wt PNPLA3 (group 1) and high TAG, wt PNPLA3 (group 3) formed distinct groups, however, normal TAG, var PNPLA3 (group 2) and high TAG, var PNPLA3 (group 4) groups were rather similar taking into account all 761 individual lipid species (Figure 1).

Table 1. Characteristics of study groups.

Characteristic	Group 1 Normal TAG, wt PNPLA3	Group 2 Normal TAG, var PNPLA3	Group 3 High TAG, wt PNPLA3	Group 4 High TAG, var PNPLA3
Age (years)	59.3 ± 12.6	60.6 ± 16.4	64.0 ± 11.8	65.1 ± 14.5
Body weight (kg)	79.3 ± 9.9	80.3 ± 13.5	86.2 ± 11.1	87.1 ± 13.1
BMI (kg/m^2)	26.1 ± 3.2	28.0 ± 5.3	31.0 ± 3.4	28.6 ± 4.0
ALT (U/L)	24.5 ± 6.5	22.0 ± 5.2	31.1 ± 9.3	35.7 ± 18.6
Liver fat (%)	1.1 ± 0.8	1.5 ± 0.7	5.9 ± 2.0 ***	7.6 ± 2.9 ***
PNPLA3 ^{148} (II/IM/MM) (n)	8/0/0	0/7/1	8/0/0	0/6/1
Sex (m/f) (n)	6/2	4/4	5/3	5/2
Number of subjects (n)	8	8	8	7

TAG: liver triacylglycerol content; PNPLA3: patatin-like phospholipase domain-containing protein 3; wt: wild-type allele with I148I; var: I148M variants, which encode I148M (heterozygous) or M148M (homozygous) variants, respectively. ALT: alanine aminotransferase, BMI: body mass index. Numbers denote averages ± standard deviations in the first five lines. *** denotes significant differences between group 3 vs. 1 or group 4 vs. 2 illustrating the effect of liver TAG content; $p < 0.001$. Significance was calculated using ANOVA with Holm-Sidak's post-hoc test and assumed as $p < 0.05$. By the comparisons of group 2 vs. 1 and group 4 vs. 3 no significant differences were found for I148M PNPLA3 variant vs. wild-type carriers.

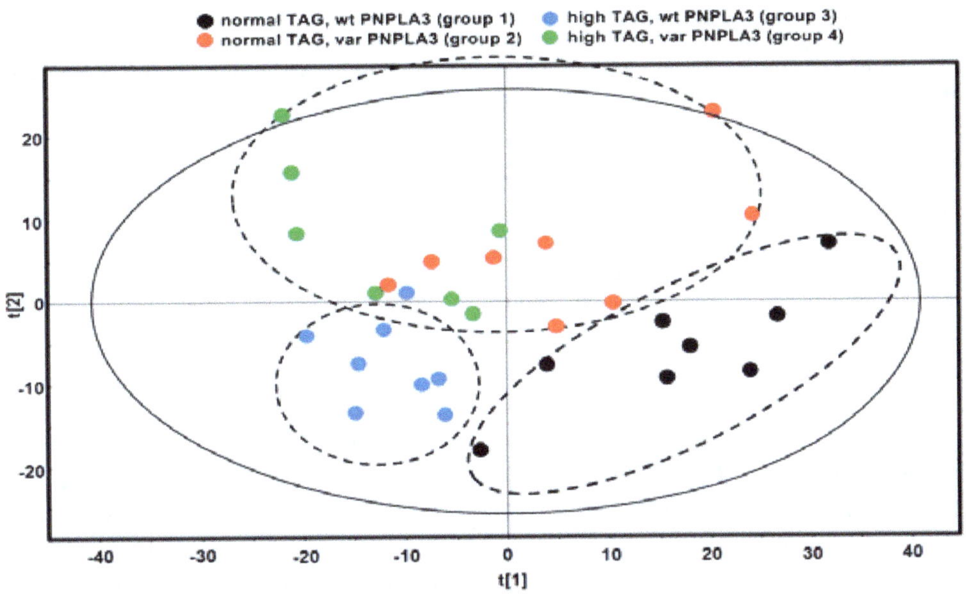

Figure 1. Partial least squares discriminant analysis (PLS-DA) score plot. Each spot represents one liver sample of the denoted group according to component 1 (x axis) and 2 (y axis). Dashed lines denote possible separation of the groups taking into account all 761 individual lipid species. TAG: liver triacylglycerol content; wt: wild-type allele with I148I; var: I148M variants, which encode I148M (heterozygous) or M148M (homozygous) variants, respectively.

3.2. I148M PNPLA3 Variant Does Not Change Relative Total Lipid Contents

As a next step, the sum of 13 lipid classes was evaluated. With increased liver TAG content, we observed significantly higher relative levels of TAG and DAG lipids (calculated as % of total lipid content, Table 2). On the other hand, the relative content of FFA, CER, DCER, HCER, PC, LPC, PE,

LPE, and SM were significantly lower in high TAG vs. normal TAG groups (Table 2). The presence of I148M PNPLA3 variant did not significantly influence the sum of lipid classes (Table 2).

Table 2. Relative lipid contents of individual classes in percent.

Lipid Class %	Group 1 Normal TAG, wt PNPLA3	Group 2 Normal TAG, var PNPLA3	Group 3 High TAG, wt PNPLA3	Group 4 High TAG, var PNPLA3
TAG	25.63 ± 12.49	35.22 ± 15.30	68.64 ± 11.26 ***	69.82 ± 11.86 ***
DAG	0.60 ± 0.30	0.57 ± 0.17	0.92 ± 0.12 *	1.02 ± 0.20 **
FFA	7.23 ± 3.57	6.07 ± 1.71	2.60 ± 1.12 ***	2.37 ± 1.01 **
CER	0.26 ± 0.04	0.25 ± 0.08	0.10 ± 0.03 ***	0.10 ± 0.05 ***
DCER	0.03 ± 0.01	0.03 ± 0.01	0.01 ± 0.00 ***	0.01 ± 0.01 ***
HCER	0.07 ± 0.02	0.05 ± 0.02	0.03 ± 0.01 ***	0.02 ± 0.01 **
LCER	0.06 ± 0.01	0.06 ± 0.03	0.04 ± 0.02	0.03 ± 0.01
PC	38.51 ± 9.74	33.06 ± 8.63	14.86 ± 6.41 ***	14.75 ± 7.83 ***
LPC	0.66 ± 0.22	0.60 ± 0.14	0.24 ± 0.14 ***	0.28 ± 0.17 **
PE	20.43 ± 5.80	17.84 ± 5.82	8.19 ± 3.24 ***	7.29 ± 3.10 ***
LPE	0.16 ± 0.05	0.15 ± 0.03	0.06 ± 0.03 ***	0.07 ± 0.04 ***
CE	2.45 ± 0.34	2.84 ± 0.45	2.73 ± 0.60	2.86 ± 0.48
SM	3.91 ± 0.81	3.28 ± 0.81	1.59 ± 0.67 ***	1.37 ± 0.60 ***

TAG: triacylglycerols, DAG: diacylglycerols, FFA: free fatty acids, CER: ceramides, DCER: dihydroceramides, HCER: hexosylceramides, LCER: lactosylceramides, PC: phosphatidylcholines, LPC: lysophosphatidylcholines, PE: phosphatidylethanolamines, LPE: lysophosphatidylethanolamines, CE: cholesterol esters, SM: sphingomyelins; wt: wild-type allele with I148I; var: I148M variants, which encode I148M (heterozygous) or M148M (homozygous) variants, respectively. Numbers denote averages ± standard deviations. * denotes significant differences between group 3 vs. 1 or group 4 vs. 2 illustrating the effect of liver TAG content; * $p < 0.05$, ** $p < 0.01$, *** $p < 0.001$. Significance was calculated using ANOVA with Holm-Sidak´s post-hoc test and assumed as $p < 0.05$. By the comparisons of group 2 vs. 1 and group 4 vs. 3 no significant differences were found for I148M PNPLA3 variant vs. wild-type carriers.

3.3. Increased Liver Fat Content Is Associated with High Proportion of DAG (FA18:1) Species in Subjects with Wild-Type PNPLA3, However, DAG (FA18:1) Remains Unchanged in I148M PNPLA3 Carriers

In order to study the combination effect of increased liver fat content and PNPLA3 variant on hepatic lipid profile, we next compared the relative proportion of lipid species in high liver fat to normal liver fat groups from subjects with wild-type (group 3 vs. 1) or with I148M PNPLA3 carriers (group 4 vs. 2) (Figure 2 and Supplementary Table S1).

Although in wild-type carriers many individual DAGs decreased with increased hepatic TAG content, the proportion of DAG (C16:0/C18:1), DAG (C18:0/C18:1), DAG (C18:1/C18:1) as well as the sum of DAG (FA18:1) were increased (Figure 2, first diagram, grey arrows). These FA18:1 containing DAGs remained however, unaltered in I148M PNPLA3 variant carriers (Figure 2, second diagram, grey arrows). Furthermore, various individual CE lipids decreased and many individual shorter TAG lipids were elevated in wild-type subjects due to increased liver TAG content; however, these lipid species remained unaltered in I148M PNPLA3 carriers (Supplementary Table S1). These results indicate that subjects, who carry the I148M PNPLA3 variant do not increase the proportion of DAG (FA18:1) lipid levels upon increased hepatic TAG, although many other lipid species altered similarly compared to wild-type carriers.

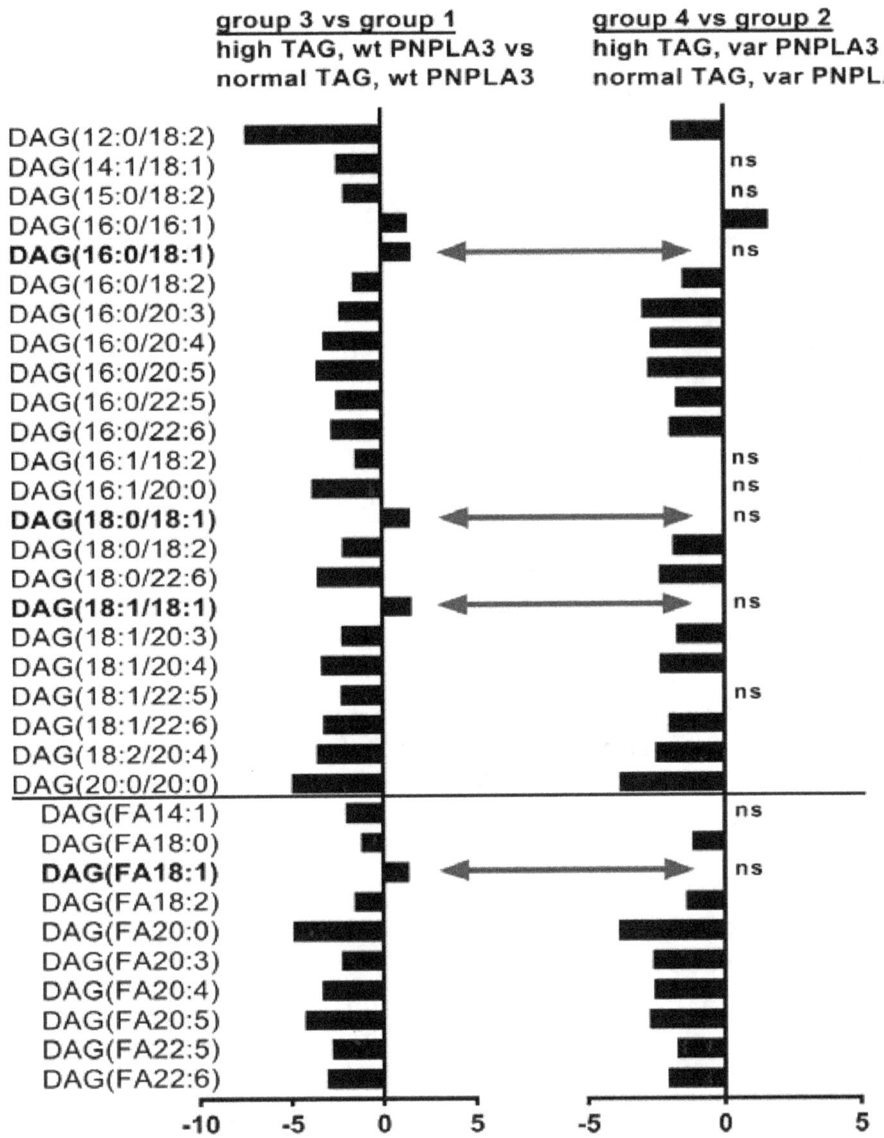

Figure 2. Individual DAGs and their sums, which are significantly changed due to high vs. normal TAG level in subjects with wild-type PNPLA3 (first diagram) and I148M PNPLA3 carriers (second diagram). Column diagrams depict linear fold changes calculated from the proportion of relative individual lipid species and sums, which were significantly altered due to increased liver TAG content in wild-type carriers (first diagram) or in I148M PNPLA3 carriers (second diagram). Positive ratios denote lipids, which are higher in subjects with high liver TAG content compared to normal TAG group, whereas negative ratios denote lipids, which are lower in subjects with high liver TAG content compared to normal TAG group. For DAGs, both fatty acid chains were determined (see as DAG(XX:X/YY:Y). First numbers denote the length of fatty acid chain and second number after ":" denote the number of double bounds. DAG(FAXX:X) depict the sum of DAGs with the denoted fatty acid chain (FA). Bold lipids depict DAG(FA18:1) lipid species, which are significantly increased in wild-type PNPLA3 carriers, but remained unchanged in I148M PNPLA3 carriers. TAG: liver triacylglycerol content; wt: wild-type allele with I148I; var: I148M variants, which encode I148M (heterozygous) or M148M (homozygous) variants, respectively. ns: non-significant differences.

4. Discussion and Conclusions

The I148M PNPLA3 variant is the best characterized and most influential determinant of NAFLD [19]. Patients with this PNPLA3 variant are also characterized with higher prevalence of NASH and hepatocellular carcinoma [19], however, they show normal insulin sensitivity [8,14].

The underlying mechanism of the dissociation between high liver fat and normal insulin sensitivity remains obscure.

To study the key lipid species, which are known to be involved in hepatic insulin resistance [21], we performed an unbiased lipidomics analysis from subjects with high and normal liver fat content with wild-type or I148M PNPLA3 variants. Our data showed, that DAG (FA18:1) lipid species were elevated in the liver of wild-type carriers upon increased liver fat content, however, these lipids remained unaltered in subjects, who carry I148M PNPLA3 variant. When the enzyme activity of wild-type PNPLA3 was characterized, PNPLA3 (as a lipase) showed hydrolytic activity against mono- (MAG), di- and triacylglycerols [16]. Interestingly, Huang et al. also observed that the wild-type PNPLA3 strongly prefers oleic acid (C18:1)-containing lipids as a substrate [16]. The I148M PNPLA3 variant was not studied for substrate preference, but it showed diminished hydrolytic activity against MAG, DAG, and TAG. Since PNPLA3 owns substrate specificity against C18:1 containing lipids and the I148M variant show diminished TAG hydrolytic activity, it is conceivable that in patients carrying I148M variant, liver TAG(FA18:1) species could be recognized by PNPLA3 in a lower extent than in wild-type carriers, hindering accumulation of DAG (FA18:1). On the other hand, PNPLA3 is not the only lipase metabolizing TAGs and some TAG(FA18:1) lipid species showed lower, but some others showed higher levels in the I148M PNPLA3 variants upon increased liver TAG content when compared to wild-type carriers (Supplementary Table S1).

Rodent studies suggested that PNPLA3 deficiency is associated with reduced hepatic DAG (FA18:1) content. High sucrose diet fed PNPLA3 knock-out mice showed only a decreased DAG (34:1) lipid content (probably consisting of DAG (C16:0/C18:1)), however, all other lipid species (phosphatidic acid, lysophosphatidic acid, TAG or other DAGs) remained unchanged compared to wild-type controls [17]. Knock-down of PNPLA3 with antisense oligonucleotides in high fat diet fed rats resulted in ameliorated hepatic steatosis, which was associated with lower total DAG, DAG (C16:0/C18:1) and DAG (C18:1/C18:1) lipid species [32]. The authors suggested that the lower levels of these DAGs led to reduction of membrane localized (activated) protein kinase C epsilon (PKCε) level, which could not interfere with insulin signaling and this mechanism was postulated to be the reason for the improved hepatic insulin sensitivity found in these PNPLA3 knock-down animals [32]. Jelenik et al. demonstrated that mice with hepatic insulin resistance showed elevated hepatic content of DAG (C16:0/C18:1) and DAG (C18:1/C18:1) lipid species, which was associated with higher PKCε activation and reduced tyrosine phosphorylation of insulin receptor substrate 2 (IRS2), which is a hallmark of impaired insulin signaling [22]. Furthermore, there are several studies [33], which reported an elevated DAG (FA18:1) content in skeletal muscle of insulin resistant patients with obesity [34] and type 2 diabetes [35]. The authors claimed that the elevated DAG levels could activate PKC theta (PKCΘ) in skeletal muscle, which in turn leads to impaired insulin signaling causing insulin resistance [35]. Moreover, elevated DAG species were also found in the liver of subjects, who showed hepatic insulin resistance [23]. From all DAG species, hepatic cytosolic level of DAG (C16:0/C18:1) and DAG (C18:1/C18:1) were two out of the three most abundant DAGs, which showed the strongest negative correlation with suppression of endogenous glucose production (EGP) [23]. Impairment in the suppression of EGP is a sign for hepatic insulin resistance [36,37]. These results indicate that elevation of DAG (FA18:1) lipid species is a characteristic of insulin resistance and impairment in PNPLA3 function is associated with lower content of hepatic DAG (FA18:1). Whether DAG (FA18:1) is attributed to specific functions in comparison with other DAG species is not clarified yet, but it is possible. Dziewulska et al. reported that mice fed with triolein diet (TAG (C18:1/C18:1/C18:1)) resulted in elevation of DAG (FA18:1) in skeletal muscle, which was associated with higher PKCΘ activation but lower serine phosphorylation of protein kinase B and diminished glucose transporter 4 translocation [38], which are signs for insulin resistance [39]. The authors also observed, that tristearin diet (TAG (C18:0/C18:0/C18:0)) feeding did not exert the former effects [38]. These results suggest that DAG (FA18:1) possibly owns a specific function among DAGs and it could serve as a strong activator of PKCs (PKCε in the liver and PKCΘ in the muscle), which, in turn, could diminish insulin signaling.

The PNPLA3 variant cohorts consisted of mainly heterozygous (I148M) and only one homozygous (M148M) carrier in each group. Previous studies also combined hetero- and homozygous carriers of the PNPLA3 variant and did not report differences in lipid composition or insulin sensitivity [8,10,15,40] suggesting that these variants are comparable. We, therefore, also analyzed all carriers of the PNPLA3 I148M/M148M genotype together in this study. The limitations of this study are the comorbidities of the subjects and the small study size, however, surgical samples were necessary to obtain sufficient tissue for the lipid analyses. Since we did not have detailed information on alcohol intake of the patients, it cannot be ruled out that some of the patients had an alcohol related cause of fatty liver rather than NAFLD. Furthermore, liver samples fulfilling the criteria of the defined groups were very limited. Therefore, further sub-analyses exceeding the initially selected groups are not possible in this study.

We found that fatty liver in subjects carrying wild-type PNPLA3 is associated with elevated hepatic DAG (FA18:1) content. These DAG (FA18:1) species were shown to disturb insulin signaling in the liver [22,23]. However, hepatic DAG (FA18:1) species remained unaltered in subjects carrying I148M PNPLA3 allele with fatty liver. Therefore, we hypothesize that I148M PNPLA3 carriers may be protected from insulin resistance via the unaltered content of DAG (FA18:1) species due to impaired PNPLA3 TAG lipase activity (Figure 3).

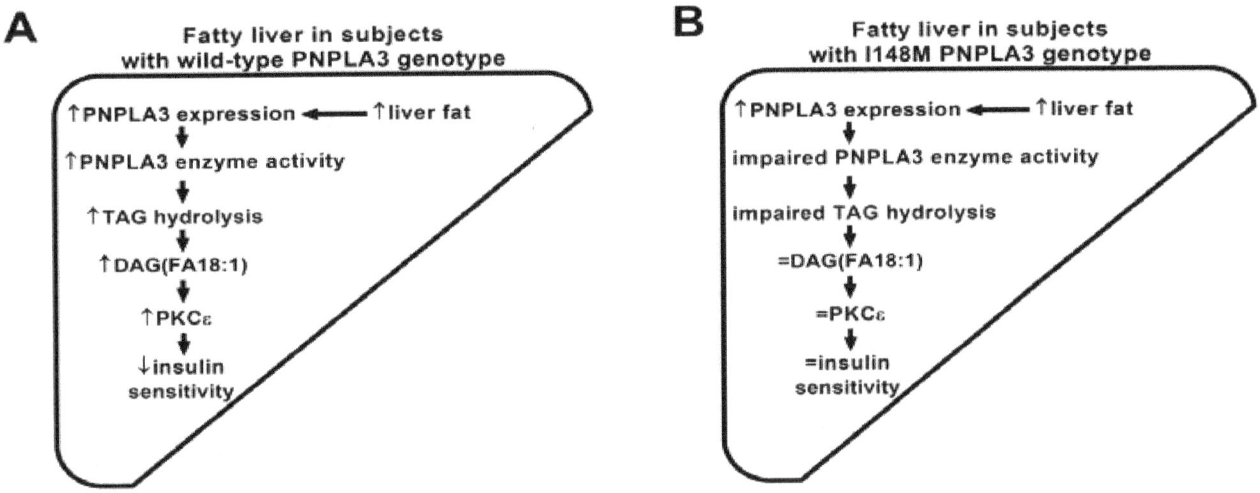

Figure 3. Hypothetical scheme showing the association between I148M PNPLA3 variant and normal insulin sensitivity. Arrows demonstrate higher (↑) or lower (↓) metabolite contents, transcript levels, enzyme activities or insulin sensitivity, respectively. Previous data shown, that liver fat content is positively associated with hepatic mRNA expression of PNPLA3, which was not altered in subjects carrying I148M PNPLA3 variant [10,14,32]. Our lipid data showed that hepatic DAG (FA18:1) species were elevated in fatty liver of wild-type PNPLA3 carriers (**A**), which was not observed in I148M PNPLA3 carriers (**B**). Elevated DAG (FA18:1) in the liver was shown to activate protein kinase c epsilon (PKCε), which, in turn, reduces tyrosin phosphorylation of insulin receptor substrate 2 (P-Tyr-IRS2) [22,23], a key molecule transmitting insulin signaling in the liver [39]. Due to the attenuated tyrosin phosphorylation of IRS2, insulin sensitivity could be impaired (as postulated earlier [22,23]) in subjects carrying wild-type PNPLA3 allele, but not in I148M PNPLA3 carriers.

Table S1. Lipids and sum of lipids, which are significantly changed due to high vs. normal TAG level in subjects.

Author Contributions: Conceptualization: S.L., A.P., H.-U.H.; methodology: D.M., C.P.; formal analysis: A.F., M.K., M.H. (Miriam Hoene); resources: B.A.J., M.H. (Martin Heni), A.K.; writing—original draft: A.F.; writing—review and editing: D.M., M.K., M.H. (Miriam Hoene), B.A.J., M.H. (Martin Heni), A.K., C.P., S.L., H.-U.H., and A.P.

Acknowledgments: We gratefully acknowledge Ines Wagener, Andreas Vosseler, Anja Dessecker, and Ellen Kollmar for their assistance in the clinical studies (Department of Internal Medicine IV, Division of Endocrinology, Diabetology, Angiology, Nephrology, and Clinical Chemistry, University Hospital Tübingen, Tübingen, Germany).

Abbreviations

DAG	Diacylglycerol
FA	Fatty acid
group 1	Subjects with normal liver fat and wild-type PNPLA3
group 2	Subjects with normal liver fat and I148M/M148M PNPLA3 variants
group 3	Subjects with high TAG and wild-type PNPLA3
group 4	Subjects with high TAG and I148M/M148M PNPLA3 variants
MAG	Monoacylglycerol
NAFLD	Nonalcoholic fatty liver disease
NASH	Nonalcoholic steatohepatitis
PKC	Protein kinase C
PNPLA3	Patatin-like phospholipase domain-containing protein 3
TAG	Triacylglycerol
var	I148M/M148M PNPLA3 variants
wt	Wild-type PNPLA3 allele

References

1. Stefan, N.; Schick, F.; Häring, H.U. Causes, characteristics, and consequences of metabolically unhealthy normal weight in humans. *Cell Metab.* **2017**, *26*, 292–300. [CrossRef] [PubMed]
2. Stefan, N.; Häring, H.U. The role of hepatokines in metabolism. *Nat. Rev. Endocrinol.* **2013**, *9*, 144–152. [CrossRef] [PubMed]
3. Younossi, Z.; Anstee, Q.M.; Marietti, M.; Hardy, T.; Henry, L.; Eslam, M.; George, J.; Bugianesi, E. Global burden of NAFLD and NASH: Trends, predictions, risk factors and prevention. *Nat. Rev. Gastroenterol. Hepatol.* **2018**, *15*, 11–20. [CrossRef] [PubMed]
4. Younossi, Z.M.; Loomba, R.; Rinella, M.E.; Bugianesi, E.; Marchesini, G.; Neuschwander-Tetri, B.A.; Serfaty, L.; Negro, F.; Caldwell, S.H.; Ratziu, V.; et al. Current and future therapeutic regimens for nonalcoholic fatty liver disease and nonalcoholic steatohepatitis. *Hepatology* **2018**, *68*, 361–371. [CrossRef] [PubMed]
5. Böhm, A.; Hoffmann, C.; Irmler, M.; Schneeweiss, P.; Schnauder, G.; Sailer, C.; Schmid, V.; Hudemann, J.; Machann, J.; Schick, F.; et al. TGF-beta contributes to impaired exercise response by suppression of mitochondrial key regulators in skeletal muscle. *Diabetes* **2016**, *65*, 2849–2861. [CrossRef] [PubMed]
6. Franko, A.; Neschen, S.; Rozman, J.; Rathkolb, B.; Aichler, M.; Feuchtinger, A.; Brachthäuser, L.; Neff, F.; Kovarova, M.; Wolf, E.; et al. Bezafibrate ameliorates diabetes via reduced steatosis and improved hepatic insulin sensitivity in diabetic TallyHo mice. *Mol. Metab.* **2017**, *6*, 256–266. [CrossRef] [PubMed]
7. Goto, T.; Itoh, M.; Suganami, T.; Kanai, S.; Shirakawa, I.; Sakai, T.; Asakawa, M.; Yoneyama, T.; Kai, T.; Ogawa, Y. Obeticholic acid protects against hepatocyte death and liver fibrosis in a murine model of nonalcoholic steatohepatitis. *Sci. Rep.* **2018**, *8*, 8157. [CrossRef] [PubMed]
8. Romeo, S.; Kozlitina, J.; Xing, C.; Pertsemlidis, A.; Cox, D.; Pennacchio, L.A.; Boerwinkle, E.; Cohen, J.C.; Hobbs, H.H. Genetic variation in PNPLA3 confers susceptibility to nonalcoholic fatty liver disease. *Nat. Genet.* **2008**, *40*, 1461–1465. [CrossRef] [PubMed]
9. Baclig, M.O.; Lozano-Kuhne, J.P.; Mapua, C.A.; Gopez-Cervantes, J.; Natividad, F.F. Genetic variation I148M in patatin-like phospholipase 3 gene and risk of non-alcoholic fatty liver disease among Filipinos. *Int. J. Clin. Exp. Med.* **2014**, *7*, 2129–2136. [PubMed]
10. Kantartzis, K.; Peter, A.; Machicao, F.; Machann, J.; Wagner, S.; Konigsrainer, I.; Konigsrainer, A.; Schick, F.; Fritsche, A.; Häring, H.U.; et al. Dissociation between fatty liver and insulin resistance in humans carrying a variant of the patatin-like phospholipase 3 gene. *Diabetes* **2009**, *58*, 2616–2623. [CrossRef] [PubMed]
11. Stojkovic, I.A.; Ericson, U.; Rukh, G.; Riddestrale, M.; Romeo, S.; Orho-Melander, M. The PNPLA3 Ile148Met interacts with overweight and dietary intakes on fasting triglyceride levels. *Genes Nutr.* **2014**, *9*, 388. [CrossRef] [PubMed]

12. Sevastianova, K.; Santos, A.; Kotronen, A.; Hakkarainen, A.; Makkonen, J.; Silander, K.; Peltonen, M.; Romeo, S.; Lundbom, J.; Lundbom, N.; et al. Effect of short-term carbohydrate overfeeding and long-term weight loss on liver fat in overweight humans. *Am. J. Clin. Nutr.* **2012**, *96*, 727–734. [CrossRef] [PubMed]
13. Scorletti, E.; West, A.L.; Bhatia, L.; Hoile, S.P.; McCormick, K.G.; Burdge, G.C.; Lillycrop, K.A.; Clough, G.F.; Calder, P.C.; Byrne, C.D. Treating liver fat and serum triglyceride levels in NAFLD, effects of PNPLA3 and TM6SF2 genotypes: Results from the WELCOME trial. *J. Hepatol.* **2015**, *63*, 1476–1483. [CrossRef] [PubMed]
14. Peter, A.; Kovarova, M.; Nadalin, S.; Cermak, T.; Konigsrainer, A.; Machicao, F.; Stefan, N.; Häring, H.U.; Schleicher, E. PNPLA3 variant I148M is associated with altered hepatic lipid composition in humans. *Diabetologia* **2014**, *57*, 2103–2107. [CrossRef] [PubMed]
15. Luukkonen, P.K.; Zhou, Y.; Sadevirta, S.; Leivonen, M.; Arola, J.; Oresic, M.; Hyotylainen, T.; Yki-Jarvinen, H. Hepatic ceramides dissociate steatosis and insulin resistance in patients with non-alcoholic fatty liver disease. *J. Hepatol.* **2016**, *64*, 1167–1175. [CrossRef] [PubMed]
16. Huang, Y.; Cohen, J.C.; Hobbs, H.H. Expression and characterization of a PNPLA3 protein isoform (I148M) associated with nonalcoholic fatty liver disease. *J. Biol. Chem.* **2011**, *286*, 37085–37093. [CrossRef] [PubMed]
17. Kumari, M.; Schoiswohl, G.; Chitraju, C.; Paar, M.; Cornaciu, I.; Rangrez, A.Y.; Wongsiriroj, N.; Nagy, H.M.; Ivanova, P.T.; Scott, S.A.; et al. Adiponutrin functions as a nutritionally regulated lysophosphatidic acid acyltransferase. *Cell Metab.* **2012**, *15*, 691–702. [CrossRef] [PubMed]
18. Mancina, R.M.; Matikainen, N.; Maglio, C.; Soderlund, S.; Lundbom, N.; Hakkarainen, A.; Rametta, R.; Mozzi, E.; Fargion, S.; Valenti, L.; et al. Paradoxical dissociation between hepatic fat content and de novo lipogenesis due to PNPLA3 sequence variant. *J. Clin. Endocrinol. Metab.* **2015**, *100*, 821–825.
19. Petaja, E.M.; Yki-Jarvinen, H. Definitions of normal liver fat and the association of insulin sensitivity with acquired and genetic NAFLD-A systematic review. *Int. J. Mol. Sci.* **2016**, *17*, 633. [CrossRef] [PubMed]
20. Li, J.Z.; Huang, Y.; Karaman, R.; Ivanova, P.T.; Brown, H.A.; Roddy, T.; Castro-Perez, J.; Cohen, J.C.; Hobbs, H.H. Chronic overexpression of PNPLA3I148M in mouse liver causes hepatic steatosis. *J. Clin. Investig.* **2012**, *122*, 4130–4144. [CrossRef] [PubMed]
21. Samuel, V.T.; Shulman, G.I. Nonalcoholic fatty liver disease as a nexus of metabolic and hepatic diseases. *Cell Metab.* **2018**, *27*, 22–41. [CrossRef] [PubMed]
22. Jelenik, T.; Kaul, K.; Sequaris, G.; Flogel, U.; Phielix, E.; Kotzka, J.; Knebel, B.; Fahlbusch, P.; Horbelt, T.; Lehr, S.; et al. Mechanisms of insulin resistance in primary and secondary nonalcoholic fatty liver. *Diabetes* **2017**, *66*, 2241–2253. [CrossRef] [PubMed]
23. Ter Horst, K.W.; Gilijamse, P.W.; Versteeg, R.I.; Ackermans, M.T.; Nederveen, A.J.; la Fleur, S.E.; Romijn, J.A.; Nieuwdorp, M.; Zhang, D.; Samuel, V.T.; et al. Hepatic diacylglycerol-associated protein kinase cepsilon translocation links hepatic steatosis to hepatic insulin resistance in humans. *Cell Rep.* **2017**, *19*, 1997–2004. [CrossRef] [PubMed]
24. Ollero, M. Methods for the study of lipid metabolites in cystic fibrosis. *J. Cyst. Fibros.* **2004**, *3*, 97–98. [CrossRef] [PubMed]
25. Lehmann, R.; Franken, H.; Dammeier, S.; Rosenbaum, L.; Kantartzis, K.; Peter, A.; Zell, A.; Adam, P.; Li, J.; Xu, G.; et al. Circulating lysophosphatidylcholines are markers of a metabolically benign nonalcoholic fatty liver. *Diabetes Care* **2013**, *36*, 2331–2338. [CrossRef] [PubMed]
26. Franko, A.; Huypens, P.; Neschen, S.; Irmler, M.; Rozman, J.; Rathkolb, B.; Neff, F.; Prehn, C.; Dubois, G.; Baumann, M.; et al. Bezafibrate improves insulin sensitivity and metabolic flexibility in STZ-induced diabetic mice. *Diabetes* **2016**, *65*, 2540–2552. [CrossRef] [PubMed]
27. Markgraf, D.F.; Al-Hasani, H.; Lehr, S. Lipidomics-reshaping the analysis and perception of type 2 diabetes. *Int. J. Mol. Sci.* **2016**, *17*, 1841. [CrossRef] [PubMed]
28. Ubhi, B.K. Direct Infusion-Tandem Mass Spectrometry (DI-MS/MS) analysis of complex lipids in human plasma and serum using the lipidyzer platform. *Methods Mol. Biol.* **2018**, *1730*, 227–236. [PubMed]
29. Peter, A.; Kantartzis, K.; Machicao, F.; Machann, J.; Wagner, S.; Templin, S.; Königsrainer, I.; Königsrainer, A.; Schick, F.; Fritsche, A.; et al. Visceral obesity modulates the impact of apolipoprotein C3 gene variants on liver fat content. *Int. J. Obes.* **2012**, *36*, 774–782. [CrossRef] [PubMed]
30. Franko, A.; Kovarova, M.; Feil, S.; Feil, R.; Wagner, R.; Heni, M.; Köngisrainer, A.; Ruoß, M.; Nüssler, A.K.; Weigert, C.; et al. cGMP-dependent protein kinase I (cGKI) modulates human hepatic stellate cell activation. *Metabolism* **2018**, *88*, 22–30. [CrossRef] [PubMed]

31. Chen, S.; Hoene, M.; Li, J.; Li, Y.; Zhao, X.; Häring, H.U.; Schleicher, E.D.; Weigert, C.; Xu, G.; Lehmann, R. Simultaneous extraction of metabolome and lipidome with methyl tert-butyl ether from a single small tissue sample for ultra-high performance liquid chromatography/mass spectrometry. *J. Chromatogr. A* **2013**, *1298*, 9–16. [CrossRef] [PubMed]
32. Kumashiro, N.; Yoshimura, T.; Cantley, J.L.; Majumdar, S.K.; Guebre-Egziabher, F.; Kursawe, R.; Vatner, D.F.; Fat, I.; Kahn, M.; Erion, D.M.; et al. Role of patatin-like phospholipase domain-containing 3 on lipid-induced hepatic steatosis and insulin resistance in rats. *Hepatology* **2013**, *57*, 1763–1772. [CrossRef] [PubMed]
33. Amati, F. Revisiting the diacylglycerol-induced insulin resistance hypothesis. *Obes. Rev.* **2012**, *13*, 40–50. [CrossRef] [PubMed]
34. Moro, C.; Galgani, J.E.; Luu, L.; Pasarica, M.; Mairal, A.; Bajpeyi, S.; Schmitz, G.; Langin, D.; Liebisch, G.; Smith, S.R. Influence of gender, obesity, and muscle lipase activity on intramyocellular lipids in sedentary individuals. *J. Clin. Endocrinol. Metab.* **2009**, *94*, 3440–3447. [CrossRef] [PubMed]
35. Szendroedi, J.; Yoshimura, T.; Phielix, E.; Koliaki, C.; Marcucci, M.; Zhang, D.; Jelenik, T.; Muller, J.; Herder, C.; Nowotny, P.; et al. Role of diacylglycerol activation of PKCtheta in lipid-induced muscle insulin resistance in humans. *Proc. Natl. Acad. Sci. USA* **2014**, *111*, 9597–9602. [CrossRef] [PubMed]
36. Franko, A.; von Kleist-Retzow, J.C.; Neschen, S.; Wu, M.; Schommers, P.; Böse, M.; Kunze, A.; Hartmann, U.; Sanchez-Lasheras, C.; Stoehr, O.; et al. Liver adapts mitochondrial function to insulin resistant and diabetic states in mice. *J. Hepatol.* **2014**, *60*, 816–823. [CrossRef] [PubMed]
37. Ayala, J.E.; Bracy, D.P.; McGuinness, O.P.; Wasserman, D.H. Considerations in the design of hyperinsulinemic-euglycemic clamps in the conscious mouse. *Diabetes* **2006**, *55*, 390–397. [CrossRef] [PubMed]
38. Dziewulska, A.; Dobrzyn, P.; Jazurek, M.; Pyrkowska, A.; Ntambi, J.M.; Dobrzyn, A. Monounsaturated fatty acids are required for membrane translocation of protein kinase C-theta induced by lipid overload in skeletal muscle. *Mol. Membr. Biol.* **2012**, *29*, 309–320. [CrossRef] [PubMed]
39. Boucher, J.; Kleinridders, A.; Kahn, C.R. Insulin receptor signaling in normal and insulin-resistant states. *Cold Spring Harb. Perspect. Biol.* **2014**, *6*, a009191. [CrossRef] [PubMed]
40. Hyysalo, J.; Gopalacharyulu, P.; Bian, H.; Hyotylainen, T.; Leivonen, M.; Jaser, N.; Juuti, A.; Honka, M.J.; Nuutila, P.; Olkkonen, V.M.; et al. Circulating triacylglycerol signatures in nonalcoholic fatty liver disease associated with the I148M variant in PNPLA3 and with obesity. *Diabetes* **2014**, *63*, 312–322. [CrossRef] [PubMed]

16

Non-Alcoholic Fatty Liver Disease in Overweight Children: Role of Fructose Intake and Dietary Pattern

Anika Nier [1], Annette Brandt [1], Ina Barbara Conzelmann [2], Yelda Özel [2] and Ina Bergheim [1,*]

[1] Department of Nutritional Sciences, Molecular Nutritional Science, University of Vienna, A-1090 Vienna, Austria; anika.nier@univie.ac.at (A.N.); annette.brandt@univie.ac.at (A.B.)

[2] Department of Nutritional Medicine, (180), University of Hohenheim, D-70599 Stuttgart, Germany; ina.conzelmann@gmx.de (I.B.C.); yelda@directbox.com (Y.Ö.)

[*] Correspondence: ina.bergheim@univie.ac.at

Abstract: The role of nutrition and diet in the development of non-alcoholic fatty liver disease (NAFLD) is still not fully understood. In the present study, we determined if dietary pattern and markers of intestinal permeability differ between overweight children with and without NAFLD. In addition, in a feasibility study, we assessed the effect of a moderate dietary intervention only focusing on nutrients identified to differ between groups on markers of intestinal barrier function and health status. Anthropometric data, dietary intake, metabolic parameters, and markers of inflammation, as well as of intestinal permeability, were assessed in overweight children ($n = 89$, aged 5–9) and normal-weight healthy controls ($n = 36$, aged 5–9). Sixteen children suffered from early signs of NAFLD, e.g., steatosis grade 1 as determined by ultrasound. Twelve children showing early signs of NAFLD were enrolled in the intervention study ($n = 6$ intervention, $n = 6$ control). Body mass index (BMI), BMI standard deviation score (BMI-SDS), and waist circumference were significantly higher in NAFLD children than in overweight children without NAFLD. Levels of bacterial endotoxin, lipopolysaccharide-binding protein (LBP), and proinflammatory markers like interleukin 6 (IL-6) and tumor necrosis factor α (TNFα) were also significantly higher in overweight children with NAFLD compared to those without. Total energy and carbohydrate intake were higher in NAFLD children than in those without. The higher carbohydrate intake mainly resulted from a higher total fructose and glucose intake derived from a significantly higher consumption of sugar-sweetened beverages. When counseling children with NAFLD regarding fructose intake (four times, 30–60 min within 1 year; one one-on-one counseling and three group counselings), neither alanine aminotransferase (ALT) nor aspartate aminotransferase (AST) activity in serum changed; however, diastolic blood pressure ($p < 0.05$) and bacterial endotoxin levels ($p = 0.06$) decreased markedly in the intervention group after one year. Similar changes were not found in uncounseled children. Our results suggest that a sugar-rich diet might contribute to the development of early stages of NAFLD in overweight children, and that moderate dietary counseling might improve the metabolic status of overweight children with NAFLD.

Keywords: children; overweight; NAFLD; fructose; dietary pattern; dietary intervention

---

1. Introduction

Non-alcoholic fatty liver disease (NAFLD) comprises a wide spectrum of diseases ranging from simple steatosis afflicted with fat accumulation to steatohepatitis, fibrosis, and even cirrhosis or hepatocellular carcinoma [1]. Results of epidemiological studies suggest that NAFLD is, by now, the most prevalent liver disease in the world [2]. Contrary to many other liver diseases, NAFLD is not a disease only found in adults, but, with a still increasing prevalence, is estimated to also affect 8% of normal-weight and up to 34% of overweight children and adolescents [3–5]. Despite intense research efforts, mechanisms underlying the onset and progression of the disease are still not fully understood, and therapies other than lifestyle interventions are not yet available. However, lifestyle interventions, be it general caloric restriction diets, or low-fat or low-carbohydrate diets with or without increased physical activity, are frequently afflicted with low compliance and high drop-out, as well as relapse rates, in both children and adults [6–8].

Similar to the results in epidemiological and clinical studies [9–12], results of animal studies analyzing the role of diet in the development of NAFLD, as well as mechanisms involved, suggest that both general overnutrition and a diet rich in certain macronutrients like saturated fat and/or sugars like fructose are critical in the onset of NAFLD [13–16]. For example, it was shown that not only obese (ob/ob) mice, but also mice fed a diet rich in saturated fats and/or fructose develop liver steatosis and early signs of hepatic inflammation within several weeks [17–19]. Furthermore, it was repeatedly shown in these dietary models that the development of NAFLD was associated with alterations of intestinal barrier function and elevated bacterial endotoxin levels. In line with these findings, results of our own group and others suggest that, in adults and children with NAFLD, the development of the disease is not only associated with general overnutriton, but also, frequently, an elevated intake of fructose and fat, as well as alterations of markers of intestinal barrier function [10,12,20–22]. However, whether or not general overnutriton or the intake of a specific dietary pattern is critical in the development of NAFLD and associated intestinal barrier dysfunction is yet to be fully clarified.

Starting from this background, the aim of the present study was to determine if the dietary pattern and lifestyle of overweight children without NAFLD differs from overweight children showing early signs of NAFLD. Accordingly, overweight children randomly recruited in primary schools, sports clubs, and kindergartens were stratified by results of liver ultrasounds in overweight children with and without NAFLD. For comparison, a group of normal-weight healthy children were enrolled in the study. Furthermore, to determine if moderate dietary counseling, focusing only on parameters identified to be critical in the dietary pattern of overweight children with NAFLD, is an approach to improve the health status of overweight children with NAFLD, some of the overweight children with NAFLD were enrolled in a feasibility study.

2. Materials and Methods

2.1. Subjects

All children were recruited from the so-called "Hohenheim Fructose Intervention (HoFI) study" registered at http://clinicaltrials.gov (NCT01306396). The ethics committee of the Landesärztekammer Baden-Württemberg (Stuttgart, Germany) approved the present study, which was then performed in accordance with the ethical standards laid down in the Declaration of Helsinki (2008). Participants were recruited between April 2009 and December 2010 primarily through elementary schools in Stuttgart and the greater area of Stuttgart, Southern Germany. All subjects and their guardians gave written informed consent to participate in the study. A total of 92 overweight children aged 5–9 years without any known signs of NAFLD or other metabolic diseases before being enrolled in the study were included, while 3 children had to be excluded from the baseline analysis due to underreporting (overweight children without NAFLD: $n = 2$; overweight children with NAFLD: $n = 1$). Of the 17 overweight children identified to suffer from early stages of NAFLD, all agreed to participate in the feasibility study detailed below. Eight of the overweight children with NAFLD were selected to be in the intervention group and nine agreed to serve as controls. Despite selecting the groups, four of the 17 children enrolled in the intervention study dropped out of the study for personal reasons (three controls and one intervention child), and one child had to be excluded from the final analysis of the feasibility study as it was identified as a case of underreporting (intervention group). In addition, data from 36 healthy normal-weight children aged 5–9 reported in previously published studies [21,23] were included in the study for comparison. None of the children included had a known history of (i) steatohepatitis, (ii) renal insufficiency, (iii) diabetes type 1 and 2, (iv) chronic diseases of the gastrointestinal tract, or (v) taking lipid-lowering drugs or drugs affecting lipid metabolism. All children enrolled in the study were prepubertal as defined by Marshall and Tanner [24,25]. Pubertal status was assessed as described by Maier et al. [26]. None of the children enrolled in the feasibility study changed pubertal status throughout the study.

2.2. Laboratory Measurements, Blood Pressure, and Abdominal Ultrasound

From all participants, the following parameters were assessed in a routine laboratory (Sindelfingen, Germany) as described previously [27]: alanine aminotransferase (ALT), aspartate aminotransferase (AST), fasting blood glucose, blood lipids, and uric acid in serum, as previously described in a fasting venous blood sample. In addition, concentrations of active plasminogen activator inhibitor 1 (PAI-1; LOXO, Dossenheim, Germany), lipopolysaccharide-binding protein (LBP; Abnova, Taipei City, Taiwan), leptin and insulin (both Hölzel GmbH, Wildberg, Germany), tumor necrosis factor α (TNFα; IBL international GmbH, Hamburg, Germany), adiponectin (TECOmedical AG, Sissach, Switzerland), c-reactive protein (CRP; DRG Instruments GmbH, Marburg, Germany), and interleukin 6 (IL-6; R&D Systems, Abingdon, UK) were determined in plasma using commercially available ELISA kits. Systolic and diastolic blood pressure, as well as liver status using ultrasound, were measured and defined as detailed previously [27].

2.3. Bacterial Endotoxin

Plasma endotoxin levels were determined by an endpoint enzymatic assay based on limulus amebocyte lysate, as detailed previously [12].

2.4. Glucose Metabolism

Glucose tolerance was determined as detailed previously [26]. The homeostasis model assessment for insulin resistance (HOMA-IR) index (HOMA-IR = (fasting insulin (μIU/mL) × fasting glucose (mmol/L))/22.5) was used to determine insulin resistance.

2.5. Assessment of Dietary Intake and Leisure Time Activities

Dietary intake using two separated 24-h recalls, including one weekend day, as well as sportive and sitting leisure time activities, was assessed as previously described [28]. For analyzing nutritional intake, the EBISpro software was used. This software contains the German Nutrient Database (in German: Bundeslebensmittelschlüssel, see also https://www.blsdb.de) which includes data of about 10,000 foods and covers average nutritional values, including free fructose (137 constituent data per food item). Dietary underreporting was determined by calculating the ratio of reported total energy intake and predicted individual basal metabolic rate, as described previously by others [29]. Only recalls with ratios above the age- and sex-specific cut-off values being 1.04 for boys and 1.01 for girls were included in the nutritional analysis [30]. Based on this calculation, three underreporters were identified (overweight children without NAFLD: n = 2, overweight children with NAFLD: n = 1) and excluded from the final analysis and the analysis of the feasibility study, respectively.

2.6. Anthropometric Measurements and Socio-Demographic Data

Anthropometric parameters were assessed by a nutritionist as detailed by Maier et al. [26]. Furthermore, socio-demographic characteristics such as age, gender, and ethnicity were recorded.

2.7. Dietary Intervention Study

In children enrolled in the feasibility study, all measurements assessing health status and anthropometry were repeated after one year. As the feasibility study required a high compliance of participants in the intervention group, e.g., attending regular meetings (one one-on-one meeting and three group meetings), and altering dietary patterns and intake throughout the year of study, study participants and their guardians were allowed to choose study arms to avoid further drop-out (for study design, see also Figure 1). Based on daily fructose intake as determined in two independently performed 24-h recalls before the study, children enrolled in the intervention group were advised to reduce their daily fructose intake by ~50% in a personal nutritional counseling taking place at the beginning of the study in the presence of their respective guardians. Counseling was then repeated every three months in small groups (see Figure 1). Children, as well as guardians, were counseled independently. Training of both children and guardians focused primarily on a change in dietary pattern and included strategies to identify fructose-rich foods, e.g., foods containing marked amounts of sucrose or fructose, such as lemonades, chocolates, cookies, cakes, and candies, as well as foods containing large amounts of free fructose, such as juices, certain fruits, and vegetables, and to replace these foods with foods containing less fructose of the same food category (e.g., exchanging cookies with rusk, replacing sucrose with glucose when making cakes or cookies, or to consume diet lemonades instead of sugar lemonades (for details, see Reference [27])). In brief, before the study, several games, quizzes, and experiments suitable for training children were developed and their feasibility was assessed in a pilot study [27]. For example, to illustrate the effect of sugar-sweetened beverages on dental health, a tooth was put into a glass containing a sugar-sweetened beverage for two days. Furthermore, children were asked to guess the number of sugar cubes contained in different foods (e.g., ketchup, chocolate bars, and sugar-sweetened beverages) by selecting glasses filled with different numbers of sugar cubes to enhance the awareness of sugar content in commercially available products. Additionally, a small supermarket with food dummies was built to practice children's behavior in the supermarket. Children were then asked to pick their favorite foods, and, together with a trained nutritionist, foods with high amounts of sugars were identified and alternative foods with lower sugar content were selected. Upon request, participants and their respective guardians enrolled in the control group received one dietary counseling based on general recommendations for a healthy nutrition as recommended by the German Nutrition Society.

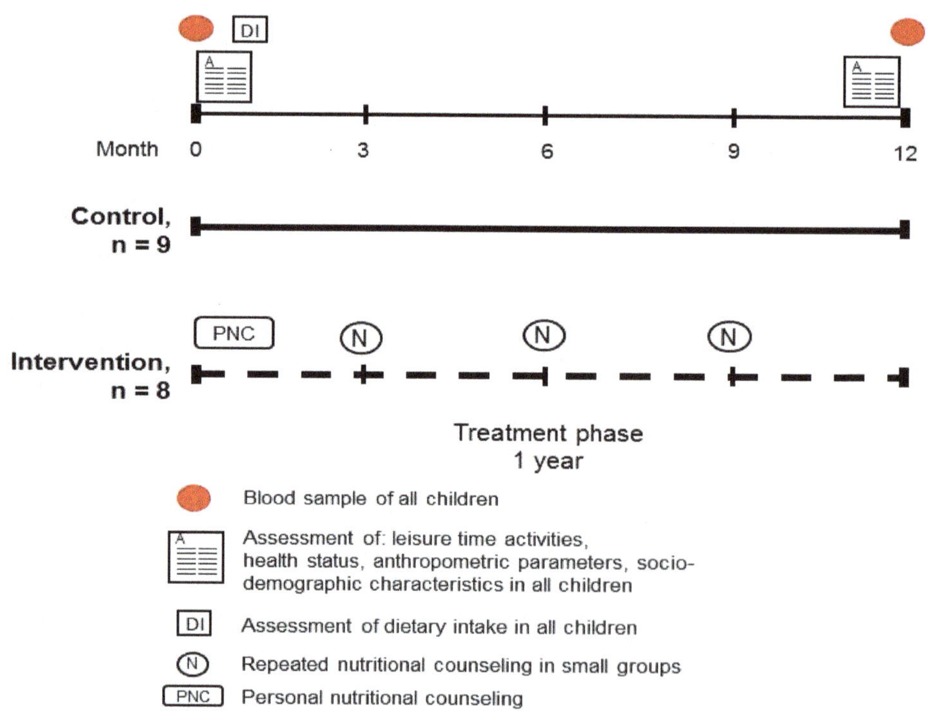

Figure 1. Study design of the feasibility study assessing the effect of a moderate dietary intervention focusing only on the reduction of fructose intake (−50%) on the health status of overweight children with non-alcoholic fatty liver disease (NAFLD).

2.8. Statistical Analyses

Data were analyzed using the *t*-test and Mann–Whitney U test for comparing overweight children with and without NAFLD and to compare baseline and end values of children enrolled in the pilot feasibility study. Healthy, normal-weight children were not included in the statistical analysis, but are shown for comparison. The Wilcoxon test was used to compare baseline and end values within the two groups enrolled in the feasibility study. Fisher's exact test was used for comparing gender and ethnicity (GraphPad Prism, version 7.03, 2017, GraphPad Software Inc., San Diego, CA, USA). Identified outliers using Grubbs' test were excluded from baseline analyses. As mentioned above, children identified as underreporters were removed from the final analyses and the analysis of the feasibility study. A p-value ≤ 0.05 was defined as the level of significance.

3. Results

3.1. Characteristics of the Study Participants

As shown in Table 1, neither age nor distribution of gender or ethnicity differed between overweight children with and without early signs of NAFLD. Body weight was significantly higher in overweight children with NAFLD than in those without, while height was similar. Accordingly, body mass index (BMI), BMI standard deviation score (BMI-SDS), and waist circumference were also significantly higher in overweight children with NAFLD (see Table 1 and Figure 2). Neither leptin nor adiponectin, nor ratio of leptin and adiponectin differed between overweight groups. Still, as expected, all of these parameters differed markedly from those of normal-weight children who were included in the study for comparison only (see Table 1).

Table 1. Characteristics of normal-weight healthy children and overweight children with and without non-alcoholic fatty liver disease (NAFLD).

	NW	OW	NAFLD
n	36	73	16
Sex (male/female)	20/16	33/40	6/10
Ethnicity (Caucasian/Asian)	27/9	54/19	8/8
Age (years)	7.3 ± 0.2	7.6 ± 0.1	7.8 ± 0.3
Weight (kg)	27 ± 1	36 ± 1	40 ± 2 *
Height (cm)	1.26 ± 0.01	1.29 ± 0.01	1.33 ± 0.02
BMI (kg/m^2)	16.7 ± 0.2	21.2 ± 0.2	22.4 ± 0.5 *
BMI-SD score	0.43 ± 0.09	1.90 ± 0.05	2.13 ± 0.11 *
Waist circumference (cm)	59 ± 1	72 ± 1	77 ± 2 *
Leptin (ng/mL)	2.3 ± 0.3	12.2 ± 1.0	9.2 ± 1.4
Adiponectin (µg/mL)	11.4 ± 0.9	10.4 ± 0.5	11.9 ± 2.2
Leptin/Adiponectin	0.3 ± 0.03	1.46 ± 0.17	1.21 ± 0.26
ALT (U/L)	19 ± 1	23 ± 1	24 ± 2
AST (U/L)	33 ± 1	31 ± 1	35 ± 2 *
Systolic blood pressure (mmHg)	103 ± 1	108 ± 1	111 ± 3
Diastolic blood pressure (mmHg)	62 ± 1	67 ± 1	70 ± 2
Triglycerides (mg/dL)	57 ± 3	81 ± 4	75 ± 6
HDL cholesterol (mg/dL)	57 ± 1	52 ± 1	48 ± 3
LDL cholesterol (mg/dL)	100 ± 3	117 ± 2	105 ± 6 *
Total cholesterol (mg/dL)	170 ± 4	185 ± 3	169 ± 6 *
Uric Acid (mg/dL)	3.6 ± 0.1	4.3 ± 0.1	4.1 ± 0.2
Insulin (µIU/mL)	9 ± 0.4	12 ± 0.6	16 ± 2.3
Fasting glucose (mg/dL)	85 ± 1	87 ± 1	85 ± 2
HOMA-IR	1.9 ± 0.1	2.5 ± 0.1	2.9 ± 0.4
Physical activity (h/week)	15 ± 1	14 ± 1	15 ± 2
Sedentary activity (h/week)	16 ± 2	22 ± 1	25 ± 4

Data are shown as absolute numbers or means ± SEM, * $p < 0.05$ compared to overweight children, NW children were not included in the statistical analysis but are shown for comparison. BMI: body mass index; BMI-SD score: BMI standard deviation score; ALT: alanine aminotransferase, AST: aspartate aminotransferase; HDL: high-density lipoprotein; LDL: low-density lipoprotein; HOMA-IR: homeostatic model assessment for insulin resistance; NW: normal-weight healthy children; OW: overweight children without NAFLD; NAFLD: overweight children with NAFLD. Underreporters were excluded from the analysis.

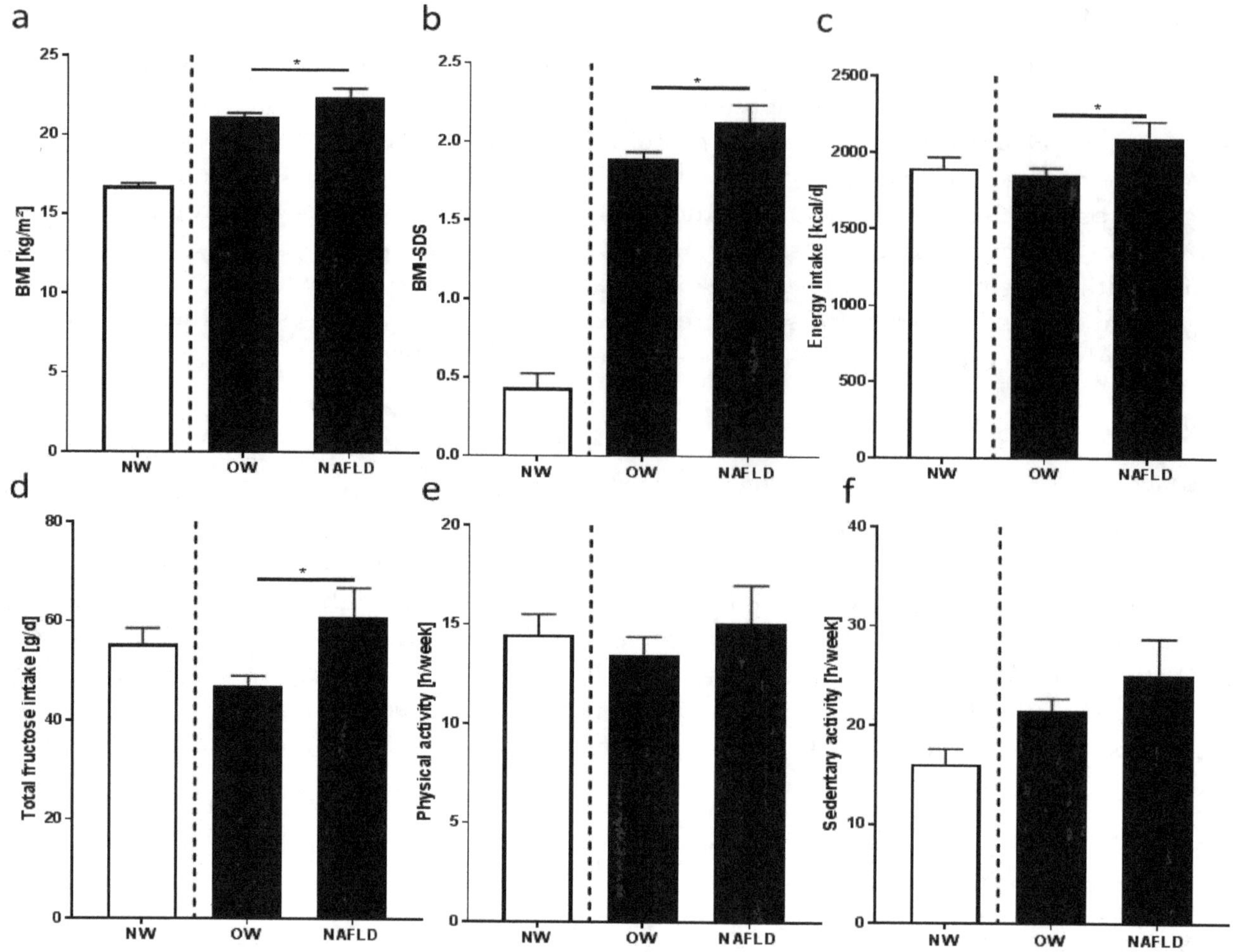

Figure 2. (**a**) Body mass index (BMI), (**b**) BMI standard deviation score (BMI-SDS), (**c**) energy, (**d**) total fructose intake (free fructose and fructose derived from sucrose), and (**e**) physical and (**f**) sedentary activities of normal-weight (NW) children, overweight children without NAFLD (OW), and overweight children with NAFLD (NAFLD). Data are means ± standard error of the mean (SEM), * $p < 0.05$ overweight children in comparison to overweight children with NAFLD; NW children were not included in the statistical analysis, but are shown for comparison. Underreporters were excluded from the analysis.

Despite showing early signs of NAFLD, e.g., fatty liver grade 1, ALT activity in serum was similar between overweight children with and without NAFLD, while AST activity in serum was significantly higher by ~4 U/L ($p < 0.05$). Systolic and diastolic blood pressures were similar between groups of overweight children. Twelve of the overweight children without NAFLD and seven of the overweight children with NAFLD were diagnosed as suffering from hypertension. Triglyceride, high-density lipoprotein (HDL), and uric acid concentrations in serum were also similar between the two overweight groups with 21 overweight children and four overweight children with NAFLD suffering from dyslipidemia. However, low-density lipoprotein (LDL) and total cholesterol were significantly higher in overweight children without NAFLD than in overweight children with NAFLD. Fasting insulin, glucose, and HOMA-IR were also similar between overweight groups. Furthermore, three overweight children and one overweight child with NAFLD suffered from an impaired glucose tolerance according to the reference levels of the German diabetes association [31]. As expected and similar to anthropometric parameters, metabolic parameters were markedly higher, or, in the case of

HDL, lower in overweight children with and without NAFLD than in normal-weight children shown for comparison (see Table 1).

3.2. Nutritional Intake, Dietary Pattern, and Leisure Time Activities

In line with the findings for body weight, BMI, and BMI-SDS, total caloric intake of overweight children with NAFLD was significantly higher than that of overweight children without NAFLD (~250 kcal/day). Total fat, protein, and fiber intakes were similar between overweight groups (see Table 2 and Figure 2). Total intake of carbohydrates was by trend higher in overweight children with NAFLD than in those without (~120 kcal/day, $p = 0.06$). As results of others and our own group suggest that intake of carbohydrates and, herein, especially mono- and disaccharides may be critical in the development of NAFLD [10,32,33], the composition of the carbohydrates was further analyzed. While the intake of complex carbohydrates was similar between overweight groups, intakes of total fructose and total glucose (free fructose and glucose, respectively, as well as fructose and glucose derived from sucrose) were significantly higher in overweight children with NAFLD than in those without (see Table 2 and Figure 2).

Table 2. Nutritional intake of normal-weight healthy children and overweight children with and without NAFLD.

	NW	OW	NAFLD
n	36	73	16
Total energy intake (kcal/day)	1900 ± 70	1853 ± 47	2101 ± 105 *
Total fat intake (g/day)	78 ± 4	77 ± 3	86 ± 6
Total protein intake (g/day)	59 ± 3	63 ± 2	68 ± 4
Total CHO intake (g/day)	242 ± 10	227 ± 7	257 ± 16
Fructose (g/day) [a]	55 ± 3	47 ± 2	61 ± 6 *
Glucose (g/day) [b]	49 ± 2	42 ± 2	53 ± 6 *
Fiber intake (g/day)	15 ± 1	14 ± 1	18 ± 2

Data are shown as means ± standard error of the mean (SEM); * $p < 0.05$ compared to overweight children; NW children were not included in the statistical analysis, but are shown for comparison. CHO: carbohydrate; NW: normal-weight healthy children; OW: overweight children without NAFLD; NAFLD: overweight children with NAFLD, [a] free fructose and fructose derived from sucrose; [b] free glucose and glucose derived from sucrose. Underreporters were excluded from the analysis.

To further determine dietary sources of higher carbohydrate, and especially, monosaccharide intake, we analyzed the dietary pattern of study participants (see Table 3). With the exception of cereals being consumed by ~47% of overweight children without NAFLD and only ~13% of overweight children with NAFLD ($p < 0.05$), the intake of food groups was similar between overweight groups (data not shown). However, when further analyzing the amount consumed of the different food groups of those children reporting consumption of these foods, overweight children with NAFLD were found to consume significantly more sweetened beverages including soft drinks and fruit juices than overweight children without NAFLD. Intake of all other food groups was similar between groups (see Table 3).

Times spent with physical and sedentary activities were similar between overweight groups. Interestingly, the intake of total calories and macronutrients, as well as time spent with physical activities, of normal-weight children was rather similar to that of overweight children with NAFLD, while time spent with sedentary activities was markedly shorter in normal-weight children than in overweight ones (see Table 1 and Figure 2). Again, underreporters were excluded from the analysis.

Table 3. Dietary pattern of normal-weight children and overweight children with and without NAFLD.

	NW	OW	NAFLD
Beverages (kcal/day)	161 ± 18	132 ± 10	208 ± 35 *
Fruits/dried fruits (kcal/day)	86 ± 12	80 ± 7	130 ± 30
Vegetables/legumes (kcal/day)	27 ± 5	30 ± 4	24 ± 5
Potatoes/pasta/rice (kcal/day)	210 ± 33	170 ± 14	201 ± 36
Bread (kcal/day)	259 ± 22	257 ± 18	262 ± 48
Spreads (kcal/day)	141 ± 23	103 ± 10	84 ± 18
Bakery goods (kcal/day)	206 ± 28	217 ± 27	167 ± 33
Cereals (kcal/day)	127 ± 35	113 ± 12	146 ± 5
Meat (kcal/day)	216 ± 24	205 ± 18	249 ± 46
Milk and dairy (kcal/day)	161 ± 16	144 ± 11	168 ± 37
Cheese and quark (kcal/day)	92 ± 15	104 ± 11	77 ± 12
Oils, margarines, and butter (kcal/day)	94 ± 12	103 ± 9	136 ± 15
Sweets and sugar (kcal/day)	154 ± 26	178 ± 15	145 ± 17
Desserts (kcal/day)	157 ± 38	111 ± 21	173 ± 80
Convenience food (kcal/day)	231 ± 28	324 ± 37	317 ± 63

Data are shown as means ± SEM; * $p < 0.05$ compared to overweight children without NAFLD; NW children were not included in the statistical analysis, but are shown for comparison. NW: normal-weight healthy children; OW: overweight children without NAFLD; NAFLD: overweight children with NAFLD.

3.3. Markers of Inflammation and Intestinal Permeability

Protein concentrations of TNFα and IL-6 were significantly higher in plasma of overweight children with NAFLD than in those without, while concentrations of CRP and active PAI-1 in plasma were similar between overweight groups (see Figure 3). Bacterial endotoxin levels in peripheral plasma and protein levels of LBP were both significantly higher in overweight children with NAFLD than in those without (see Figure 3).

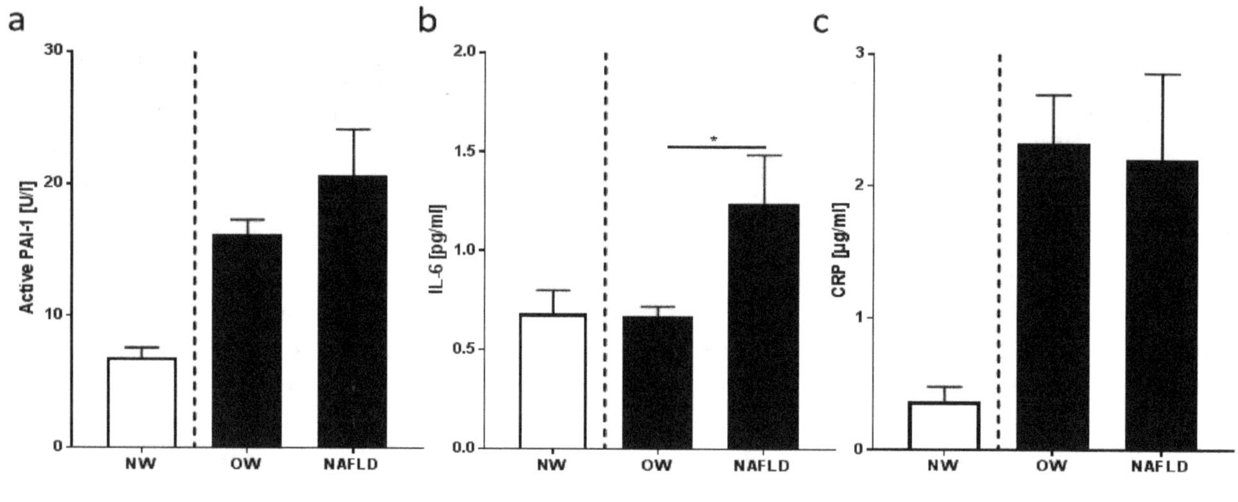

Figure 3. *Cont.*

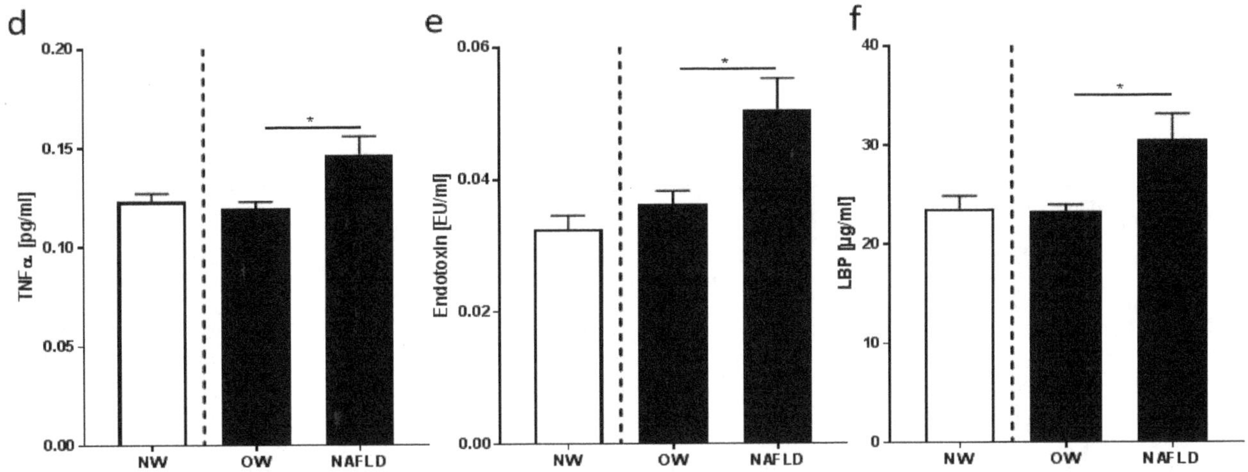

Figure 3. (**a**) Plasma active plasminogen activator inhibitor 1 (PAI-1), (**b**) interleukin 6 (IL-6), (**c**) serum c-reactive protein (CRP), (**d**) tumor necrosis factor α (TNFα), (**e**) endotoxin, (**f**) lipopolysaccharide-binding protein (LBP) plasma concentrations of normal-weight (NW) children, overweight children without NAFLD (OW), and overweight children with NAFLD (NAFLD). Data are means ± SEM; * $p < 0.05$ overweight children in comparison to overweight children with NAFLD; NW children were not included in the statistical analysis, but are shown for comparison. Underreporters were excluded from the analysis.

3.4. Feasibility Study: Characteristics of Study Participants, Nutritional Intake, and Metabolic Parameters

Four children dropped out of the feasibility study due to personal reasons, and one child was excluded as an underreporter. Therefore, only six children in the control group and six children in the intervention group were included in the final analysis. Despite being allowed to select study arms to enhance compliance and to avoid the loss of children, at baseline, none of the parameters assessed differed between the overweight children with NAFLD selecting the intervention arm and those who chose to participate in the feasibility study as controls, with the exception of TNFα levels in plasma (see Figure 4). TNFα levels in plasma were significantly higher in children in the intervention group than in controls. Additionally, total intakes of energy, macronutrients, and sugars (total fructose and total glucose) per day were similar between groups (see Supplementary Materials, Table S1) at baseline. Data of normal-weight children in Table 4 and Figure 4 are shown for comparison, but were not included in the statistical analysis. While both groups had lower BMI-SDS at the end of the study compared to the beginning of the study (control: $p < 0.05$; intervention: $p = 0.16$), waist circumference was significantly higher in the intervention group at the end of the study (see Table 4). A similar increase in waist circumference was not found in the controls. Nonetheless, waist circumference did not differ between groups at the end of the study. In line with the findings for waist circumference, neither adiponectin nor leptin plasma concentrations nor leptin/adiponectin ratio differed at baseline. While leptin levels remained unchanged, adiponectin concentrations in the plasma of children in the intervention group were by trend lower ($p = 0.06$) at the end of the study when compared to baseline, whereas leptin/adiponectin ratio was significantly higher in these children.

Table 4. Anthropometric and metabolic parameters of overweight children with NAFLD before and after dietary intervention.

	Healthy Children	NAFLD Children			
	NW (n = 36)	Control (n = 6)		Intervention (n = 7)	
		Baseline	After 1 Year	Baseline	After 1 Year
Sex (male/female)	20/16	3/3		4/2	
Ethnicity (Caucasian/Asian)	27/9	2/4		5/1	
Age (years)	7.3 ± 0.2	8.0 ± 0.3	9.0 ± 0.5 *	7.5 ± 0.4	8.7 ± 0.4 *
BMI-SD score	0.43 ± 0.09	1.9 ± 0.1	1.6 ± 0.2 *	2.2 ± 0.2	2.0 ± 0.3
Waist circumference (cm)	59 ± 1	77 ± 4	77 ± 4	76 ± 3	83 ± 3 *
Leptin (ng/mL)	2.3 ± 0.3	9.5 ± 3.0	16.6 ± 4.8	8.8 ± 2.5	17.5 ± 5.7
Adiponectin (μg/mL)	11.4 ± 0.9	7.6 ± 1.4	6.9 ± 0.7	18.5 ± 4.3	8.3 ± 1.9
Leptin/adiponectin	0.3 ± 0.03	1.6 ± 0.6	2.5 ± 0.8	0.7 ± 0.3	2.0 ± 0.3 *
LBP (μg/mL)	23.6 ± 1.3	28.3 ± 4.0	30.2 ± 3.2	28.8 ± 4.5	25.6 ± 2.6
Active PAI-1 (U/L)	6.8 ± 0.8	18.2 ± 5.6	18.2 ± 8.6	17.0 ± 4.0	9.6 ± 1.4
ALT (U/L)	19 ± 1	26 ± 4	26 ± 3	20 ± 1	23 ± 3
AST (U/L)	33 ± 1	38 ± 5	30 ± 2	32 ± 3	33 ± 3
Systolic blood pressure (mmHg)	103 ± 1	111 ± 5	113 ± 5	107 ± 4	105 ± 5
Diastolic blood pressure (mmHg)	62 ± 1	69 ± 3	70 ± 6	69 ± 4	65 ± 4 *
Triglycerides (mg/dL)	57 ± 3	80 ± 7	85 ± 13	74 ± 15	89 ± 27
HDL cholesterol (mg/dL)	57 ± 1	48 ± 3	52 ± 4	56 ± 4	57 ± 5
LDL cholesterol (mg/dL)	100 ± 3	109 ± 8	115 ± 10	102 ± 13	116 ± 11 *
Total cholesterol (mg/dL)	160 ± 4	176 ± 7	174 ± 12	170 ± 12	187 ± 10 *
Insulin (μIU/mL)	9 ± 0.4	13 ± 1	15 ± 3	13 ± 4	16 ± 4
Fasting glucose (mg/dL)	85 ± 1	78 ± 4	86 ± 3	85 ± 2	86 ± 3
HOMA-IR	1.9 ± 0.1	2.5 ± 0.3	3.3 ± 0.8	2.8 ± 0.9	3.4 ± 0.9
Physical activity (h/week)	15 ± 1	17 ± 4	17 ± 5	14 ± 2	14 ± 2
Sedentary activity (h/week)	16 ± 2	23 ± 7	25 ± 4	24 ± 4	18 ± 4

Data are shown as absolute numbers or means ± SEM; * $p < 0.05$ compared to the respective baseline value. BMI-SD score: BMI standard deviation score; LBP: lipopolysaccharide binding protein; PAI-1: plasminogen activator inhibitor-1; ALT: alanine aminotransferase; AST: aspartate aminotransferase; HDL: high-density lipoprotein; LDL: low-density lipoprotein; HOMA-IR: homeostatic model assessment for insulin resistance. NW children were not included in the statistical analysis, but are shown for comparison. Underreporters were excluded from the analysis.

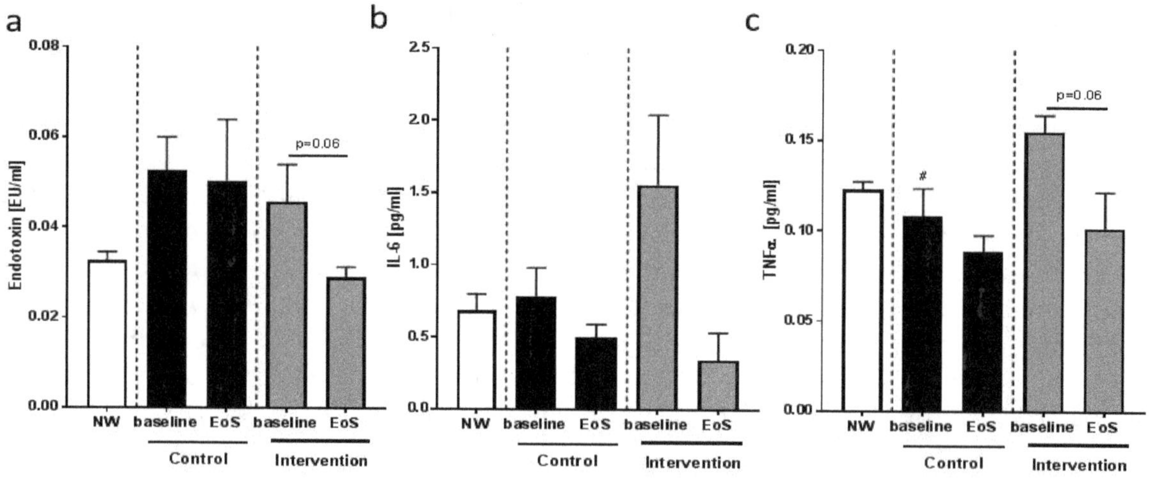

Figure 4. (**a**) Plasma endotoxin, (**b**) serum IL-6, and (**c**) plasma TNFα concentrations of children with NAFLD enrolled in the control (Control) and intervention (Intervention) group at baseline (baseline) and at the end of the study (EoS). Data are means ± SEM; # $p < 0.05$ values at baseline between both groups; NW children were not included in the statistical analysis, but are shown for comparison. Underreporters were excluded from the analysis.

ALT and AST activities, as well as concentrations of triglycerides and HDL in serum, were not altered throughout the intervention study and did not differ between NAFLD groups. Fasting insulin and glucose concentrations, as well as HOMA-IR, were also similar between groups at the beginning of the study and were not changed throughout the study (see Table 4). However, LDL and total cholesterol levels increased significantly throughout the study in the sera of children in the intervention group.

LDL concentrations in serum also increased in the control group; however, as data varied considerably within these groups, differences did not reach statistical significance. The systolic blood pressure of children was similar between groups at the beginning of the study and was also not changed. In contrast, diastolic blood pressure being similar between groups at baseline was significantly lower in children in the intervention group at the end of the study, whereas a similar decrease was not found in control NAFLD children (see Table 4).

3.5. Feasibility Study: Inflammatory Markers and Indices of Intestinal Permeability

Concentrations of active PAI-1 and IL-6 were similar between groups at the beginning of the study and were not altered. While changes in concentration of these inflammatory markers were not significant within groups or between groups, at the end of the feasibility study, concentrations of most parameters were at the level of normal-weight children (see Table 4 and Figure 4). In contrast, plasma TNFα levels, being significantly higher in the intervention group at baseline compared to controls, decreased markedly ($p = 0.06$) throughout the study almost to the level of normal-weight control children (see Figure 4). Bacterial endotoxin and LBP concentrations in plasma were also similar between groups at the beginning of the study. LBP concentration in plasma was unchanged in both groups at the end of the study (see Table 4), whereas the concentration of bacterial endotoxin in the peripheral blood of children in the intervention group was lower by trend at the end of the study ($p = 0.06$; see Figure 4).

4. Discussion

With a still increasing prevalence, NAFLD is, by now, thought to be the most prevalent liver disease worldwide [2]. Overweight and insulin resistance are among the key risk factors for the development of NAFLD [34,35]; however, despite intense research efforts, the question as to why some overweight individuals develop NAFLD and others do not is yet to be fully answered. In the present study, employing a cohort of randomly selected overweight children with no known signs of liver disease or other metabolic diseases before the study, it was shown that children with early signs of NAFLD, e.g., fatty liver grade 1 as assessed by ultrasound, had a higher BMI, BMI-SDS, and waist circumference than overweight children without NAFLD. Also, while still being within the normal range, AST activity was higher in the sera of overweight children with NAFLD, whereas neither ALT activity nor markers of glucose metabolism nor other metabolic markers, such as blood pressure and triglycerides, differed between groups. Somewhat contrasting the findings for waist circumference, the ratio of adiponectin to leptin, suggested to be indicative of visceral fat volume and NAFLD in obese adolescents [36], was similar between overweight groups. However, results of a recently published study by Dhaliwal et al. [37] using computed tomography to assess hepatic steatosis and the abdominal fat area suggest that, while abdominal subcutaneous adipose tissue per se is greater in children with hepatic steatosis than in those without, increases in visceral adipose tissue area seem to be related to the presence of steatosis in older children ($\geq$9.8 years). Therefore, the apparent lack of relation of waist circumference and the ratio of adiponectin to leptin might be related to the rather young age of study participants (<9 years) and to differences in subcutaneous adipose tissue mass rather than visceral adipose tissue. Furthermore, results of others also suggested that overweight children with hepatic steatosis have a higher BMI and waist circumference when compared to overweight children without signs of NAFLD [5,38,39]. Previous studies of others also reported that transaminase activities in the sera of overweight children were also similar to those of overweight children serving as controls [38]; however, in contrast to the findings of the present study, in studies of others, a strong association of the presence of NAFLD in overweight children with increased markers of insulin resistance, dyslipidemia, and the presence of metabolic abnormalities was found [5,38,39]. Indeed, in the present study, total cholesterol in serum was even found to be higher in overweight children without NAFLD than in those with NAFLD. Differences between the results of these studies (>9 years old) and the present study (<9 years old) might have resulted from differences in the age of study participants, as well as in the severity of steatosis (in the present study, only grade I vs. minimal-to-severe fatty liver or even beginning non-alcoholic steatohepatitis (NASH) in other studies) and obesity of participants enrolled [5,38]. The study setting (here, children recruited in schools vs. hospitals in most other studies) and markers used to assess insulin resistance (in the present study, fasting glucose and insulin vs. oral glucose tolerance tests) were also markedly different between these studies and the present study [5,38,39]. Reasons for the significantly higher levels of total cholesterol and LDL cholesterol in the sera of overweight children without NAFLD have to be delineated in future studies.

Also, while overweight children with NAFLD only showed very early signs of the disease, IL-6 and TNFα levels in plasma were both higher in children with NAFLD than in overweight controls, whereas CRP and active PAI-1 levels in plasma—both markedly higher than in normal-weight controls—did not differ between overweight groups. In line with these findings, others showed that concentrations of IL-6 and TNFα in serum are closely related to the prevalence of NALFD [40]. Results of others also suggest that, in overweight children, CRP and active PAI-1 levels may be elevated independently of the presence of NAFLD [41,42]. Indeed, while active PAI-1 levels were shown to be related to severe stages of the disease, e.g., manifest steatosis or NASH [43], this acute-phase protein was also shown to be related to HOMA-IR by others [44], and it was similarly higher in both overweight groups in the present study when compared to controls. Taken together, results of the present study suggest that, in overweight children, very early stages of NAFLD are associated with higher body weight, greater waist circumference, and elevated proinflammatory cytokine levels while, markers of insulin resistance are not different. However, the results of the present study by no means preclude that an impaired glucose tolerance or insulin resistance contributes to the onset of NAFLD. Indeed, in adults and mouse models, it was shown that both fasting insulin and glucose levels can still be within the normal range in peripheral blood, while, in liver tissue, the expressions of insulin receptor and insulin receptor substrate were markedly lower [45,46]. Therefore, it could be that, in the present study, overweight children with NAFLD may have suffered from impairments of insulin signaling and glucose metabolism in liver tissue, while fasting glucose and insulin concentrations in peripheral blood were still within the normal range. This needs to be addressed in future studies.

4.1. Absolute Energy Intake, Nutritional Intake, and Dietary Pattern of Overweight Children with and without NAFLD Differ

Results of animal studies suggest that not only general overnutrition, but also the composition of the diet, e.g., the proportion of saturated fatty acids and sugars, and herein, especially of fructose, may be critical in the development of NAFLD [19,47]. In a cohort of children with NAFLD, Mosca et al. [33] recently showed that dietary fructose intake is independently associated with NASH. Furthermore, it was shown that children with NAFLD absorb and metabolize fructose more effectively than normal-weight children [48]. In the present study, overweight children with early signs of NAFLD had a significantly higher mean daily total energy intake when compared to overweight children without NAFLD (~250 kcal/day) which mainly seemed to result from a higher daily total fructose (free fructose and fructose derived from sucrose) and total glucose (free glucose and glucose derived from sucrose) intake originating from a markedly higher soft-drink and juice intake. Results of the present study are in line with the findings of others, showing that both children and adults with NAFLD have a higher mean fructose intake mainly resulting from a higher consumption of soft drinks and fruit juices [10,49–51]; however, in most of these studies, normal-weight healthy individuals were compared with overweight patients with NAFLD [10,12]. Indeed, the number of human studies comparing the nutritional intake and dietary pattern of overweight individuals, and even more so, weight-matched individuals with and without NAFLD is rather limited. In line with the findings of the present study, Ouyang et al. and Assy et al. [52,53] showed that adult patients with NAFLD drank more soft drinks and juices.

Interestingly, normal-weight children enrolled for comparison almost had similar daily total energy, monosaccharide, and disaccharide intakes without showing any signs of NAFLD or other metabolic diseases when compared to overweight children with NAFLD. Yet, normal weight children, on average, were ~16 h/week (~140 min/day) sedentarily active doing handcrafting, drawing, reading, and watching TV or playing video games, while overweight children with NAFLD, on average, spent 25 h/week (~215 min/day) with these activities. Indeed, results of Felix et al. [54] suggest that, in overweight children, the intake of refined carbohydrates and the lack of physical activity were associated with a higher risk of developing NAFLD, further suggesting that protection against the development of NAFLD, and probably, overweight in normal-weight children was strongly dependent upon their physical activity in the present study. In support of this hypothesis, lifestyle changes not only focusing on changes in dietary habits, but also on increasing aerobic exercise were suggested to improve aminotransferase activity levels in children and adolescents with NAFLD [50,55].

4.2. Overweight Children with NAFLD Have Higher Bacterial Endotoxin and LBP Levels in Peripheral Blood Than Overweight Children without NAFLD, Which Were Lowered by Moderate Dietary Counseling

In the present study, both bacterial endotoxin and LBP levels were significantly higher in overweight children with NAFLD than in those without. These findings are in line with the results of several human and animal studies, suggesting that alterations of intestinal barrier function, and subsequently, an increased translocation of bacterial endotoxin are critical in the development of NAFLD [10,12,17,21,56–58]. While data derived from animal studies suggest that these alterations may be related to the intake of fructose [14,19,58], results of human studies are somewhat contradictory. Indeed, in some studies, it was shown that both the intake of dietary fructose and bacterial endotoxin levels in peripheral blood were elevated in patients with NAFLD; however, frequently, not only fructose intake, but also total caloric intake of patients was significantly higher than that of controls [49,53]. So far, studies focusing on a reduction of fructose intake suggest that, in adults with steatosis and steatohepatitis, this kind of counseling is associated with an improvement in liver status, a reduction in bacterial endotoxin levels, and improved intestinal barrier function [59]. In the present feasibility study, while only slightly affecting overall weight and metabolic status, the moderate dietary counseling focusing only on a reduction in dietary fructose intake was associated with a reduction in bacterial endotoxin and TNFα levels, almost to the level of normal-weight controls, in overweight children with NAFLD. The apparent reduction in adiponectin levels from baseline to the end of study in children with NAFLD enrolled in the intervention arm might have resulted from the slightly, but not significantly, younger age of these children when compared to controls at baseline (7.5 vs. 8.0 years). Indeed, it was shown before that adiponectin plasma levels decrease between the ages of five and eight years [60]. Furthermore, studies of Murphy et al. [60] also showed that total cholesterol plasma levels increase over time in children aged between five and eight years, in line with findings of the present study. In contrast, despite lowering their BMI-SDS and maintaining their waist circumference, the bacterial endotoxin levels of overweight controls with NAFLD were unchanged. Taken together, these data suggest that the total intake of sugar-rich foods and bacterial endotoxin levels both may be critical in the development of NAFLD in overweight children. However, our results do not preclude that other factors such as genetic predisposition, intake of other nutrients, and sedentary lifestyle are also critical in the development of NAFLD. Rather, our data suggest that, at least in some children, targeting intestinal barrier function through dietary fructose intake may be beneficial in the prevention and therapy of this liver disease.

4.3. Limitations

Our study is not without limitations which have to be considered when interpreting the results. Overweight children with and without NAFLD were not weight-matched; however, children were randomly recruited and enrolled in non-clinical settings, and, at the time of recruitment, had no known history of metabolic or liver diseases. Therefore, both overweight groups included metabolically healthy and unhealthy children. Thus, results might differ in larger and more homogeneous clinical studies. Nonetheless, as we aimed to study the early onset of the disease, this approach seemed to be the most feasible. Furthermore, the sample size of the intervention study was rather small, as the intervention focused only on children with NAFLD and five children were lost due to personal reasons or underreporting. Furthermore, as the focus of the intervention study was to show feasibility of this kind of moderate dietary intervention, no power calculation was performed to determine the number of subjects needed to be included for statistically significant outcomes. Thus, the characteristics of the feasibility study are rather explorative, and the effect of a moderate dietary intervention on metabolic and inflammatory markers needs to be assured in a larger randomized population. However, despite the small sample size, our findings are in line with others showing that dietary counseling might be beneficial in improving metabolic parameters in children [61]. Furthermore, a selection bias cannot be ruled out as control and intervention groups were self-selected due to incompliance of many guardians for randomization. Indeed, due to drop out and underreporting, the number of Asian participants deciding to undergo nutritional counseling was lower than the number of Asian children in the control group. However, as we were highly dependent upon the willingness of parents and children to attend the regular counseling meetings, from our perspective, this was the most feasible way of avoiding an even higher drop-out rate. Indeed, when enrolling children into the study, guardians repeatedly pointed out their unwillingness to participate in regular meetings, suggesting that it felt too straining. Accordingly, it was also not possible to obtain valid data regarding nutritional intake and dietary pattern at the end of the intervention. Therefore, it is not clear if the beneficial effects on bacterial endotoxin levels found at the end of the study resulted from a change in fructose intake or dietary pattern, or other factors. The role and impact of fructose on the beneficial effects found in the intervention group will have to be addressed in future studies. Reasons for this incompliance to participate in meetings might have been that our study was not situated in a clinical setting, and that children were thought to be healthy with the exception of being overweight/ obese before the study. Another limitation is the reduction of BMI-SDS in both groups of the intervention study. This, in part, might have resulted from the fact that guardians became aware of the potential health issues of their children. Indeed, some of the families might have changed additional dietary habits, and prolonged time spent physically active, while time spent sedentary active was reduced, without bringing this to our attention. Furthermore, in the region of Germany where our study was situated, "healthy" nutrition is part of the curriculum in elementary school and sometimes even in kindergarten. Therefore, it cannot be ruled out that at least some of the children in the intervention study and probably also their parents, e.g., during parent–teacher conferences and school enrollment, might have received additional training in regards to avoiding sugar-rich foods and to following a healthy lifestyle. Furthermore, in the present study, physical and sedentary activities were only acquired by questionnaires rather than activity monitors. Additionally, no follow-up was carried out to assess sustainability of the intervention on weight status, metabolic disorders, and associated proinflammatory alterations. However, we thought that the length of the study would be sufficient to test the principal hypothesis that, in children, a diet focusing only on a reduction in fructose intake may be a sufficient measure for reducing bacterial endotoxin levels and concentrations of proinflammatory cytokines. Long-term effects will have to be determined in larger randomized studies with a longer duration and follow-up.

5. Conclusions

Taken together, results of the present study suggest that body weight, dietary pattern, and especially, the intake of sweetened beverages may be critical in the development of NAFLD in overweight children. Our data also suggest that changes in intestinal barrier function are also associated with the development of NAFLD in children. Results of the present study also suggest that targeting sugar or fructose intake even with moderate measures may be beneficial for overall health status of overweight children with NAFLD. Still, the concept of moderate lifestyle interventions only focusing on a limited number of changes and the long-term effects of interventions like the one used in the present study need to be assessed in larger randomized studies in the future, as, in the present study, the sample size was quite small and participants were allowed to self-select their groups. Also, future studies should maybe aim to include more family members in the intervention, so as to improve the motivation to participate in and attend regular meetings, as well as to translate information and advice provided during the counseling and regular meetings to daily life, subsequently leading to a better compliance and greater health effects. In addition, employing new dietary counseling tools not requiring physical presence in a study center may also be an option for future studies. Furthermore, mechanisms underlying the elevated bacterial endotoxin levels found in the present study, as well as other studies, remain to be determined.

Author Contributions: Conceptualization, I.B. Data curation, A.N., A.B., I.B.C., and Y.Ö. Formal analysis, A.N., A.B., I.B.C., and Y.Ö. Funding acquisition, I.B. Investigation, I.B.C. and Y.Ö. Project administration, I.B. Supervision, I.B. Validation, I.B. Visualization, A.N. Writing—original draft, A.N. and I.B. Writing—review and editing, I.B.

References

1. Angulo, P.; Lindor, K.D. Non-alcoholic fatty liver disease. *J. Gastroenterol. Hepatol.* **2002**, *17*, S186–S190. [CrossRef] [PubMed]
2. Younossi, Z.; Anstee, Q.M.; Marietti, M.; Hardy, T.; Henry, L.; Eslam, M.; George, J.; Bugianesi, E. Global burden of nafld and nash: Trends, predictions, risk factors and prevention. *Nat. Rev. Gastroenterol. Hepatol.* **2018**, *15*, 11–20. [CrossRef] [PubMed]
3. Alkassabany, Y.M.; Farghaly, A.G.; El-Ghitany, E.M. Prevalence, risk factors, and predictors of nonalcoholic fatty liver disease among schoolchildren: A hospital-based study in alexandria, egypt. *Arab. J. Gastroenterol.* **2014**, *15*, 76–81. [CrossRef] [PubMed]
4. Anderson, E.L.; Howe, L.D.; Jones, H.E.; Higgins, J.P.T.; Lawlor, D.A.; Fraser, A. The prevalence of non-alcoholic fatty liver disease in children and adolescents: A systematic review and meta-analysis. *PLoS ONE* **2015**, *10*, e0140908. [CrossRef] [PubMed]
5. Denzer, C.; Thiere, D.; Muche, R.; Koenig, W.; Mayer, H.; Kratzer, W.; Wabitsch, M. Gender-specific prevalences of fatty liver in obese children and adolescents: Roles of body fat distribution, sex steroids, and insulin resistance. *J. Clin. Endocrinol. Metab.* **2009**, *94*, 3872–3881. [CrossRef] [PubMed]
6. Denzer, C.; Reithofer, E.; Wabitsch, M.; Widhalm, K. The outcome of childhood obesity management depends highly upon patient compliance. *Eur. J. Pediatr.* **2004**, *163*, 99–104. [CrossRef] [PubMed]
7. McManus, K.; Antinoro, L.; Sacks, F. A randomized controlled trial of a moderate-fat, low-energy diet compared with a low fat, low-energy diet for weight loss in overweight adults. *Int. J. Obes. Relat. Metab. Disord.* **2001**, *25*, 1503–1511. [CrossRef] [PubMed]
8. Reinehr, T. Effectiveness of Lifestyle Intervention in Overweight Children. *Proc. Nutr. Soc.* **2011**, *70*, 494–505. [CrossRef] [PubMed]
9. Sullivan, S. Implications of diet on nonalcoholic fatty liver disease. *Curr. Opin. Gastroenterol.* **2010**, *26*, 160–164. [CrossRef] [PubMed]
10. Thuy, S.; Ladurner, R.; Volynets, V.; Wagner, S.; Strahl, S.; Konigsrainer, A.; Maier, K.P.; Bischoff, S.C.; Bergheim, I. Nonalcoholic fatty liver disease in humans is associated with increased plasma endotoxin and plasminogen activator inhibitor 1 concentrations and with fructose intake. *J. Nutr.* **2008**, *138*, 1452–1455. [CrossRef] [PubMed]
11. Toshimitsu, K.; Matsuura, B.; Ohkubo, I.; Niiya, T.; Furukawa, S.; Hiasa, Y.; Kawamura, M.; Ebihara, K.; Onji, M. Dietary habits and nutrient intake in non-alcoholic steatohepatitis. *Nutrition* **2007**, *23*, 46–52. [CrossRef] [PubMed]
12. Volynets, V.; Kuper, M.A.; Strahl, S.; Maier, I.B.; Spruss, A.; Wagnerberger, S.; Konigsrainer, A.; Bischoff, S.C.; Bergheim, I. Nutrition, intestinal permeability, and blood ethanol levels are altered in patients with nonalcoholic fatty liver disease (nafld). *Dig. Dis. Sci.* **2012**, *57*, 1932–1941. [CrossRef] [PubMed]
13. Ackerman, Z.; Oron-Herman, M.; Grozovski, M.; Rosenthal, T.; Pappo, O.; Link, G.; Sela, B.A. Fructose-induced fatty liver disease: Hepatic effects of blood pressure and plasma triglyceride reduction. *Hypertension* **2005**, *45*, 1012–1018. [CrossRef] [PubMed]

14. Bergheim, I.; Weber, S.; Vos, M.; Kramer, S.; Volynets, V.; Kaserouni, S.; McClain, C.J.; Bischoff, S.C. Antibiotics protect against fructose-induced hepatic lipid accumulation in mice: Role of endotoxin. *J. Hepatol.* **2008**, *48*, 983–992. [CrossRef] [PubMed]
15. Kanuri, G.; Spruss, A.; Wagnerberger, S.; Bischoff, S.C.; Bergheim, I. Fructose-induced steatosis in mice: Role of plasminogen activator inhibitor-1, microsomal triglyceride transfer protein and nkt cells. *Lab. Investig.* **2011**, *91*, 885–895. [CrossRef] [PubMed]
16. Spruss, A.; Bergheim, I. Dietary fructose and intestinal barrier: Potential risk factor in the pathogenesis of nonalcoholic fatty liver disease. *J. Nutr. Biochem.* **2009**, *20*, 657–662. [CrossRef] [PubMed]
17. Brandt, A.; Jin, C.J.; Nolte, K.; Sellmann, C.; Engstler, A.J.; Bergheim, I. Short-term intake of a fructose-, fat- and cholesterol-rich diet causes hepatic steatosis in mice: Effect of antibiotic treatment. *Nutrients* **2017**, *9*. [CrossRef] [PubMed]
18. Kanuri, G.; Bergheim, I. In vitro and in vivo models of non-alcoholic fatty liver disease (nafld). *Int. J. Mol. Sci.* **2013**, *14*, 11963–11980. [CrossRef] [PubMed]
19. Sellmann, C.; Priebs, J.; Landmann, M.; Degen, C.; Engstler, A.J.; Jin, C.J.; Garttner, S.; Spruss, A.; Huber, O.; Bergheim, I. Diets rich in fructose, fat or fructose and fat alter intestinal barrier function and lead to the development of nonalcoholic fatty liver disease over time. *J. Nutr. Biochem.* **2015**, *26*, 1183–1192. [CrossRef] [PubMed]
20. Hashemi Kani, A.; Alavian, S.M.; Esmaillzadeh, A.; Adibi, P.; Azadbakht, L. Dietary quality indices and biochemical parameters among patients with non alcoholic fatty liver disease (nafld). *Hepat. Mon.* **2013**, *13*, e10943. [CrossRef] [PubMed]
21. Nier, A.; Engstler, A.J.; Maier, I.B.; Bergheim, I. Markers of intestinal permeability are already altered in early stages of non-alcoholic fatty liver disease: Studies in children. *PLoS ONE* **2017**, *12*, e0183282. [CrossRef] [PubMed]
22. Shi, L.; Liu, Z.W.; Li, Y.; Gong, C.; Zhang, H.; Song, L.J.; Huang, C.Y.; Li, M. The prevalence of nonalcoholic fatty liver disease and its association with lifestyle/dietary habits among university faculty and staff in chengdu. *Biomed. Environ. Sci.* **2012**, *25*, 383–391. [CrossRef] [PubMed]
23. Engstler, A.J.; Aumiller, T.; Degen, C.; Durr, M.; Weiss, E.; Maier, I.B.; Schattenberg, J.M.; Jin, C.J.; Sellmann, C.; Bergheim, I. Insulin resistance alters hepatic ethanol metabolism: Studies in mice and children with non-alcoholic fatty liver disease. *Gut* **2016**, *65*, 1564–1571. [CrossRef] [PubMed]
24. Marshall, W.A.; Tanner, J.M. Variations in pattern of pubertal changes in girls. *Arch. Dis. Child.* **1969**, *44*, 291–303. [CrossRef] [PubMed]
25. Marshall, W.A.; Tanner, J.M. Variations in the pattern of pubertal changes in boys. *Arch. Dis. Child.* **1970**, *45*, 13–23. [CrossRef] [PubMed]
26. Maier, I.B.; Ozel, Y.; Engstler, A.J.; Puchinger, S.; Wagnerberger, S.; Hulpke-Wette, M.; Bischoff, S.C.; Bergheim, I. Differences in the prevalence of metabolic disorders between prepubertal boys and girls from 5 to 8 years of age. *Acta Paediatr.* **2014**, *103*, e154–e160. [CrossRef] [PubMed]
27. Maier, I.B.; Stricker, L.; Ozel, Y.; Wagnerberger, S.; Bischoff, S.C.; Bergheim, I. A low fructose diet in the treatment of pediatric obesity: A pilot study. *Pediatr. Int.* **2011**, *53*, 303–308. [CrossRef] [PubMed]
28. Maier, I.B.; Ozel, Y.; Wagnerberger, S.; Bischoff, S.C.; Bergheim, I. Dietary pattern and leisure time activity of overweight and normal weight children in germany: Sex-specific differences. *Nutr. J.* **2013**, *12*, 14. [CrossRef] [PubMed]
29. Schofield, W.N. Predicting basal metabolic rate, new standards and review of previous work. *Hum. Nutr. Clin. Nutr.* **1985**, *39* (Suppl. 1), 5–41. [PubMed]
30. Sichert-Hellert, W.; Kersting, M.; Schoch, G. Underreporting of energy intake in 1 to 18 year old german children and adolescents. *Z. Ernahrungswiss.* **1998**, *37*, 242–251. [CrossRef] [PubMed]
31. DDG. Evidenzbasierte Leitlinie der Deutschen Diabetes-Gesellschaft. Available online: www.deutsche-diabetes-gesellschaft.de (accessed on 20 July 2018).
32. Mager, D.R.; Patterson, C.; So, S.; Rogenstein, C.D.; Wykes, L.J.; Roberts, E.A. Dietary and physical activity patterns in children with fatty liver. *Eur. J. Clin. Nutr.* **2010**, *64*, 628–635. [CrossRef] [PubMed]
33. Mosca, A.; Nobili, V.; De Vito, R.; Crudele, A.; Scorletti, E.; Villani, A.; Alisi, A.; Byrne, C.D. Serum uric acid concentrations and fructose consumption are independently associated with nash in children and adolescents. *J. Hepatol.* **2017**, *66*, 1031–1036. [CrossRef] [PubMed]

34. D'Adamo, E.; Impicciatore, M.; Capanna, R.; Loredana Marcovecchio, M.; Masuccio, F.G.; Chiarelli, F.; Mohn, A.A. Liver steatosis in obese prepubertal children: A possible role of insulin resistance. *Obesity* **2008**, *16*, 677–683. [CrossRef] [PubMed]
35. Nath, P.; Singh, S.P. Nonalcoholic fatty liver disease: Time to take the bull by the horns. *Eur. J. Hepatol.-Gastroenterol.* **2018**, *8*, 47–51. [CrossRef] [PubMed]
36. Angin, Y.; Arslan, N.; Kuralay, F. Leptin-to-adiponectin ratio in obese adolescents with nonalcoholic fatty liver disease. *Turk. J. Pediatr.* **2014**, *56*, 259–266. [PubMed]
37. Dhaliwal, J.; Chavhan, G.B.; Lurz, E.; Shalabi, A.; Yuen, N.; Williams, B.; Martincevic, I.; Amirabadi, A.; Wales, P.W.; Lee, W.; et al. Hepatic steatosis is highly prevalent across the paediatric age spectrum, including in pre-school age children. *Aliment. Pharmacol. Ther.* **2018**. [CrossRef] [PubMed]
38. Papandreou, D.; Karavetian, M.; Karabouta, Z.; Andreou, E. Obese children with metabolic syndrome have 3 times higher risk to have nonalcoholic fatty liver disease compared with those without metabolic syndrome. *Int. J. Endocrinol.* **2017**, *2017*, 2671692. [CrossRef] [PubMed]
39. Prokopowicz, Z.; Malecka-Tendera, E.; Matusik, P. Predictive value of adiposity level, metabolic syndrome, and insulin resistance for the risk of nonalcoholic fatty liver disease diagnosis in obese children. *Can. J. Gastroenterol. Hepatol.* **2018**, *2018*, 9465784. [CrossRef] [PubMed]
40. Alisi, A.; Manco, M.; Devito, R.; Piemonte, F.; Nobili, V. Endotoxin and plasminogen activator inhibitor-1 serum levels associated with nonalcoholic steatohepatitis in children. *J. Pediatr. Gastroenterol. Nutr.* **2010**, *50*, 645–649. [CrossRef] [PubMed]
41. Assuncao, S.N.F.; Sorte, N.; Alves, C.A.D.; Mendes, P.S.A.; Alves, C.R.B.; Silva, L.R. Inflammatory cytokines and non-alcoholic fatty liver disease (nafld) in obese children and adolescents. *Nutr. Hosp.* **2018**, *35*, 78–83. [CrossRef] [PubMed]
42. Estelles, A.; Dalmau, J.; Falco, C.; Berbel, O.; Castello, R.; Espana, F.; Aznar, J. Plasma pai-1 levels in obese children—Effect of weight loss and influence of pai-1 promoter 4g/5g genotype. *Thromb. Haemost.* **2001**, *86*, 647–652. [PubMed]
43. Fitzpatrick, E.; Dew, T.K.; Quaglia, A.; Sherwood, R.A.; Mitry, R.R.; Dhawan, A. Analysis of adipokine concentrations in paediatric non-alcoholic fatty liver disease. *Pediatr. Obes.* **2012**, *7*, 471–479. [CrossRef] [PubMed]
44. Masquio, D.C.; de Piano, A.; Campos, R.M.; Sanches, P.L.; Corgosinho, F.C.; Carnier, J.; Oyama, L.M.; do Nascimento, C.M.; de Mello, M.T.; Tufik, S.; et al. Saturated fatty acid intake can influence increase in plasminogen activator inhibitor-1 in obese adolescents. *Horm. Metab. Res.* **2014**, *46*, 245–251. [CrossRef] [PubMed]
45. Jin, C.J.; Sellmann, C.; Engstler, A.J.; Ziegenhardt, D.; Bergheim, I. Supplementation of sodium butyrate protects mice from the development of non-alcoholic steatohepatitis (nash). *Br. J. Nutr.* **2015**, *114*, 1745–1755. [CrossRef] [PubMed]
46. Kanuri, G.; Ladurner, R.; Skibovskaya, J.; Spruss, A.; Konigsrainer, A.; Bischoff, S.C.; Bergheim, I. Expression of toll-like receptors 1-5 but not tlr 6-10 is elevated in livers of patients with non-alcoholic fatty liver disease. *Liver. Int.* **2015**, *35*, 562–568. [CrossRef] [PubMed]
47. Kim, T.H.; Choi, D.; Kim, J.Y.; Lee, J.H.; Koo, S.H. Fast food diet-induced non-alcoholic fatty liver disease exerts early protective effect against acetaminophen intoxication in mice. *BMC Gastroenterol.* **2017**, *17*, 124. [CrossRef] [PubMed]
48. Sullivan, J.S.; Le, M.T.; Pan, Z.; Rivard, C.; Love-Osborne, K.; Robbins, K.; Johnson, R.J.; Sokol, R.J.; Sundaram, S.S. Oral fructose absorption in obese children with non-alcoholic fatty liver disease. *Pediatr. Obes.* **2015**, *10*, 188–195. [CrossRef] [PubMed]
49. Abdelmalek, M.F.; Suzuki, A.; Guy, C.; Unalp-Arida, A.; Colvin, R.; Johnson, R.J.; Diehl, A.M.; Clini, N.S. Increased fructose consumption is associated with fibrosis severity in patients with nonalcoholic fatty liver disease. *Hepatology* **2010**, *51*, 1961–1971. [CrossRef] [PubMed]
50. Utz-Melere, M.; Targa-Ferreira, C.; Lessa-Horta, B.; Epifanio, M.; Mouzaki, M.; Mattos, A.A. Non-alcoholic fatty liver disease in children and adolescents: Lifestyle change—A systematic review and meta-analysis. *Ann. Hepatol.* **2018**, *17*, 345–354. [CrossRef] [PubMed]
51. Zelber-Sagi, S.; Nitzan-Kaluski, D.; Goldsmith, R.; Webb, M.; Blendis, L.; Halpern, Z.; Oren, R. Long term nutritional intake and the risk for non-alcoholic fatty liver disease (nafld): A population based study. *J. Hepatol.* **2007**, *47*, 711–717. [CrossRef] [PubMed]

52. Assy, N.; Nasser, G.; Kamayse, I.; Nseir, W.; Beniashvili, Z.; Djibre, A.; Grosovski, M. Soft drink consumption linked with fatty liver in the absence of traditional risk factors. *Can. J. Gastroenterol.* **2008**, *22*, 811–816. [CrossRef] [PubMed]
53. Ouyang, X.; Cirillo, P.; Sautin, Y.; McCall, S.; Bruchette, J.L.; Diehl, A.M.; Johnson, R.J.; Abdelmalek, M.F. Fructose consumption as a risk factor for non-alcoholic fatty liver disease. *J. Hepatol.* **2008**, *48*, 993–999. [CrossRef] [PubMed]
54. Félix, D.R.; Costenaro, F.; Gottschall, C.B.A.; Coral, G.P. Non-alcoholic fatty liver disease (nafld) in obese children- effect of refined carbohydrates in diet. *BMC Pediatr.* **2016**, *16*, 187. [CrossRef] [PubMed]
55. Medrano, M.; Cadenas-Sanchez, C.; Alvarez-Bueno, C.; Cavero-Redondo, I.; Ruiz, J.R.; Ortega, F.B.; Labayen, I. Evidence-based exercise recommendations to reduce hepatic fat content in youth- a systematic review and meta-analysis. *Prog. Cardiovasc. Dis.* **2018**. [CrossRef] [PubMed]
56. Guercio Nuzio, S.; Di Stasi, M.; Pierri, L.; Troisi, J.; Poeta, M.; Bisogno, A.; Belmonte, F.; Tripodi, M.; Di Salvio, D.; Massa, G.; et al. Multiple gut-liver axis abnormalities in children with obesity with and without hepatic involvement. *Pediatr. Obes.* **2016**. [CrossRef]
57. Harte, A.L.; da Silva, N.F.; Creely, S.J.; McGee, K.C.; Billyard, T.; Youssef-Elabd, E.M.; Tripathi, G.; Ashour, E.; Abdalla, M.S.; Sharada, H.M.; et al. Elevated endotoxin levels in non-alcoholic fatty liver disease. *J. Inflamm.* **2010**, *7*, 15. [CrossRef] [PubMed]
58. Ouelaa, W.; Jegatheesan, P.; M'Bouyou-Boungou, J.; Vicente, C.; Nakib, S.; Nubret, E.; De Bandt, J.P. Citrulline decreases hepatic endotoxin-induced injury in fructose-induced non-alcoholic liver disease: An ex vivo study in the isolated perfused rat liver. *Br. J. Nutr.* **2017**, *117*, 1487–1494. [CrossRef] [PubMed]
59. Volynets, V.; Machann, J.; Kuper, M.A.; Maier, I.B.; Spruss, A.; Konigsrainer, A.; Bischoff, S.C.; Bergheim, I. A moderate weight reduction through dietary intervention decreases hepatic fat content in patients with non-alcoholic fatty liver disease (nafld): A pilot study. *Eur. J. Nutr.* **2013**, *52*, 527–535. [CrossRef] [PubMed]
60. Murphy, M.J.; Hosking, J.; Metcalf, B.S.; Voss, L.D.; Jeffery, A.N.; Sattar, N.; Williams, R.; Jeffery, J.; Wilkin, T.J. Distribution of adiponectin, leptin, and metabolic correlates of insulin resistance: A longitudinal study in british children; 1: Prepuberty (earlybird 15). *Clin. Chem.* **2008**, *54*, 1298–1306. [CrossRef] [PubMed]
61. Chen, A.K.; Roberts, C.K.; Barnard, R.J. Effect of a short-term diet and exercise intervention on metabolic syndrome in overweight children. *Metabolism* **2006**, *55*, 871–878. [CrossRef] [PubMed]

17

Soybean Oil-Derived Poly-Unsaturated Fatty Acids Enhance Liver Damage in NAFLD Induced by Dietary Cholesterol

Janin Henkel [1,*], Eugenia Alfine [2,3], Juliana Saín [1,4], Korinna Jöhrens [5], Daniela Weber [6], José P. Castro [6,7], Jeannette König [6], Christin Stuhlmann [1], Madita Vahrenbrink [1], Wenke Jonas [3,8], André Kleinridders [2,3] and Gerhard P. Püschel [1]

1 Department of Nutritional Biochemistry, Institute of Nutritional Science, University of Potsdam, D-14558 Nuthetal, Germany; jsain@fbcb.unl.edu.ar (J.S.); stuhlman@uni-potsdam.de (C.S.); vahrenbrink@uni-potsdam.de (M.V.); gpuesche@uni-potsdam.de (G.P.P.)

2 German Institute of Human Nutrition, Junior Research Group Central Regulation of Metabolism; D-14558 Nuthetal, Germany; Eugenia.Alfine@dife.de (E.A.); Andre.Kleinridders@dife.de (A.K.)

3 German Center for Diabetes Research (DZD), D-85764 München-Neuherberg, Germany; Wenke.Jonas@dife.de

4 Department of Biological Sciences, Food Science and Nutrition, Faculty of Biochemistry and Biological Sciences, National University of the Litoral (UNL), Santa Fe S3000, Argentina

5 Institute of Pathology, Carl Gustav Carus University Hospital Dresden; D-01307 Dresden, Germany; korinna.joehrens@uniklinikum-dresden.de

6 Department of Molecular Toxicology, German Institute of Human Nutrition; D-14558 Nuthetal, Germany; Daniela.Weber@dife.de (D.W.); Jose.Castro@dife.de (J.P.C.); Jeannette.Koenig@dife.de (J.K.)

7 Department of Medicine, Division of Genetics, Brigham and Women's Hospital and Harvard Medical School, Boston, MA 02115, USA

8 Department of Experimental Diabetology, German Institute of Human Nutrition; D-14558 Nuthetal, Germany

* Correspondence: jhenkel@uni-potsdam.de

Abstract: While the impact of dietary cholesterol on the progression of atherosclerosis has probably been overestimated, increasing evidence suggests that dietary cholesterol might favor the transition from blunt steatosis to non-alcoholic steatohepatitis (NASH), especially in combination with high fat diets. It is poorly understood how cholesterol alone or in combination with other dietary lipid components contributes to the development of lipotoxicity. The current study demonstrated that liver damage caused by dietary cholesterol in mice was strongly enhanced by a high fat diet containing soybean oil-derived ω6-poly-unsaturated fatty acids (ω6-PUFA), but not by a lard-based high fat diet containing mainly saturated fatty acids. In contrast to the lard-based diet the soybean oil-based diet augmented cholesterol accumulation in hepatocytes, presumably by impairing cholesterol-eliminating pathways. The soybean oil-based diet enhanced cholesterol-induced mitochondrial damage and amplified the ensuing oxidative stress, probably by peroxidation of poly-unsaturated fatty acids. This resulted in hepatocyte death, recruitment of inflammatory cells, and fibrosis, and caused a transition from steatosis to NASH, doubling the NASH activity score. Thus, the recommendation to reduce cholesterol intake, in particular in diets rich in ω6-PUFA, although not necessary to reduce the risk of atherosclerosis, might be sensible for patients suffering from non-alcoholic fatty liver disease.

Keywords: NASH; non-alcoholic fatty liver disease (NAFLD); cholesterol; PUFA; inflammation; oxidative stress

1. Introduction

The poor reputation of dietary cholesterol traces back to its supposed promoting role in the development of atherosclerosis [1]. However, the impact of dietary cholesterol on atherosclerosis has apparently been largely overestimated [2,3] and more recent recommendations for cardio-protective diets do not include the previously suggested radical reduction of cholesterol intake [4]. Although from the point of view of atherosclerosis, dietary cholesterol might be less relevant than previously assumed, it has reentered the focus of interest because of its potential role in the progression of non-alcoholic fatty liver disease (NAFLD) [5,6].

NAFLD describes a range of liver pathologies that have in common a lipid accumulation in hepatocytes in the absence of significant alcohol intake. NAFLD is a major and growing health problem [7]. While in recent years the prevalence of NAFLD in the general population has attained a level of 25%, it is present in the vast majority of overweight or obese patients and is considered the hepatic manifestation of the metabolic syndrome [8]. The disease pattern ranges from fully reversible blunt steatosis (NAFL) to a chronically progressive disease (non-alcoholic steatohepatitis, NASH) that is characterized by varying degrees of hepatocyte death, inflammation, and fibrosis and may ultimately result in liver cirrhosis, hepatocellular carcinoma, and terminal organ failure [9]. The transition from steatosis to the more severe forms of the disease occurs in roughly one third of affected patients, but it is still unclear what triggers this progression. However, there is evidence that dietary cholesterol might impact this transition. A number of independent animal experimental studies showed that enrichment of a high fat diet with 0.2 to 2% cholesterol resulted in a rapid progression from blunt steatosis to a NASH-like phenotype with ballooning, infiltration with inflammatory cells, and fibrosis [10–14]. Similarly, animal experiments [15] and clinical studies [16] using the cholesterol uptake inhibitor ezitimibe suggest that inhibition of cholesterol uptake from the gut might protect against NASH development. The mechanisms of how dietary cholesterol might trigger the transition to NASH have so far not been fully elucidated. The supposed mechanisms include activation of ER-stress response in hepatocytes, impairment of mitochondrial function resulting in oxidative stress, and the activation of resident or infiltrating macrophages by danger-associated molecular patterns (DAMPs) released from cholesterol-laden dying hepatocytes [17,18].

Our current study supports the view that dietary cholesterol can trigger NASH-development by causing mitochondrial dysfunction and oxidative stress and shows that these patho-mechanisms are severely aggravated by the presence of poly-unsaturated fatty acids (PUFA) in dietary fat.

2. Materials and Methods

All chemicals were of analytical or higher grade and obtained from local providers unless otherwise stated.

Animals and experimental design. Male C57BL/6JRj mice (own breeding) were housed in type II-cages at 20 ± 2 °C with a 12 h light/dark-cycle. Mice were randomly assigned to one of the following diet groups with free access to food and drinking water for 20 weeks: standard chow diet (V153 R/M-H; Ssniff, Soest, Germany) (STD), 0.75% cholesterol on a standard diet (CHO + STD), 0.75% cholesterol in a high fat diet containing ω6-PUFA-rich soybean oil (CHO + SOY; Altromin, Lage, Germany) or 0.75% cholesterol in a high fat diet containing mainly lard as fat source (CHO + LAR, D12451; Research Diets, New Brunswick, NJ, USA). Detailed diet composition is shown in Table 1. Mice had access to wooden gnawing sticks to avoid excessive teeth growth. Body weight was measured weekly. Mice were killed by cervical dislocation after isoflurane anesthesia. Serum and organs were snap-frozen in liquid nitrogen and stored at −70 °C for biochemical analysis, aliquots of the organs were fixed for histological examination. Animal experiments were performed according to the ARRIVE guidelines. Treatment of the animals followed the German animal protection laws and was performed with approval of the state animal welfare committee (LUGV Brandenburg, V3 2347).

Table 1. Diet composition. Mice diets used in the feeding experiment. Standard chow diet (STD), 0.75% cholesterol in a Standard diet (CHO + CHO), 0.75% cholesterol in a high fat diet containing ω6-PUFA-rich soybean oil (CHO + SOY), 0.75% cholesterol in a high fat diet containing mainly lard as fat source (CHO + LAR).

	STD	CHO + STD	CHO + SOY	CHO + LAR
Metabolizing energy (kcal/g)	3.06	3.06	4.64	4.73
Energy from carbohydrates (%)	65	65	35	35
Energy from protein (%)	25	25	16	20
Energy from fat (%)	10	10	49	45
Cholesterol (%)	0.00	0.75	0.75	0.75
Fatty acid composition				
Saturated fatty acids (g/100g)	0.55	0.55	4.00	7.26
Mono-unsaturated fatty acids (g/100g)	0.64	0.64	5.75	8.69
Poly-unsaturated fatty acids (g/100g)	2.01	2.01	14.50	6.36

In vivo experiments. Body fat content was measured at the beginning and at the end of the diet intervention by nuclear magnetic resonance spectroscopy (EchoMRI 2012 Body Composition Analyzer, Houston, TX, USA). The oral glucose tolerance test was performed in week 18 after an overnight fast by oral gavage of glucose (2 mg/kg body weight). Glucose and insulin levels were measured at the times indicated by a glucose sensor (Breeze2, Bayer; Berlin, Germany) or an insulin ELISA kit (Crystall Chem; Downers Grove, IL, USA).

Serum and tissue analysis. Serum parameters were quantified by an automated analyzer (Cobas Mira S, Hoffmann-La Roche, Basel, Switzerland) with the appropriate commercially available reagent kits. Liver triglycerides were determined by TRIGS-assay (Randox; Crumlin, UK). Total and free cholesterol in liver tissue was determined by a modified version of a protocol described previously [19]. Briefly, frozen tissues were homogenized by sonication using phosphate buffer (10 mM, pH 7.4) containing 1% polyoxyehylen-10-tridecylether. Homogenates were heated (5 min at 70 °C) to inactivate enzymes and then centrifuged for 10 min at 4 °C. Aliquots of supernatant were incubated in the presence or absence of 0.5 U/mL of cholesterol esterase to quantify the total and free cholesterol, respectively. The reaction buffer contained 100 mmol/L Tris (pH 7.7); 6 mmol/l phenol, 1 mmol/L 4-aminoantipyrine, 4 mmol/L 3,4-dichlorophenol, 10 mmol/L sodium cholate, 3 g/L fatty alcohol polyglycol ether, 50 mmol/L $MgCl_2$, 0.2 U/mL cholesterol oxidase, and 0.4 U/mL peroxidase. The quinoneimine dye formed after 30 min is proportional to the quantity of cholesterol and was detected at 500 nm. A calibration curve was performed using a cholesterol solution 200 mg% (m/v) in fatty alcohol polyglycol ether (3 g/L). The esterified cholesterol was quantified by the difference between total and free cholesterol. Malondialdehyde was quantified by HPLC with fluorescence detection as described previously [11].

Histology. Formalin-fixed and paraffin-embedded liver sections (2–3 μm) were stained with Hematoxylin & Eosin or Sirius Red (both Sigma-Aldrich, Taufkirchen, Germany). Immunohistochemistry analyses were performed with anti-F4/80 antibody (AbD Serotec, Bio-Rad, Munich, Germany). Terminal deoxynucleotidyl transferase dUTP Nick End Labeling (TUNEL) assay was achieved with the Click-iT™ TUNEL Colorimetric IHC Detection Kit (Thermo Fisher Scientific, Berlin, Germany). Histological steatosis, inflammation and fibrosis were graded according to the NASH activity score (NAS) [20,21] by a liver pathologist (KJ) blinded to the diet. Quantification of histological staining of Sirius Red, F4/80, and TUNEL-positive cells was performed by using ImageJ software (version ImageJ 1.51j8, Wayne Rasband, National Institutes of Health, USA) in images of five randomly chosen fields of each liver. Details are described in the Methods section of the Supplementary Material.

Real-time RT-PCR analysis. RNA isolation, reverse transcription, and qPCR were performed as previously described [22]. Results are expressed as relative gene expression normalized to expression levels of reference genes (Hprt, Eef2 and Srsf4) according to the formula: fold induction =

$2^{(a\,-\,b)\ \text{gene of interest}}/2^{(a\,-\,b)\ \text{reference genes}}$. Parameter "a" is the arithmetic mean of all Ct-values from samples of the STD group and parameter "b" is the Ct-value of every single sample. For calculations with more than one reference gene the geometric mean of the difference (a − b) of each reference gene was used.

Western blot and Oxyblot analysis. Western blot was performed as described previously [23] with anti-PGC-1α antibody and oxidative phosphorylation cocktail for Western blot (both abcam, Cambridge, UK), as well as Ponceau S-staining (Sigma-Aldrich, Taufkirchen, Germany) as a loading control. Oxyblot analysis was done as described [11] with anti-DNP antibody (Sigma-Aldrich, Taufkirchen, Germany). Visualization of immune complexes was performed by using a chemoluminescence reagent in the ChemiDoc™ Imaging System with ImageLab software (Bio-Rad, Munich, Germany).

Statistical analysis. The statistical significance of differences was determined by one-way-ANOVA with Tukey's post hoc test for multiple comparisons or Krukal-Wallis test for non-parametric samples as detailed in the legends to the figures using GraphPad Prism version 6 for Windows (GraphPad Software, La Jolla, California, CA, USA). Differences with a $p \leq 0.05$ were considered statistically significant.

3. Results

3.1. Diet-Induced Weight Gain, Insulin Resistance and NAFLD

Mice received either standard chow diet (STD), chow diet enriched with 0.75% cholesterol (CHO + STD), a soybean oil-based high fat diet with 0.75% cholesterol (CHO + SOY) or a lard-based high fat diet with 0.75% cholesterol (CHO + LAR) for 20 weeks, as described in Table 1. Animals on both high fat diets gained more weight than animals fed either chow diet or cholesterol-enriched chow diet (Figure 1A). The high fat diet-induced weight gain could be attributed to an increase in fat mass (Figure 1B) while the fat-free mass remained largely unaltered. Despite similar weight gain and increase in fat mass, animals fed the CHO + LAR diet were significantly more insulin resistant than animals receiving CHO + SOY diet (Figure 1C). As expected from the body weight data, CHO + STD-fed animals showed no signs of insulin resistance.

Serum cholesterol levels increased only slightly (20%) in animals receiving the CHO + STD diet (Figure 2A). By contrast, serum cholesterol concentrations were doubled in comparison to the control in animals receiving either one of the high fat diets with cholesterol. Notably, no difference in serum cholesterol levels was observed between CHO + SOY- and CHO + LAR-fed animals (Figure 2A).

Unexpectedly, but in keeping with data of many independent studies in the literature [11,24,25], serum triglyceride levels were not elevated but instead were decreased in animals receiving either one of the cholesterol-enriched diets, irrespective of their fat content (Figure 2B). Total cholesterol was increased in livers of all animals receiving cholesterol-enriched diets. However, whereas CHO + STD and CHO + LAR-fed animals showed a similar approximately 2 to 3-fold increase in hepatic cholesterol content, animals receiving CHO + SOY diet exhibited a 6-fold increase in hepatic total cholesterol content (Figure 2C). Notably, free cholesterol was not significantly increased in CHO + STD-fed or CHO + LAR-fed animals in comparison to STD-fed animals, whereas free cholesterol content was doubled in CHO + SOY-fed mice (Figure 2C). In line with this, high amounts of cholesterol crystals could be detected only in livers of CHO + SOY-fed mice whereas only few or no cholesterol crystals were visible in livers of CHO + STD or CHO + LAR-fed mice (own observation).

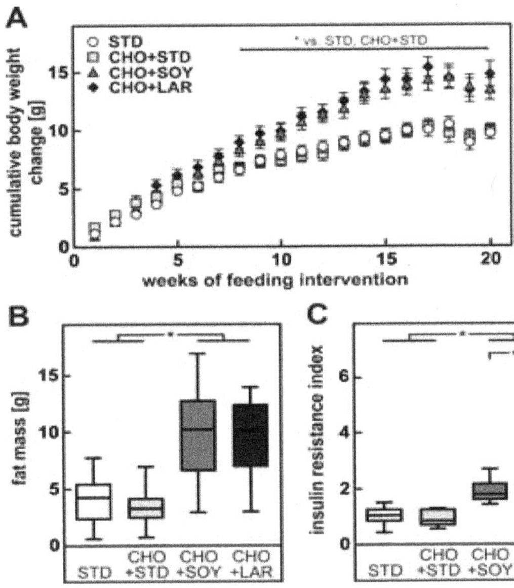

Figure 1. Increase in body weight, fat mass and insulin resistance in mice fed a CHO + SOY or CHO + LAR diet for 20 weeks. (**A**) Cumulative body weight change. (**B**) Fat mass in week 20. (**C**) Insulin resistance index was calculated by the sum of the products of insulin concentration × glucose concentration during the oral glucose tolerance test. Values are median (line), upper- and lower quartile (box) and extremes (whiskers) of 17–35 (**A**,**B**) or 8–10 (**C**) mice per group. Statistics: Multiple Student's *t*-test for unpaired samples (**A**) or one-way-ANOVA with Tukey's post hoc test for multiple comparisons (**B**,**C**). * $p < 0.05$.

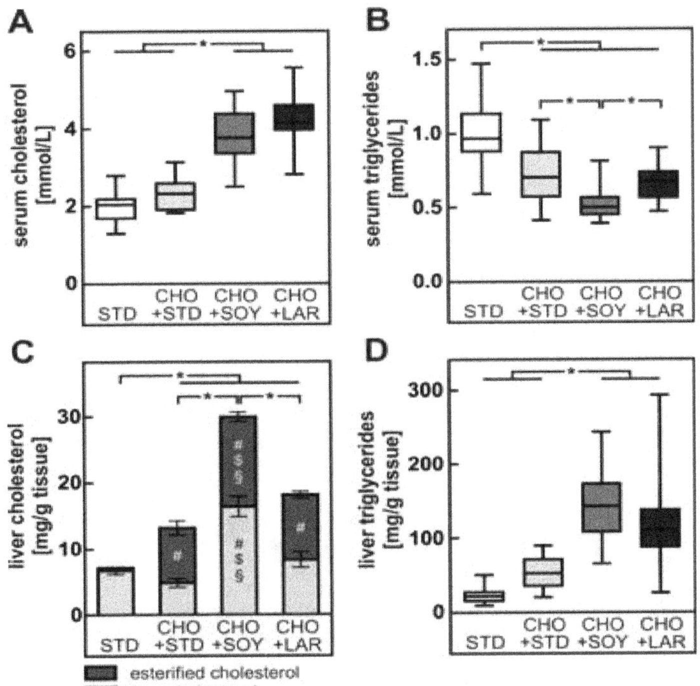

Figure 2. Diet-induced changes in serum and liver lipids after 20 weeks. (**A**) Cholesterol concentrations in serum. (**B**) Triglyceride concentrations in serum. (**C**) Levels of free and esterified cholesterol in liver. (**D**) Triglyceride levels in liver. Values are median (line), upper- and lower quartile (box) and extremes (whiskers) (**A**,**B**,**D**) or mean and sem (**C**) of 17–35 mice per group. Statistics: One-way-ANOVA with Tukey's post hoc test for multiple comparisons. *: $p < 0.05$. Separate statistic for free and esterified cholesterol (**C**): #: vs. STD, $: vs. CHO + STD, §: vs. CHO+ LAD with $p < 0.05$.

Although weight gain was unaltered in animals receiving CHO + STD diet, these animals had a pronounced hepatic steatosis (see below, Figure 4). Hepatic triglyceride content increased more than twofold in comparison to chow-fed animals (Figure 2D). Hepatic triglyceride accumulation was more pronounced in animals receiving cholesterol-enriched high fat diets. Livers of CHO + SOY-fed and CHO + LAR-fed animals contained 7-fold or 5-fold more triglycerides than STD-fed animals, respectively (Figure 2D). The difference between the two high fat diets was, however, not significant.

In summary, mice fed a CHO + SOY diet accumulated significantly higher amounts of free and esterified cholesterol in the liver compared to mice fed one of the other cholesterol-containing diets. Since the CHO + STD, CHO + SOY and CHO + LAD diets contained equal amounts of cholesterol, the combination of dietary cholesterol and ω6-PUFA-rich soybean oil may favor hepatic cholesterol accumulation.

The more pronounced increase in hepatic cholesterol content can either be the consequence of an enhanced uptake or a diminished excretion or conversion of cholesterol. In accordance with the latter hypothesis, the expression of the cholesterol export pump Abcg5 was induced more than fourfold in animals receiving either CHO + STD or CHO + LAR diet (Figure 3A). By contrast, the export pump was induced merely twofold, and hence significantly less, in animals receiving CHO + SOY diet than in either of the other two cholesterol containing diets (Figure 3A). Gene expression of Abcg8, the heterodimerization partner of Abcg5, was similar, yet it did not reach significance (Figure 3B). In comparison to the standard chow diet, Abca1, another cholesterol transporter mainly expressed in macrophages, was induced approximately 1.32-fold in livers of mice fed any of the cholesterol-containing diets. The increase was significant only in the CHO + STD diet group and no significant differences between the cholesterol-fed groups were observed.

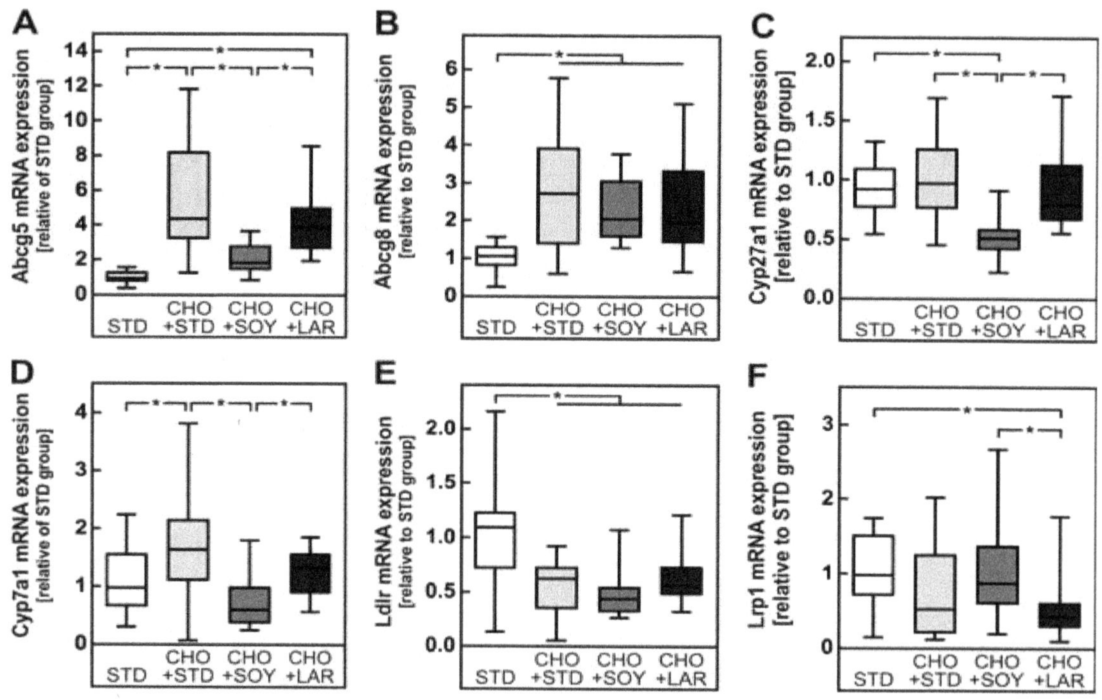

Figure 3. Markers of cholesterol metabolism in mice fed a cholesterol-containing diet for 20 weeks. Relative mRNA expression of the cholesterol transporters ATP-binding cassette sub-family G (Abcg) member 5 (**A**) and 8 (**B**), the cholesterol- metabolizing enzymes cytochrome P450 family 27 a1 (Cyp27a1, **C**) and family 7 a1 (Cyp7a1, **D**) as well as the transporters for the cholesterol intake LDL receptor (Ldlr, **E**) and LDL receptor related protein 1 (Lrp1, **F**) in mice liver. Values are median (line), upper- and lower quartile (box) and extremes (whiskers) of 17–35 mice per group. Statistics: One-way-ANOVA with Tukey's post hoc test for multiple comparisons. *: $p < 0.05$.

In addition, the expression of Cyp27a1, a key enzyme for the conversion of cholesterol into bile acids, was significantly repressed in livers of CHO + SOY-fed mice (Figure 3C). Similarly, Cyp7a1 was repressed in CHO + SOY-fed animals, whereas it was unaffected or even induced in CHO + LAR diet and CHO + STD diet-fed animals, respectively (Figure 3D). Gene expression of the LDL receptor was repressed to a similar extent in livers of animals receiving any of the three cholesterol-containing diets (Figure 3E). By contrast, the expression of the LDL receptor related protein 1 (Lrp1) was slightly or significantly reduced in livers of animals receiving the CHO + STD or CHO + LAR diets, whereas expression was unaltered in livers of CHO + SOY-fed animals (Figure 3F).

In conclusion, the enhanced cholesterol accumulation in livers of CHO + SOY-fed mice can be explained by a decreased Abcg5-mediated cholesterol export, reduced Cyp27a1-dependent conversion of cholesterol into bile acids, as well as impaired repression of Lrp1-related cholesterol uptake into hepatocytes.

Following, livers were examined histologically to determine the NASH activity score (NAS) (Table 2 and Figure 4). No signs of NAFLD were detected in livers of STD-fed control animals. By contrast, all animals receiving cholesterol-enriched diets had a positive NAS. However, while the average NAS for CHO + STD-fed and CHO + LAR-fed animals reached a maximum of 4 and hence indicated the presence of blunt steatosis, the average NAS of CHO + SOY-fed mice was above 7, clearly indicating the presence of active NASH (Table 2).

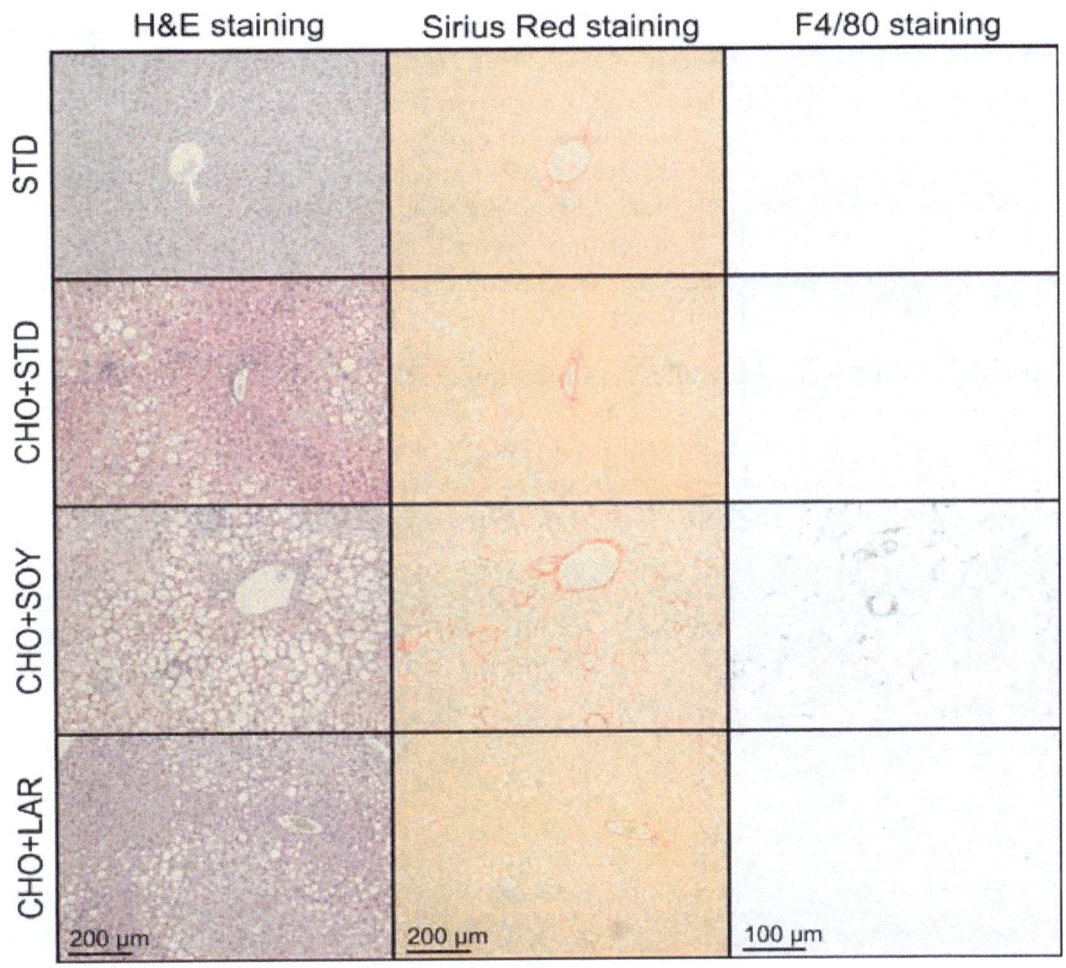

Figure 4. CHO + SOY diet induced steatohepatitis with steatosis, fibrosis, and macrophage infiltration. Mice received the diets for 20 weeks. Representative microphotographs of liver sections, magnification 10× or 20×.

Table 2. NASH activity score grading steatosis, ballooning (hepatocyte hypertrophy), inflammation, and fibrosis. Values are mean ± SEM of 17–35 mice per group. Statistics: Kruskal-Wallis test with Dunn's post hoc test for multiple comparisons. #: vs. STD, $: vs. CHO + STD, §: vs. CHO + LAD with $p < 0.05$.

Scoring Parameter	STD	CHO + STD	CHO + SOY	CHO + LAR
Steatosis	0.00 ± 0.00	1.53 ± 0.37 (#)	3.77 ± 0.08 (#,$,§)	2.41 ± 0.33 (#)
Hepatocyte hypertrophy	0.00 ± 0.00	0.35 ± 0.15	1.73 ± 0.10 (#,$,§)	0.76 ± 0.18 (#)
Inflammation	0.10 ± 0.05	0.53 ± 0.15	1.50 ± 0.13 (#,$,§)	0.41 ± 0.12
Fibrosis	0.26 ± 0.08	0.59 ± 0.12	0.80 ± 0.07 (#)	0.47 ± 0.12
NASH activity score (NAS)	0.36 ± 0.10	3.00 ± 0.59 (#)	7.80 ± 0.20 (#,$,§)	4.06 ± 0.49 (#)

3.2. Diet-Induced Inflammation and Fibrosis

All cholesterol-containing diets apparently triggered an inflammatory response in the liver. However, in accordance with the higher NAS, animals receiving the CHO + SOY diet showed more pronounced signs of inflammation (Figure 4 right panel, quantification in Figure 5B). The expression of the chemotactic cytokine Ccl2 (Mcp-1) was increased about two-fold in animals receiving CHO + STD or CHO + LAR diets, whereas an almost 10-fold increase was observed in CHO + SOY diet-fed animals (Figure 5A). Consequently, the expression of the macrophage markers F4/80, Cd68, and Cd11b was increased by all cholesterol-containing diets, but was significantly higher in CHO + SOY-fed animals than in animals receiving any of the other diets (Figure 5B–D). Similarly, the induction of the pro-inflammatory cytokine TNF-α was two-fold higher in livers of CHO + SOY-fed mice than in animals that received the CHO + STD or CHO + LAR diet (Figure 5E). Inducible nitric oxide synthase (Nos2, iNos), a key enzyme in inflammation-dependent NO production was only induced in livers of CHO + SOY-fed animals (Figure 5F). Furthermore, a significantly higher amount of TUNEL-positive hepatocytes were detected in livers of CHO + SOY-fed mice compared to mice fed any of the other diets, showing increased hepatic apoptosis (Figure 5G).

In order to assess fibrosis, liver slices were stained with Sirius Red (Figure 4). A significant increase in fibrosis was only observed in animals receiving CHO + SOY diet, whereas all other animals only showed minor age-appropriate positive staining for Sirius Red (Figure 5H). In accordance with these histological data, collagen 1a1 expression was slightly induced in animals fed CHO + STD or CHO + LAR diets, whereas a more than 10-fold induction was observed in livers of CHO + SOY-fed mice (Figure 5I).

These results show that only mice fed a CHO + SOY diet developed clear signs of hepatic inflammation with macrophage infiltration and increased expression of pro-inflammatory cytokines as well as hepatocyte apoptosis and liver fibrosis.

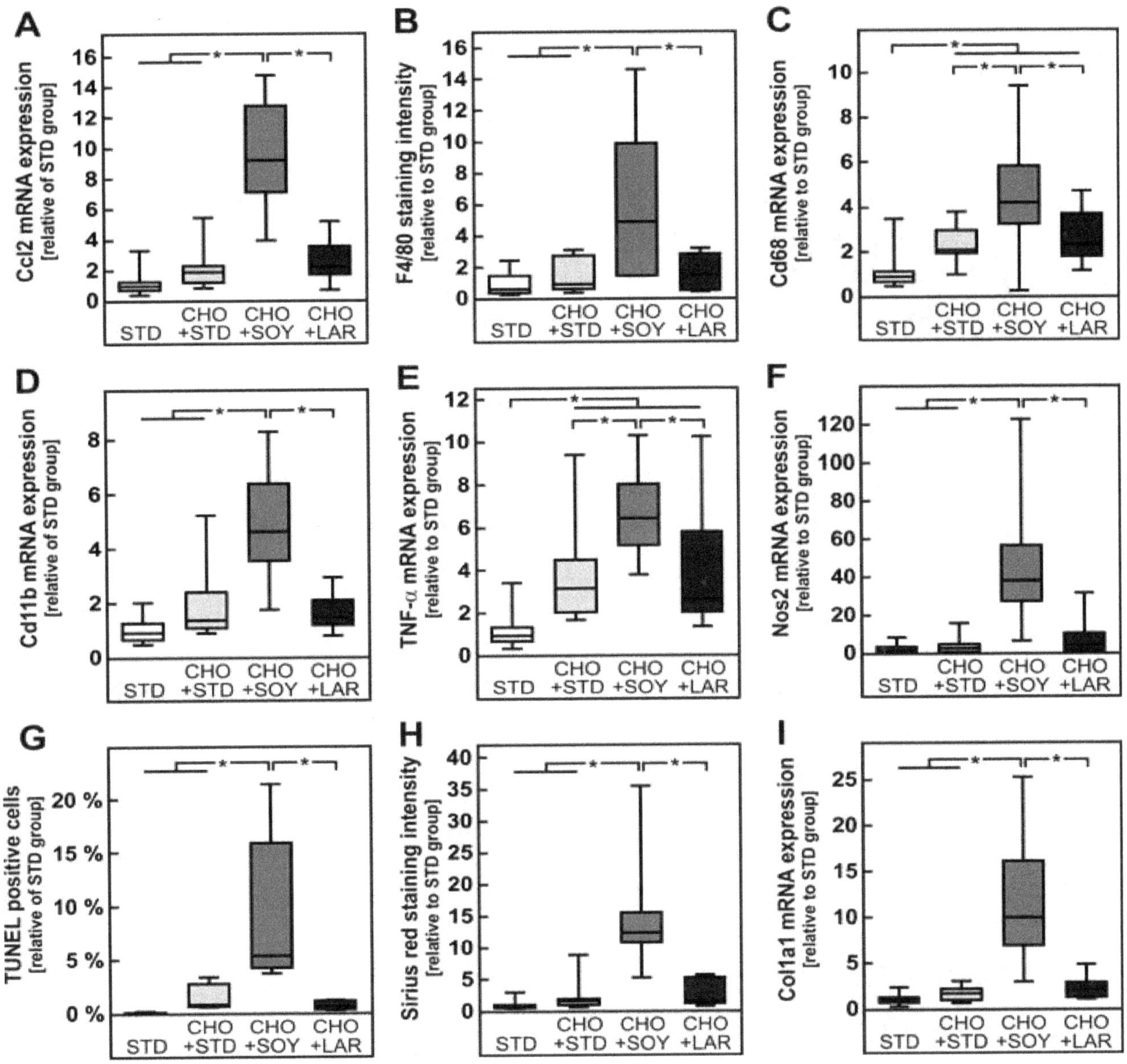

Figure 5. Enhanced macrophage infiltration, inflammation, apoptosis and fibrosis in mice fed a CHO + SOY diet. Mice received the diets for 20 weeks. (**A**) Relative mRNA expression of the chemokine Ccl2 (alternative name Mcp-1) in mice liver. (**B**) Quantification of F4/80-stained microphotographs of the liver. (**C**,**D**,**E**,**F**) Relative mRNA expression of the macrophage markers Cd68 (**C**) and Cd11b (**D**, gene name *Itgam*), the cytokine tumor necrosis factor α (TNF- α, **E**) and the enzyme inducible nitric oxide synthase 2 (**F**, alternative name iNos) in mice liver. (**G**) Quantification of hepatocyte apoptosis by TUNEL assay. (**H**) Quantification of Sirius Red-stained microphotographs of the liver calculated by dense intensity of Sirius Red relative to the amount of cytosolic background per field in 5 randomly chosen microphotographs per liver section. (**I**) Relative mRNA expression of the fibrosis marker collagen 1a1 (Col1a1) in mice liver. Values are median (line), upper- and lower quartile (box) and extremes (whiskers) of 17–35 (**A**,**C**,**D**,**E**,**F**,**I**), 4–7 (**B**,**G**) or 13–16 (**H**) mice per group. Statistics: One-way-ANOVA with Tukey's post hoc test for multiple comparisons. *: $p < 0.05$.

3.3. Diet-Induced Mitochondrial Damage and Oxidative Stress

The cholesterol-dependent induction of liver damage has previously been attributed to mitochondrial damage resulting from cholesterol accumulation in mitochondrial membranes. However, judging from the expression of complex I, II, and IV of the respiratory chain, dietary cholesterol alone apparently did cause low but no severe mitochondrial damage in our model

(Figure 6A). A mild reduction of complex I, II, and IV content was also observed in livers from animals receiving CHO + LAR diet. In stark contrast, complex I, II, and IV proteins were dramatically reduced in livers of CHO + SOY-fed animals, indicating severe mitochondrial damage in only this group (Figure 6A). In keeping with these data, the amount of PGC-1α protein was strongly reduced in livers of animals receiving the CHO + SOY diet (Figure 6B).

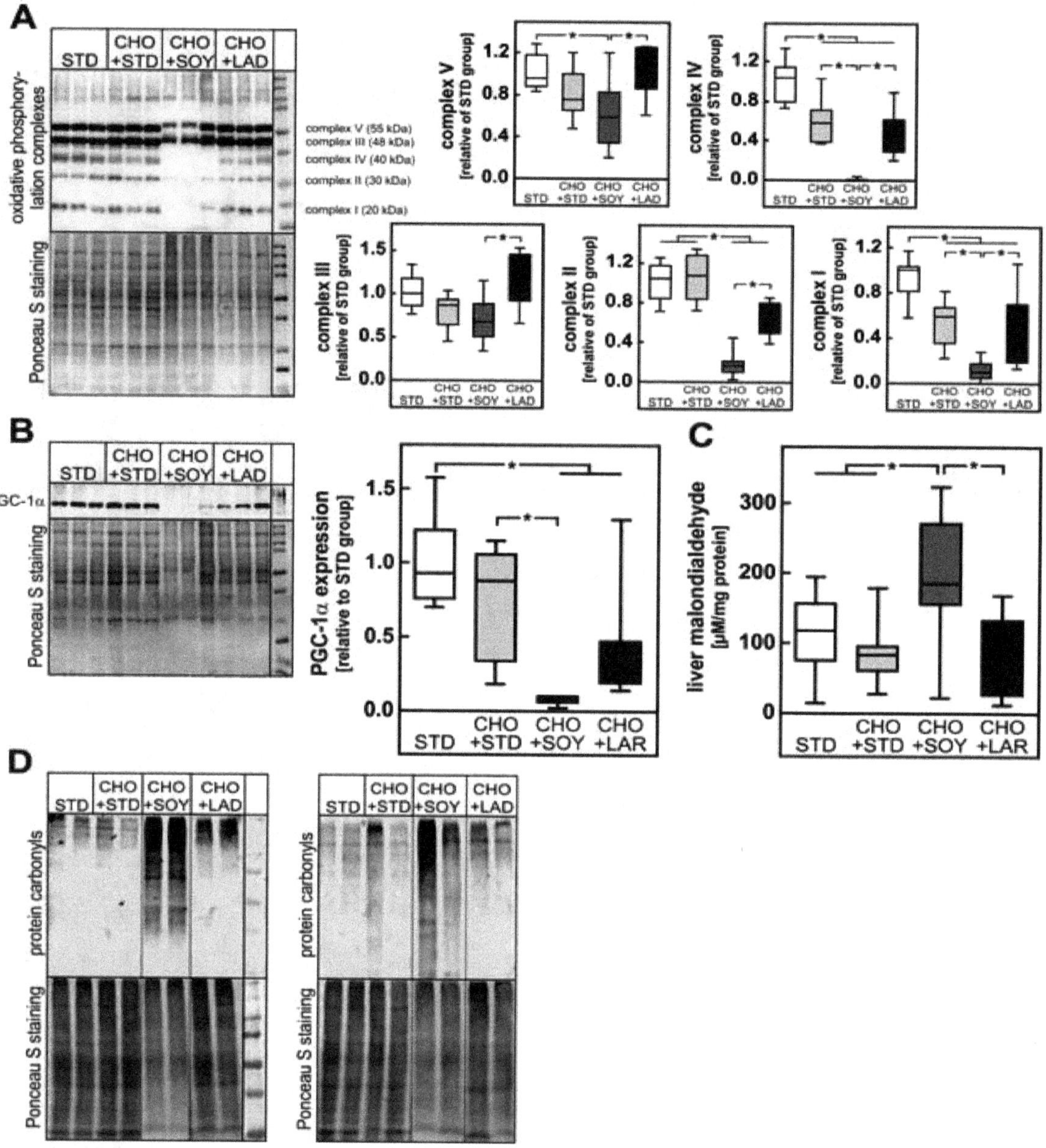

Figure 6. Increased mitochondrial damage and oxidative stress in mice fed a CHO + SOY diet for 20 weeks. (**A**,**B**) Hepatic protein expression of the oxidative phosphorylation complexes (**A**) and PGC-1α (**B**). Dense intensity was normalized to Ponceau S staining, which was verified on the same Western blot membrane as a loading control and calculated relative to the STD group in each gel. A representative blot is shown. All original blots are provided in the Supplementary Material, Figures S1 and S2. (**C**) Concentration of malondialdehyde in liver as a marker of lipid peroxidation. (**D**) Determination of protein carbonyls in liver homogenates verified by oxyblot with Ponceau staining as a loading control. Blots were cut at the dotted lines. Original blots are shown in the Supplementary Material, Figure S3. Values are median (line), upper- and lower quartile (box) and extremes (whiskers) of 8–10 (**A**,**B**) or 9–28 (**C**) mice per group. Statistics: One-way-ANOVA with Tukey's post hoc test for multiple comparisons. *: $p < 0.05$.

Impairment of mitochondrial respiration causes severe oxidative stress. Accordingly, levels of malondialdehyde, a reaction product of lipid peroxidation of unsaturated fatty acids, and protein carbonyls were only increased in livers of CHO + SOY-fed mice (Figure 6C,D).

Thus, cholesterol-induced mitochondrial damage and oxidative stress was clearly enhanced by soybean oil-derived PUFA probably due to augmented lipid peroxidation.

3.4. Oxidative Stress Preceding Inflammation

In order to elucidate whether oxidative stress in livers of CHO + SOY-fed animals was the cause or consequence of the inflammation observed in the livers of these animals, the CHO + SOY diet was fed for a shorter period, i.e., 19 days. While liver steatosis, a reduction of PGC-1α, a reduction of complexes of the respiratory chain as well as signs of oxidative stress were already present after 19 days of feeding, no increase in inflammatory markers was detectable, indicating that mitochondrial damage and oxidative stress precede the development of inflammation (Figure 7, Figure S4 in Supplementary Material).

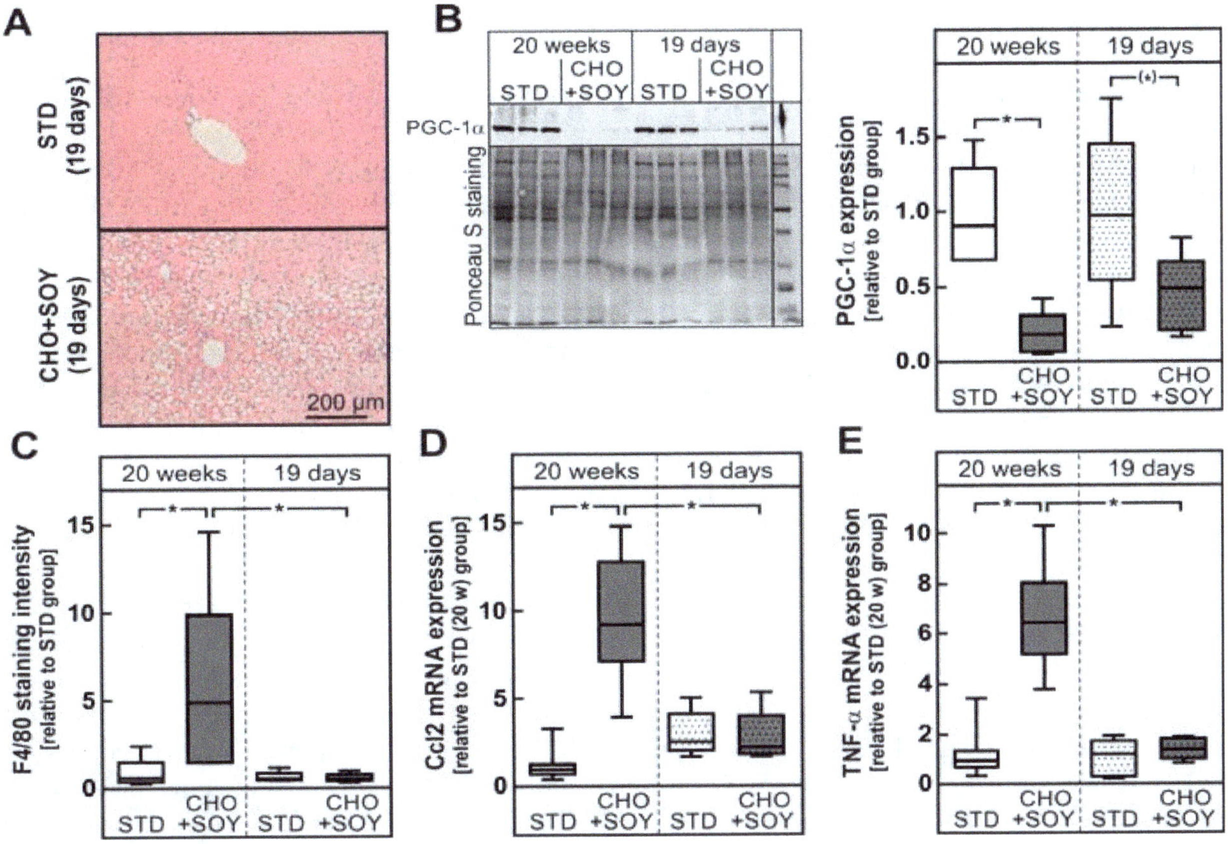

Figure 7. Enhanced mitochondrial damage but no signs of inflammation in mice fed a CHO + SOY diet for 19 days. Mice received the STD CHO + SOY diet for 20 weeks or 19 days. (**A**) Representative H&E-stained microphotographs of the liver. (**B**) Hepatic protein expression of PGC-1α after 20 week and 19 days feeding intervention. Dense intensity was normalized to Ponceau S staining, which was verified on the same Western blot membrane as a loading control and calculated relative to the STD group in each gel. A representative blot is shown. All original blots are provided in the Supplementary Material, Figure S4. (**C**) Quantification of F4/80-stained microphotographs of the liver calculated by dense intensity of F4/80 relative to the amount of cytosolic background per field in 5 randomly chosen microphotographs per liver section. (**D**,**E**) Relative mRNA expression of Ccl2 (**D**, alternative name Mcp-1) and tumor necrosis factor α (TNF-α, E) in mice liver. Values are median (line), upper- and lower quartile (box) and extremes (whiskers) of 6 (**B**,**C**) or 6–7 (**D**,**E**) mice per group. Statistics: One-way-ANOVA with Tukey's post hoc test for multiple comparisons. *: $p < 0.05$.

4. Discussion

In our current study we showed that dietary cholesterol induced hepatic steatosis and NAFLD independent of the accompanying lipid content of the diet. However, histological signs of progression to NASH, hepatocyte apoptosis, infiltration with inflammatory cells, and fibrosis only developed when dietary cholesterol was combined with a soybean oil-based high fat diet rich in ω6-PUFA. Our results indicate the contribution of two potentially cooperating mechanisms to this transition: (1) soybean oil-derived PUFA increased hepatic cholesterol accumulation, most likely by repression of pathways that are responsible for the elimination of cholesterol via the bile. (2) soybean oil-derived PUFA augmented cholesterol-induced mitochondrial damage and oxidative stress presumably via lipid peroxidation.

4.1. PUFA-Dependent Increase in Cholesterol Accumulation

An increase in hepatic cholesterol accumulation by a soybean oil-based high fat diet has been observed previously in a study that compared the tissue distribution of cholesterol in rats fed a soybean oil-based or tallow-based high fat diet [26]. Yet, the underlying mechanisms were not analyzed in this early study. Hepatic cholesterol accumulation in the presence of dietary PUFA could result either from increased hepatic uptake or decreased removal.

Since dietary cholesterol is absorbed via the chylomicron pathway, an increase in hepatic cholesterol uptake should most likely be mediated by an augmented hepatic clearance of remnant particles or absorption of HDL cholesterol. Both processes involve the LDL receptor, the LDL-receptor-related protein 1, and the scavenger receptor class B type1. While the LDL receptor, as expected, was downregulated in animals fed any of the cholesterol-containing diets, gene expression of the LDL receptor related protein 1 (Lrp1) was reduced only in animals receiving CHO + STD or CHO + LAR diets, but not in the CHO + SOY-fed animals (Figure 3E,F). These differences were however rather small and unlikely to account for the two-fold increase in hepatic cholesterol observed in CHO + SOY-fed animals (Figure 2C). In the literature, a PUFA-induced increase in SR-B1 expression was described in a genetically obese rat strain [27] that was supposed to result in a more efficient hepatic uptake of cholesterol from HDL and hence might contribute to hepatic cholesterol accumulation and at the same time contribute to the anti-atherogenic effect of dietary PUFA.

The current data indicate that a dietary PUFA-dependent inhibition of cholesterol removal from the liver either as free cholesterol or after conversion into bile acids is the more likely explanation for the pronounced cholesterol accumulation in livers of CHO + SOY-fed animals. Cholesterol can be excreted directly into the bile by the ABCG5/ABCG8 export pump [28]. The expression of Abcg5 was induced four- to sixfold in CHO + LAR- or CHO + STD-fed animals, respectively. By contrast a significantly lower twofold induction was observed in livers of CHO + SOY-fed animals (Figure 3A,B). Similarly, the expression of the genes for enzymes involved in bile acid formation was repressed by CHO + SOY diet feeding. The CHO + SOY diet is rich in ω6-PUFA whereas the content in ω3-fatty acids is relatively low. In contrast to ω6-PUFA, ω3-PUFA appeared to increase the expression both of cholesterol export pumps and key enzymes of bile acid synthesis [29]. Interestingly, whereas ω6-fatty acids favor accumulation of cholesterol in the liver, long chain ω3-poly-unsaturated fatty acids seem to counteract this effect. Thus, hamsters fed a diet that contained 38% linoleic acid (18:2(ω6)) accumulated almost twice as much cholesterol ester in the liver as animals fed a similar diet in which half of the linoleic acid was replaced by long chain ω3-fatty acids, mainly eicosapentaenoic acid (20:5(ω3)) and docosahexaenoic acid (22:6(ω3)) [30]. Similarly, hepatic cholesterol content was reduced by long chain ω3-PUFA supplementation in mice fed a high fat high cholesterol diet rich in ω6-fatty acids [31]. This might in part explain why supplementation with ω3-fatty acids has repeatedly been reported to protect from NAFLD or NASH development [32,33] while depletion of ω3-PUFA increased hepatic steatosis [34].

Also highly unlikely, it cannot be entirely excluded that apart from the pronounced differences in the fatty acid composition minor differences in the protein composition between the two high fat diets also contributed to the different phenotypes observed in particular to hepatic lipid accumulation, since diets extremely rich in protein appear to protect from hepatic steatosis [35].

4.2. PUFA-Dependent Enhancement of Oxidative Stress

Dietary cholesterol initially accumulates in the hepatocyte. This results in an increase in cholesterol content in the membranes of different cellular compartments and the subsequent impairment of their function. Thus, it has been shown that an increment in the cholesterol content of the ER membrane may result in the inhibition of the ER calcium pump, a drop in ER calcium concentration, impaired protein folding, and ER stress ([18] and references therein). It has, however, been questioned, whether this mechanism is relevant for NASH development [36]. Similarly, accumulation of cholesterol in the outer phospholipid monolayer of lipid droplets has been assumed to impair lipid turnover and may result in the formation of cholesterol crystals in lipid droplets [12]. Most importantly, however, excessive incorporation of cholesterol in mitochondrial membranes has been shown to impair the function of the α-ketoglutarate carrier that is responsible for the import of reduced glutathione from the cytosol into the mitochondrion [37]. As a consequence, the quenching of reactive oxygen species formed in the respiratory chain is impaired and oxidative stress ensues [38]. The oxidative stress further impairs mitochondrial function and may sensitize the hepatocyte to other death-inducing signals. Apparently, this mechanism was further aggravated by the presence of PUFA in the CHO + SOY diet, since only the combination of cholesterol with soybean oil-based high fat diet resulted in a reduction of mitochondrial respiratory chain proteins and PGC-1α, the master regulator of mitochondrial biogenesis (Figure 6A,B), as well as profound oxidative stress leading to the formation of large amounts of protein carbonyls (Figure 6D). Apart from enhancing cholesterol accumulation in the hepatocyte (see above), PUFA might amplify cholesterol-dependent oxidative stress by lipid peroxidation chain reactions resulting, among others, in the formation of malondialdehyde (Figure 6C). Lipid peroxides have been shown to decrease the content of mitochondrial respiratory chain proteins [39] and cause mitochondrial dysfunction. A reduction in the content of mitochondrial respiratory chain proteins in the liver of NASH patients has been described [25]. Lipid peroxidation also favors the non-enzymatic formation of oxysterols. While oxysterols at low concentrations activate liver X receptor (LXR) and may initiate pathways that protect against consequences of a cholesterol overload, high oxysterol concentrations induce apoptosis by triggering the mitochondrial apoptotic pathway [40] in hepatoma cells or primary rat hepatocytes, in particular if cells were exposed to a combination of oxysterols and fatty acids. In addition, oxysterols at high concentrations appear to contribute to cell death by antagonizing Akt-dependent survival pathways [41]. Oxysterols are elevated in NAFLD patients [42] and may be causative in NASH development [43].

The oxidative stress-induced death of the cholesterol laden hepatocytes might then trigger the subsequent inflammatory response and the initiation of the development of fibrosis. Notably, signs of mitochondrial damage and oxidative stress preceded the development of inflammation (Figure 7). Hepatocyte detritus may be taken up by Kupffer cells and infiltrating macrophages that have been shown to form crown-like structures around dying hepatocytes [44]. Since cholesterol cannot be removed by macrophages, this results in a self-perpetuating chronic inflammation that triggers scar formation and fibrosis (Figure 4). Activation of macrophages and stellate cells by cholesterol or cholesterol crystals [11,12,45] and oxysterols [46] has been shown to promote this process.

4.3. Possible Clinical Impact

There is evidence that dietary cholesterol may also favor NASH development in humans [47–49] and the interruption of intestinal cholesterol absorption by ezetimibe has been shown to be beneficial in NAFLD patients in a meta-analysis of several clinical studies [16]. Notably, in one study ezetimibe reduced the NASH activity score without affecting steatosis [50]. A possible interaction between dietary cholesterol and fatty acid composition of the diet apparently was not systematically analyzed in human studies. However, meta-analysis of several clinical studies showed that supplementation with long chain ω3-PUFA caused a more or less pronounced reduction in the plasma levels of alanine aminotransferase (ALAT), aspartate aminotransferase (ASAT), and γ-glutamyltransferase (GGT), indicating a reduction of liver damage. However, the actual NASH activity score was not determined [51].

5. Conclusions

A direct translation of the results of the current study to a dietary recommendation for humans is beyond any doubt inappropriate. However, the data suggest that the recommendation to replace saturated fat by fat from sources rich in ω6-PUFA without a simultaneous reduction of cholesterol intake may be sensible from the point of view of protection against cardiovascular diseases and possibly other consequences of the metabolic syndrome, however, may not be advisable from the point of view of NASH development.

Supplementary Materials:
Supplementary Methods: Quantification of immunohistochemistry analysis; Supplementary Figure S1: Expression of oxidative phosphorylation complexes in liver homogenates; Supplementary Figure S2: Expression of PGC-1α in liver homogenates; Supplementary Figure S3: Detection of protein carbonyls by oxyblot analysis in liver homogenates; Supplementary Figure S4: Increased mitochondrial damage and oxidative stress in mice fed a CHO + SOY diet for 19 days.

Author Contributions: Conceptualization, J.H. and G.P.P.; Data curation, J.H.; Formal analysis, J.H.; Funding acquisition, J.H.; Investigation, J.H. and G.P.P.; Methodology, J.H., E.A., J.S., K.J., D.W., J.P.C., J.K., C.S., and M.V.; Resources, W.J. and A.K.; Supervision, G.P.P.; Validation, J.H., E.A., J.S., W.J., and A.K.; Visualization, J.H.; Writing and original draft, J.H. and G.P.P.; Writing, review and editing, A.K.

Acknowledgments: The outstandingly skillful technical work of Manuela Kuna as well as the technical assistance of Fabian Gellert, Ines Kahnt, Elisabeth Meyer, and Susann Richter is gratefully acknowledged. The excellent proof-reading competence of Brit-Maren Schjeide is highly appreciated. We further acknowledge the support of Deutsche Forschungsgemeinschaft (German Research Foundation) and Open Access Publication Fund of the University of Potsdam.

References

1. Lee, Y.T.; Laxton, V.; Lin, H.Y.; Chan, Y.W.F.; Fitzgerald-Smith, S.; To, T.L.O.; Yan, B.P.; Liu, T.; Tse, G. Animal models of atherosclerosis. *Biomed. Rep.* **2017**, *6*, 259–266. [CrossRef] [PubMed]
2. McNamara, D.J. Dietary cholesterol, heart disease risk and cognitive dissonance. *Pro. Nut. Soc.* **2014**, *73*, 161–166. [CrossRef] [PubMed]
3. Berger, S.; Raman, G.; Vishwanathan, R.; Jacques, P.F.; Johnson, E.J. Dietary cholesterol and cardiovascular disease: A systematic review and meta-analysis. *Am. J. Clin. Nutr.* **2015**, *102*, 276–294. [CrossRef] [PubMed]
4. Brownawell, A.M.; Falk, M.C. Cholesterol: Where science and public health policy intersect. *Nutr. Rev.* **2010**, *68*, 355–364. [CrossRef] [PubMed]
5. Vinué, Á.; Herrero-Cervera, A.; González-Navarro, H. Understanding the impact of dietary cholesterol on chronic metabolic diseases through studies in rodent models. *Nutrients* **2018**, *10*, 939. [CrossRef] [PubMed]
6. Jahn, D.; Kircher, S.; Hermanns, H.M.; Geier, A. Animal models of NAFLD from a hepatologist's point of view. *BBA-Mol. Basis. Dis.* **2018**. [CrossRef] [PubMed]
7. Estes, C.; Razavi, H.; Loomba, R.; Younossi, Z.; Sanyal, A.J. Modeling the epidemic of nonalcoholic fatty liver disease demonstrates an exponential increase in burden of disease. *Hepatology* **2018**, *67*, 123–133. [CrossRef] [PubMed]
8. Andronescu, C.I.; Purcarea, M.R.; Babes, P.A. Nonalcoholic fatty liver disease: Epidemiology, pathogenesis and therapeutic implications. *J. Med. Life* **2018**, *11*, 20–23. [PubMed]
9. Brunt, E.M.; Wong, V.W.S.; Nobili, V.; Day, C.P.; Sookoian, S.; Maher, J.J.; Bugianesi, E.; Sirlin, C.B.; Neuschwander-Tetri, B.A.; Rinella, M.E. Nonalcoholic fatty liver disease. *Nat. Rev. Dis. Primers* **2015**, *1*, 15080. [CrossRef] [PubMed]

10. Subramanian, S.; Goodspeed, L.; Wang, S.; Kim, J.; Zeng, L.; Ioannou, G.N.; Haigh, W.G.; Yeh, M.M.; Kowdley, K.V.; O'Brien, K.D.; et al. Dietary cholesterol exacerbates hepatic steatosis and inflammation in obese LDL receptor-deficient mice. *J. Lipid Res.* **2011**, *52*, 1626–1635. [CrossRef] [PubMed]
11. Henkel, J.; Coleman, C.D.; Schraplau, A.; Jöhrens, K.; Weber, D.; Castro, J.P.; Hugo, M.; Schulz, T.J.; Krämer, S.; Schürmann, A.; et al. Induction of steatohepatitis (NASH) with insulin resistance in wildtype B6 mice by a western-type diet containing soybean oil and cholesterol. *Mol. Med.* **2017**, *23*, 70. [CrossRef] [PubMed]
12. Ioannou, G.N.; Subramanian, S.; Chait, A.; Haigh, W.G.; Yeh, M.M.; Farrell, G.C.; Lee, S.P.; Savard, C. Cholesterol crystallization within hepatocyte lipid droplets and its role in murine NASH. *J. Lipid Res.* **2017**, *58*, 1067–1079. [CrossRef] [PubMed]
13. Buettner, R.; Ascher, M.; Gäbele, E.; Hellerbrand, C.; Kob, R.; Bertsch, T.; Bollheimer, L.C. Olive oil attenuates the cholesterol-induced development of nonalcoholic steatohepatitis despite increased insulin resistance in a rodent model. *Horm. Metab. Res.* **2013**, *45*, 795–801. [CrossRef] [PubMed]
14. Hansen, H.H.; Feigh, M.; Veidal, S.S.; Rigbolt, K.T.; Vrang, N.; Fosgerau, K. Mouse models of nonalcoholic steatohepatitis in preclinical drug development. *Drug Discov. Today* **2017**, *22*, 1707–1718. [CrossRef] [PubMed]
15. Wang, X.; Ren, Q.; Wu, T.; Guo, Y.; Liang, Y.; Liu, S. Ezetimibe prevents the development of non-alcoholic fatty liver disease induced by high-fat diet in C57BL/6J mice. *Mol. Med. Rep.* **2014**, *10*, 2917–2923. [CrossRef] [PubMed]
16. Nakade, Y.; Murotani, K.; Inoue, T.; Kobayashi, Y.; Yamamoto, T.; Ishii, N.; Ohashi, T.; Ito, K.; Fukuzawa, Y.; Yoneda, M. Ezetimibe for the treatment of non-alcoholic fatty liver disease: A meta-analysis. *Hepatol. Res.* **2017**, *47*, 1417–1428. [CrossRef] [PubMed]
17. Tirosh, O. Hypoxic signaling and cholesterol lipotoxicity in fatty liver disease progression. *Oxid. Med. Cell. Longev.* **2018**, *7*, 1–15. [CrossRef] [PubMed]
18. Ioannou, G.N. The Role of Cholesterol in the Pathogenesis of NASH. *Trends Endocrinol. Metab.* **2016**, *27*, 84–95. [CrossRef] [PubMed]
19. Siedel, J.; Rollinger, W.; Röschlau, P.; Ziegenhorn, J.; Bergmeyer, H.U. Total cholesterol, end-point and kinetic method. In *Methods of Enzymatic Analysis*; Verlag Chemie GmbH: Weinheim, Germany, 1984; pp. 139–148.
20. Kleiner, D.E.; Brunt, E.M.; van Natta, M.; Behling, C.; Contos, M.J.; Cummings, O.W.; Ferrell, L.D.; Liu, Y.-C.; Torbenson, M.S.; Unalp-Arida, A.; et al. Design and validation of a histological scoring system for nonalcoholic fatty liver disease. *Hepatology* **2005**, *41*, 1313–1321. [CrossRef] [PubMed]
21. Liang, W.; Menke, A.L.; Driessen, A.; Koek, G.H.; Lindeman, J.H.; Stoop, R.; Havekes, L.M.; Kleemann, R.; van den Hoek, A.M. Establishment of a general NAFLD scoring system for rodent models and comparison to human liver pathology. *PLoS ONE* **2014**, *9*, e115922. [CrossRef] [PubMed]
22. Manowsky, J.; Camargo, R.G.; Kipp, A.P.; Henkel, J.; Püschel, G.P. Insulin-induced cytokine production in macrophages causes insulin resistance in hepatocytes. *Am. J. Physiol. Endocrin. Met.* **2016**, *310*, E938–E946. [CrossRef] [PubMed]
23. Henkel, J.; Neuschäfer-Rube, F.; Pathe-Neuschäfer-Rube, A.; Püschel, G.P. Aggravation by prostaglandin E2 of interleukin-6-dependent insulin resistance in hepatocytes. *Hepatology* **2009**, *50*, 781–790. [CrossRef] [PubMed]
24. Xu, Z.J.; Fan, J.G.; Ding, X.D.; Qiao, L.; Wang, G.L. Characterization of high-fat, diet-induced, non-alcoholic steatohepatitis with fibrosis in rats. *Digest. Dis. Sci.* **2010**, *55*, 931–940. [CrossRef] [PubMed]
25. Matsuzawa, N.; Takamura, T.; Kurita, S.; Misu, H.; Ota, T.; Ando, H.; Yokoyama, M.; Honda, M.; Zen, Y.; Nakanuma, Y.; et al. Lipid-induced oxidative stress causes steatohepatitis in mice fed an atherogenic diet. *Hepatology* **2007**, *46*, 1392–1403. [CrossRef] [PubMed]
26. Wiggers, K.D.; Richard, M.J.; Stewart, J.W.; Jacobson, N.L.; Berger, P.J. Type and amount of dietary fat affect relative concentration of cholesterol in blood and other tissues of rats. *Atherosclerosis* **1977**, *27*, 27–34. [CrossRef]
27. Sheril, A.; Jeyakumar, S.M.; Jayashree, T.; Giridharan, N.V.; Vajreswari, A. Impact of feeding polyunsaturated fatty acids on cholesterol metabolism of dyslipidemic obese rats of WNIN/GR-Ob strain. *Atherosclerosis* **2009**, *204*, 136–140. [CrossRef] [PubMed]
28. Schumacher, T.; Benndorf, R.A. ABC transport proteins in cardiovascular disease—A brief summary. *Molecules* **2017**, *22*, 589. [CrossRef] [PubMed]
29. Pizzini, A.; Lunger, L.; Demetz, E.; Hilbe, R.; Weiss, G.; Ebenbichler, C.; Tancevski, I. The role of omega-3 fatty acids in reverse cholesterol transport: A review. *Nutrients* **2017**, *9*, 1099. [CrossRef] [PubMed]

30. Lu, S.C.; Lin, M.H.; Huang, P.C. A high cholesterol, (n-3) polyunsaturated fatty acid diet induces hypercholesterolemia more than a high cholesterol (n-6) polyunsaturated fatty acid diet in hamsters. *J. Nutr.* **1996**, *126*, 1759–1765. [PubMed]
31. Wang, S.; Matthan, N.R.; Wu, D.; Reed, D.B.; Bapat, P.; Yin, X.; Grammas, P.; Shen, C.L.; Lichtenstein, A.H. Lipid content in hepatic and gonadal adipose tissue parallel aortic cholesterol accumulation in mice fed diets with different omega-6 PUFA to EPA plus DHA ratios. *Clin. Nutr.* **2014**, *33*, 260–266. [CrossRef] [PubMed]
32. Jump, D.B.; Depner, C.M.; Tripathy, S.; Lytle, K.A. Impact of dietary fat on the development of non-alcoholic fatty liver disease in Ldlr−/− mice. *Proc. Nutr. Soc.* **2016**, *75*, 1–9. [CrossRef] [PubMed]
33. Shang, T.; Liu, L.; Zhou, J.; Zhang, M.; Hu, Q.; Fang, M.; Wu, Y.; Yao, P.; Gong, Z. Protective effects of various ratios of DHA/EPA supplementation on high-fat diet-induced liver damage in mice. *Lipids Health Dis.* **2017**, *16*, 65. [CrossRef] [PubMed]
34. Pachikian, B.D.; Essaghir, A.; Demoulin, J.B.; Neyrinck, A.M.; Catry, E.; de Backer, F.C.; Dejeans, N.; Dewulf, E.M.; Sohet, F.M.; Portois, L.; et al. Hepatic n-3 polyunsaturated fatty acid depletion promotes steatosis and insulin resistance in mice: Genomic analysis of cellular targets. *PLoS ONE* **2011**, *6*, e23365. [CrossRef] [PubMed]
35. Schwarz, J.; Tomé, D.; Baars, A.; Hooiveld, G.J.; Müller, M. Dietary protein affects gene expression and prevents lipid accumulation in the liver in mice. *PLoS ONE* **2012**, *7*, e47303. [CrossRef] [PubMed]
36. Legry, V.; van Rooyen, D.M.; Lambert, B.; Sempoux, C.; Poekes, L.; Español-Suñer, R.; Molendi-Coste, O.; Horsmans, Y.; Farrell, G.C.; Leclercq, I.A. Endoplasmic reticulum stress does not contribute to steatohepatitis in obese and insulin-resistant high-fat-diet-fed foz/foz mice. *Clin. Sci.* **2014**, *127*, 507–518. [CrossRef] [PubMed]
37. Ribas, V.; García-Ruiz, C.; Fernández-Checa, J.C. Glutathione and mitochondria. *Front. Pharmacol.* **2014**, *5*, 151. [CrossRef] [PubMed]
38. Marí, M.; Caballero, F.; Colell, A.; Morales, A.; Caballeria, J.; Fernandez, A.; Enrich, C.; Fernandez-Checa, J.C.; García-Ruiz, C. Mitochondrial free cholesterol loading sensitizes to TNF- and Fas-mediated steatohepatitis. *Cell Metab.* **2006**, *4*, 185–198. [CrossRef] [PubMed]
39. Schrauwen, P.; Schrauwen-Hinderling, V.; Hoeks, J.; Hesselink, M.K.C. Mitochondrial dysfunction and lipotoxicity. *BBA-Mol. Cell Biol. Lipids* **2010**, *1801*, 266–271. [CrossRef] [PubMed]
40. Bellanti, F.; Mitarotonda, D.; Tamborra, R.; Blonda, M.; Iannelli, G.; Petrella, A.; Sanginario, V.; Iuliano, L.; Vendemiale, G.; Serviddio, G. Oxysterols induce mitochondrial impairment and hepatocellular toxicity in non-alcoholic fatty liver disease. *Free Radic. Biol. Med.* **2014**, *75*, S16–S17. [CrossRef] [PubMed]
41. Vejux, A.; Guyot, S.; Montange, T.; Riedinger, J.M.; Kahn, E.; Lizard, G. Phospholipidosis and down-regulation of the PI3-K/PDK-1/Akt signalling pathway are vitamin E inhibitable events associated with 7-ketocholesterol-induced apoptosis. *J. Nutr. Biochem.* **2009**, *20*, 45–61. [CrossRef] [PubMed]
42. Ikegami, T.; Hyogo, H.; Honda, A.; Miyazaki, T.; Tokushige, K.; Hashimoto, E.; Inui, K.; Matsuzaki, Y.; Tazuma, S. Increased serum liver X receptor ligand oxysterols in patients with non-alcoholic fatty liver disease. *J. Gastroenterol.* **2012**, *47*, 1257–1266. [CrossRef] [PubMed]
43. Serviddio, G.; Blonda, M.; Bellanti, F.; Villani, R.; Iuliano, L.; Vendemiale, G. Oxysterols and redox signaling in the pathogenesis of non-alcoholic fatty liver disease. *Free Radic. Res.* **2013**, *47*, 881–893. [CrossRef] [PubMed]
44. Ioannou, G.N.; Haigh, W.G.; Thorning, D.; Savard, C. Hepatic cholesterol crystals and crown-like structures distinguish NASH from simple steatosis. *J. Lipid Res.* **2013**, *54*, 1326–1334. [CrossRef] [PubMed]
45. Tsuchida, T.; Friedman, S.L. Mechanisms of hepatic stellate cell activation. *Nat. Rev. Gastroenterol. Hepat.* **2017**, *14*, 397–411. [CrossRef] [PubMed]
46. Ferré, N.; Martínez-Clemente, M.; López-Parra, M.; González-Périz, A.; Horrillo, R.; Planagumà, A.; Camps, J.; Joven, J.; Tres, A.; Guardiola, F.; et al. Increased susceptibility to exacerbated liver injury in hypercholesterolemic ApoE-deficient mice: Potential involvement of oxysterols. *Am. J. Physiol. Gastr. Liver Physiol.* **2009**, *296*, G553–G562. [CrossRef] [PubMed]
47. Ioannou, G.N.; Morrow, O.B.; Connole, M.L.; Lee, S.P. Association between dietary nutrient composition and the incidence of cirrhosis or liver cancer in the United States population. *Hepatology* **2009**, *50*, 175–184. [CrossRef] [PubMed]
48. Musso, G.; Gambino, R.; de Michieli, F.; Cassader, M.; Rizzetto, M.; Durazzo, M.; Fagà, E.; Silli, B.;

Pagano, G. Dietary habits and their relations to insulin resistance and postprandial lipemia in nonalcoholic steatohepatitis. *Hepatology* **2003**, *37*, 909–916. [CrossRef] [PubMed]

49. Yasutake, K.; Nakamuta, M.; Shima, Y.; Ohyama, A.; Masuda, K.; Haruta, N.; Fujino, T.; Aoyagi, Y.; Fukuizumi, K.; Yoshimoto, T.; et al. Nutritional investigation of non-obese patients with non-alcoholic fatty liver disease: The significance of dietary cholesterol. *Scand. J. Gastroenterol.* **2009**, *44*, 471–477. [CrossRef] [PubMed]
50. Lee, H.Y.; Jun, D.W.; Kim, H.J.; Oh, H.; Saeed, W.K.; Ahn, H.; Cheung, R.C.; Nguyen, M.H. Ezetimibe decreased nonalcoholic fatty liver disease activity score but not hepatic steatosis. *Korean J. Int. Med.* **2018**. [CrossRef] [PubMed]
51. He, X.X.; Wu, X.L.; Chen, R.P.; Chen, C.; Liu, X.G.; Wu, B.J.; Huang, Z.M. Effectiveness of omega-3 polyunsaturated fatty acids in non-alcoholic fatty liver disease: A meta-analysis of randomized controlled trials. *PLoS ONE* **2016**, *11*, e0162368. [CrossRef] [PubMed]

18

ChREBP Rather than SHP Regulates Hepatic VLDL Secretion

Hiroyuki Niwa [1], Katsumi Iizuka [1,2,*], Takehiro Kato [1], Wudelehu Wu [1], Hiromi Tsuchida [1], Ken Takao [1], Yukio Horikawa [1] and Jun Takeda [1]

[1] Department of Diabetes and Endocrinology, Graduate School of Medicine, Gifu University, Gifu 501-1194, Japan; hiroyu760202@yahoo.co.jp (H.N.); bado_aberu@yahoo.co.jp (T.K.); wudelehu100@126.com (W.W.); Gif095@gifu-u.ac.jp (H.T.); lamgerrpard@yahoo.co.jp (K.T.); yhorikaw@gifu-u.ac.jp (Y.H.); jtakeda@gifu-u.ac.jp (J.T.)

[2] Gifu University Hospital Center for Nutritional Support and Infection Control, Gifu 501-1194, Japan

* Correspondence: kiizuka@gifu-u.ac.jp

Abstract: The regulation of hepatic very-low-density lipoprotein (VLDL) secretion plays an important role in the pathogenesis of dyslipidemia and fatty liver diseases. VLDL is controlled by hepatic microsomal triglyceride transfer protein (MTTP). *Mttp* is regulated by carbohydrate response element binding protein (ChREBP) and small heterodimer partner (SHP). However, it is unclear whether both coordinately regulate *Mttp* expression and VLDL secretion. Here, adenoviral overexpression of ChREBP and SHP in rat primary hepatocytes induced and suppressed *Mttp* mRNA, respectively. However, *Mttp* induction by ChREBP was much more potent than suppression by SHP. Promoter assays of *Mttp* and the liver type pyruvate kinase gene revealed that SHP and ChREBP did not affect the transcriptional activity of each other. *Mttp* mRNA and protein levels of $Shp^{-/-}$ mice were similar to those of wild-types; however, those of $Chrebp^{-/-}Shp^{-/-}$ and $Chrebp^{-/-}$ mice were significantly much lower. Consistent with this, the VLDL particle number and VLDL secretion rates in $Shp^{-/-}$ mice were similar to wild-types but were much lower in $Chrebp^{-/-}$ and $Chrebp^{-/-}Shp^{-/-}$ mice. These findings suggest that ChREBP, rather than SHP, regulates VLDL secretion under normal conditions and that ChREBP and SHP do not affect the transcriptional activities of each other.

Keywords: carbohydrate response element binding protein; small heterodimer partner; microsomal triglyceride transfer protein; very-low-density lipoprotein

1. Introduction

Nonalcoholic fatty liver disease (NAFLD) is the most common chronic liver disease in the world [1,2]. High fat diets and high carbohydrate diets are responsible in the development of NAFLD [3–5]. High carbohydrate diets cause fatty liver by increasing hepatic de novo lipogenesis [3]. High fat diets increase hepatic fat content [4]. Therefore, lifestyle modifications, including hypocaloric diets, are critical for the prevention and treatment of NAFLD. Non-alcoholic fatty liver disease (NAFLD) is associated with hepatic insulin resistance and hepatic fibrosis and can lead to the development of diabetes mellitus, dyslipidemia, non-alcoholic steatohepatitis, and hepatocellular carcinoma [1,2]. Hepatic lipid accumulation is regulated by the free fatty acid (FFA) supply from adipose tissue, and de novo lipogenesis from the secretion of glucose, acyl CoA oxidation, and very-low-density lipoprotein (VLDL) in the liver [6]. Visceral adipose tissue is the primary source of hepatic fat in adults, contributing 59% of the triglycerides found in the liver [6]. Glucose and insulin signals regulate hepatic de novo lipogenesis through the carbohydrate response element binding protein (ChREBP) and sterol response element binding protein 1c (SREBP1c), respectively [7]. Moreover, altered VLDL secretion also contributes to the pathogenesis of NAFLD [8,9]. VLDL secretion is controlled by microsomal triglyceride transfer protein (MTTP) [8,9]. MTTP is essential for the assembly and secretion of apolipoprotein B-containing lipoproteins. In humans and mice, *Mttp* deficiency causes hypolipidemia and fatty liver [8,9]. Thus, *Mttp* is involved in the pathogenesis of NAFLD.

Mttp regulation depends on a few highly-conserved *cis*-elements in its promoter. The *Mttp* promoter sequence contains critical positive (hepatic nuclear factor [HNF]-1, HNF-4, direct repeat 1, and FOX) and negative regulatory sterol and insulin response elements [8,9]. Small heterodimer partner (SHP, also known as NR0B2) is a unique nuclear receptor (NR) that contains the dimerization and ligand-binding domain found in other family members but lacks the conserved DNA-binding domain [10]. We previously reported that human *SHP* genetic variations appear to cause mild obesity and type 2 diabetes mellitus [11,12]. As a co-repressor, SHP represses the activities of HNF-4α and the retinoid X receptor liver receptor homolog-1 (LRH-1) by interacting with these factors [13,14]. However, it is not certain whether SHP affects the VLDL secretion rate [15,16].

As with the effects of nutritional conditions on Mttp expression, high fat diets and high carbohydrate diets induce Mttp expression, resulting in hyperlipidemia [17,18]. High fat diets increase hepatic *Mttp* expression through decreased binding of sterol regulatory element-binding proteins to the *Mttp* promoter [17]. High sucrose and high fructose consumption also increase Mttp expression [18]; however, the mechanisms of this are unclear. Recently, we reported that *Mttp* mRNA levels and VLDL secretion rates were lower in the livers of Carbohydrate Response Element Binding Protein [ChREBP] knockout (Chrebp$^{-/-}$) mice [19]. ChREBP is a glucose-activated transcription factor that regulates hepatic de novo lipogenesis in the liver [20–23]. ChREBP transcriptional activities are regulated by phosphorylation/dephosphorylation, nuclear translocation, and conformational changes [20–23]. It was recently proposed that ChREBP transcriptional activity is regulated through interactions with nuclear factors, such as farnesoid X receptor (FXR) and HNF4a [24–28]. Moreover, computer analysis revealed that ChREBP contains a nuclear receptor binding motif [29]. Considering that SHP represses the activities of many transcription factors by interacting with these factors [10], we speculated that SHP might also affect *Mttp* transcription in cooperation with ChREBP.

ChREBP and SHP control the regulation of *Mttp* expression. Using rat hepatocytes and knockout mice, we therefore evaluated the following: (1) whether ChREBP and SHP affect the transcriptional activities of each other; (2) whether ChREBP and SHP coordinately affect *Mttp* expression and thereby VLDL secretion; and (3) if ChREBP or SHP regulate VLDL secretion more potently. An appreciation of the roles of ChREBP and SHP in regulating *Mttp* and VLDL secretion will be beneficial for understanding the role of nutritional signals in the development of NAFLD and dyslipidemia.

2. Materials and Methods

2.1. Establishment of Chrebp$^{-/-}$ Shp$^{-/-}$ Double Knockout (DKO) Mice

Animal experiments were carried out in accordance with the National Institute of Health Guide for the Care and Use of Laboratory Animals (NIH Publications No. 8023, revised 1978). All animal care was approved by the animal care committee of the University of Gifu (No. 27-30, approval date: 4 June 2015). Mice were housed at 23 °C on a 12-h light/dark cycle. Chrebp$^{-/-}$ mice were backcrossed for at least 10 generations onto the C57BL/6J background [19,30]. Shp$^{-/-}$ mice were purchased from Lexicon Genetics Inc. (The Woodlands, TX, USA). Shp$^{+/-}$ mice were backcrossed for at least 12 generations onto the C57BL/6J background. Male mice were used for all studies. Chrebp$^{-/-}$Shp$^{-/-}$ (DKO) mice were intercrossed with Chrebp$^{-/-}$ and Shp$^{-/-}$ mice.

Mice had free access to water and were fed an autoclaved CE-2 diet (CLEA Japan, Tokyo, Japan). Wild-type (WT), Chrebp$^{-/-}$, Shp$^{-/-}$, and DKO mice were housed separately with a total of three mice per cage. Body weight was measured weekly between 7 and 21 weeks of age. Mice were sacrificed at 21 weeks of age by cervical dislocation. All tissue samples were immediately placed into liquid nitrogen and stored at −80 °C until further analysis for hepatic triacylglycerol and cholesterol contents and for quantitative polymerase chain reaction (PCR).

2.2. *Liver Triglyceride and Cholesterol Content and Plasma Profile Measurements*

Liver lipids were extracted using the Bligh and Dyer method [31]; they were measured using triglyceride (Wako Pure Chemicals, Osaka, Japan) and cholesterol E-tests (Wako). Blood plasma was collected from the retro–orbital venous plexus, following ad libitum feeding or after a 6-h fast. Blood glucose and beta-hydroxybutyrate (β-OHB) levels were measured using a FreeStyle Freedom monitoring system (Nipro, Osaka, Japan). Plasma insulin, FFA, fibroblast growth factor 21 (FGF21), triglyceride, and total cholesterol levels were determined using commercial assay kits, as follows: mouse insulin enzyme-linked immunosorbent assay (ELISA) (H type) (Shibayagi, Gunma, Japan), NEFA C-test (Wako Pure Chemicals, Tokyo, Japan), mouse/rat Fgf21 ELISA (R&D Systems, Minneapolis, MN, USA), triglyceride E-test (Wako), and the cholesterol E-test (Wako), respectively.

2.3. *RNA Isolation and Quantitative Real-Time PCR*

Total RNA isolation, cDNA synthesis, and real-time PCR analysis were performed as previously described [13]. Real-time PCR primers for mouse/rat Chrebp, liver type pyruvate kinase (Pklr), Fgf21, Mttp, and RNA polymerase II (Pol2) have been previously reported [31–33]. All amplifications were performed in triplicate. The relative amounts of mRNA were calculated using the comparative CT method. Pol2 expression was used as an internal control.

2.4. *VLDL Secretion Test and MTTP Protein Contents*

VLDL secretion tests were performed as previously reported [19]. Briefly, 500 mg/kg body weight tyloxapol was administered intraperitoneally to 5 h fasted mice. Blood sampling was performed at the indicated times. The triglyceride (TG) content in lipoprotein fractions and the VLDL particle numbers were analyzed using gel-permeation high-performance liquid chromatography (LipoSEARCH®) at Skylight Biotech Inc. (Akita, Japan) [34]. Serum samples obtained from six mice after 6 h fasting were pooled and measured. Liver MTTP protein contents were measured by an MTTP ELISA kit (Cloud-Clone Corp Inc., Houston, TX, USA).

2.5. *Adenoviral Delivery into Rat Primary Hepatocytes*

Rat primary hepatocytes were isolated as previously described [32,33]. Isolated hepatocytes were suspended in DMEM, supplemented with 10% fetal calf serum, 100 nM insulin, 100 nM dexamethasone, 10 nM triiodothronine (T3), and 100 μg/mL penicillin/streptomycin. Cells were seeded in 6-well plates or 10-cm dishes and grown in a humidified atmosphere of 5% CO_2 and 95% air at 37 °C. After the cells had been incubated for 4 h, the medium was replaced with DMEM containing 10 nM T3. Adenoviruses harboring dominant active rat Chrebp lacking 1–196 a.a. (Ad-daChREBP) and mouse SHP full length (Ad-SHP) were constructed according to the manufacturer's protocol (Invitrogen, Carlsbad, CA, USA). After 4 h infection with Ad-daChREBP and/or Ad-SHP, rat hepatocytes were incubated for 20 h. *Mttp* mRNA levels were detected by real-time PCR.

2.6. *Transfections and Luciferase Reporter Assay*

Reporter plasmids pGL3 3×LPK ChoRE, pcDNA-daChrebp, and pcDNA-empty have been previously reported [32,33]. pcDNA-SHP and pcDNA-FXR were constructed using the pcDNA™3.2-DEST Mammalian Expression Vector (Invitrogen) according to the manufacturer's protocol (Invitrogen). pGL3-Mttp (−211 bp) was constructed as follows: mouse Mttp promoter regions (−211 bp to +77 bp) amplified by PrimSTAR MAX DNA Polymerase (Takara Bio, Kusatsu, Japan) were inserted into the pGL3 basic vector (Promega, Madison, WI, USA). Then, 1.0 μg of pGL3 MTTP (−211 bp), 0.1 μg pRL-TK vector, pcDNA-empty + pcDNA-daChREBP + pcDNA-SHP (total 1.0 μg), and 3 μL of Lipofectamine 2000 (Invitrogen) were transfected into primary rat hepatocytes. After incubation for 24 h, cells were collected and used in luciferase assays.

2.7. Statistical Analysis

All values are presented as means ± standard deviations. Data were analyzed using Tukey's test. A p-value < 0.05 was considered to be statistically significant.

3. Results

3.1. Adenoviral Overexpression of ChREBP and SHP Respectively Increased and Decreased Mttp Expression

Adenoviral ChREBP caused an increase in *Mttp* and *Pklr* mRNA expression, while SHP suppressed only *Mttp* expression in primary rat hepatocytes (Figure 1A,B). Moreover, overexpressing SHP by more than 70-fold (above physiological levels) was found to suppress ChREBP-mediated *Mttp* induction (Figure 1A). In contrast, SHP overexpression failed to suppress ChREBP-mediated *Pklr* induction (Figure 1B). This suggested that ChREBP induced *Mttp* expression more potently than SHP suppressed it.

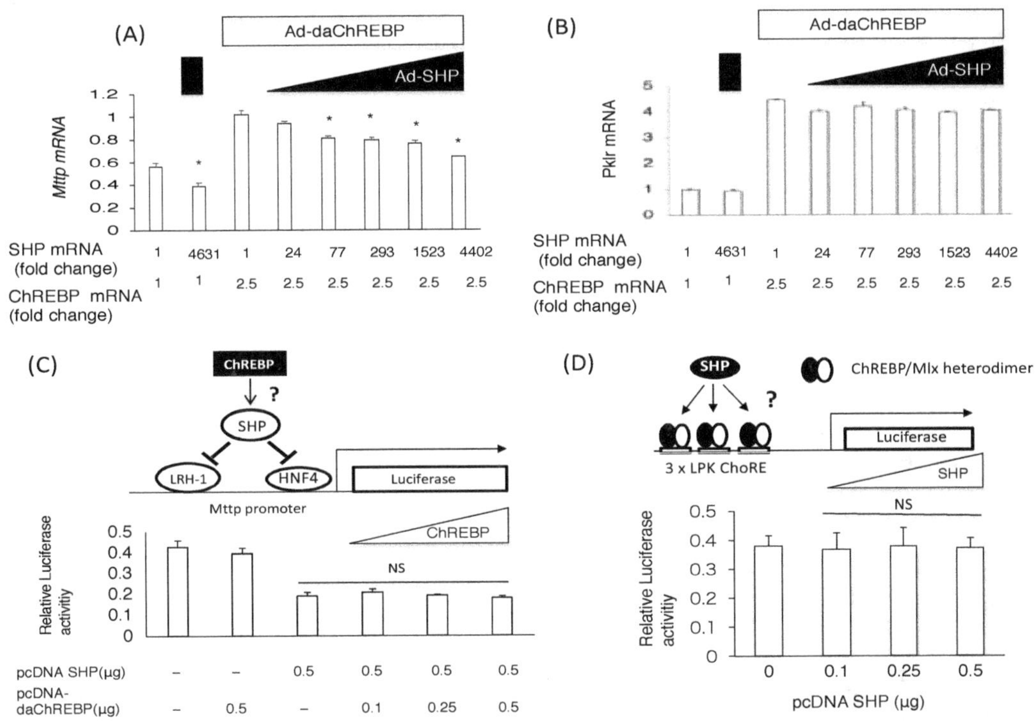

Figure 1. The coordinated effects of carbohydrate response element binding protein (ChREBP) and small heterodimer partner (SHP) on *Mttp* expression. (**A**) and (**B**) The effects of SHP on ChREBP-mediated *Mttp* (**A**) and *Pklr* (**B**) mRNA induction. After 4 h infection with Ad-daChREBP and/or Ad-SHP in hepatocytes, cells were incubated for 20 h. *Mttp* mRNA levels were detected by real-time Polymerase chain reaction method. Open symbols and closed symbols indicated adenoviral overexpression of daChREBP and SHP, respectively. The x-axis indicates *Shp and Chrebp* mRNA levels (fold change). Adenoviral overexpression of ChREBP caused a 2.5-fold increase in Chrebp mRNA levels. Adenoviral SHP expression caused an indicated fold increase in Shp expresssion. Pol2 expression was used as an internal control. $n = 4$ per group. * $p < 0.05$; (**C**) Reporter assay using pGL3-Mttp (−211 bp). The indicated amounts of pcDNA-daChREBP and pcDNA-SHP were transfected with pGL3-Mttp (−211 bp) and pRL-TK vectors and Lipofectamine 2000 reagent into primary rat hepatocytes. After 24 h incubation, cells were collected for the dual luciferase assay. Luciferase activity was normalized to Renilla luciferase activity. N.S., not significant. $n = 6$ per group; (**D**) Reporter assay using pGL3 3×LPK ChoRE. The indicated amount of pcDNA-SHP was cotransfected with pGL3-3×LPK ChoRE, PRL-TK, pcDNA daChREBP, and Lipofectamine 2000 into primary rat hepatocytes. After 24 h incubation, cells were collected for the dual luciferase assay. Luciferase activity was normalized to Renilla luciferase activity. NS, not significant vs control. $n = 6$ per group.

SHP is known to suppress HNF4/HNF1/LRH-1-mediated *Mttp* expression [13,35]. Accordingly, transfection of the PGL3 basic vector containing 211 bp of the *Mttp* promoter region (pcDNA-SHP), including the HNF4/HNF1/LRH-1 binding site, successfully suppressed PGL3-*Mttp* (−211 bp) luciferase activity. However, co-transfection of pcDNA-daChREBP did not reverse this effect (Figure 1C). In contrast, the transfection of the pcDNA SHP vector could not suppress pGL3 *Pklr* luciferase activities induced by pcDNA-daChREBP (Figure 1D). This suggested that SHP and ChREBP did not affect the transcriptional activities of each other

3.2. *Chrebp Shp DKO Mice Resembled Chrebp$^{-/-}$ Mice*

We next assessed the effects of ChREBP and SHP on the mouse metabolic phenotype in vivo. *Chrebp$^{-/-}$* mice displayed characteristically higher liver weights, lower white adipose tissue weights, higher plasma FFA, FGF-21, and β-OHB levels, and elevated liver glycogen contents compared with those of WT mice. Chrebp$^{-/-}$Shp$^{-/-}$ double knockout (DKO) mice also displayed similar characteristics (Table 1).

Table 1. Phenotypic comparison between WT, ChREBP$^{-/-}$, SHP$^{-/-}$, ChREBP$^{-/-}$SHP$^{-/-}$ (DKO) mice.

	WT	ChREBP$^{-/-}$	SHP$^{-/-}$	DKO
BW (g)	29.50 ± 0.71	30.40 ± 1.92	28.57 ± 2.98	30.2 ± 2.51
Liver (%BW)	5.02 ± 0.08	5.37 ± 0.27 *	5.01 ± 0.14	5.52 ± 0.24 *
Epidydimal fat (%BW)	2.41 ± 0.30	1.68 ± 0.62 *	2.07 ± 0.33	1.41 ± 0.24 *
Mesenteric fat (%BW)	1.16 ± 0.13	0.77 ± 0.16 *	1.02±0.28	0.55 ± 0.11 *
Brown adipose tissue (%BW)	0.30 ± 0.07	0.27 ± 0.10	0.36 ± 0.12	0.49 ± 0.15
Plasma glucose (mg/dL)	132.3 ± 17.3	128.4 ± 13.2	118.7 ± 21.5	117.2 ± 11.5
Plasma insulin (ng/dL)	0.86 ± 0.26	1.01 ± 0.33	0.91 ± 0.41	0.65 ± 0.17
HOMA-R	0.28 ± 0.08	0.32 ± 0.12	0.27 ± 0.15	0.19 ± 0.03
Plasma triglyceride (mg/dL)	66.1 ± 10.1	56.2 ± 11.5	65.2 ± 12.6	67.3 ± 19.8
Plasma FGF21 (pg/mL)	802.1 ± 365.8	150.2 ± 51.1 *	584.1 ± 268.6	124.0 ± 61.8 *
Plasma β-hydroxybutyrate (mM)	2.05 ± 0.24	1.32 ± 0.11	2.37 ± 0.40	1.49 ± 0.22
Liver glycogen content (mg/g liver)	40.5 ± 12.4	80.8 ± 20.2 *	33.4 ± 10.5	78.0 ± 22.7 *
Liver cholesterol content (mg/g liver)	8.82 ± 1.63	9.54 ± 1.02	8.98 ± 1.53	7.17 ± 1.66
Liver triglyceride content (mg/g liver)	17.3 ± 4.2	16.0 ± 3.77	17.2 ± 5.14	15.7 ± 3.17

BW, body weight; EP, epidydimal fat weight; VS, visceral fat weight; BAT, brown adipose tissue weights; FGF21, fibroblast growth factor 21. * $p < 0.05$ vs. WT.

Chrebp and *Shp* mRNA levels were unaffected by *Shp* and *Chrebp* deletions, respectively (Figure 2A,B). Consistent with these phenotypes, the expression levels of ChREBP target genes, such as *Pklr* and *Fgf21*, were significantly lower in Chrebp$^{-/-}$and DKO mice (Figure 2C,D). In contrast, the expression of *Cyp7a1*, a SHP target gene, was significantly higher in Shp$^{-/-}$ and DKO mice but was unchanged in Chrebp$^{-/-}$ mice (Figure 2E). Many phenotypes seen in DKO mice were similar to those of Chrebp$^{-/-}$ mice, suggesting that SHP had little effect on ChREBP target gene expression.

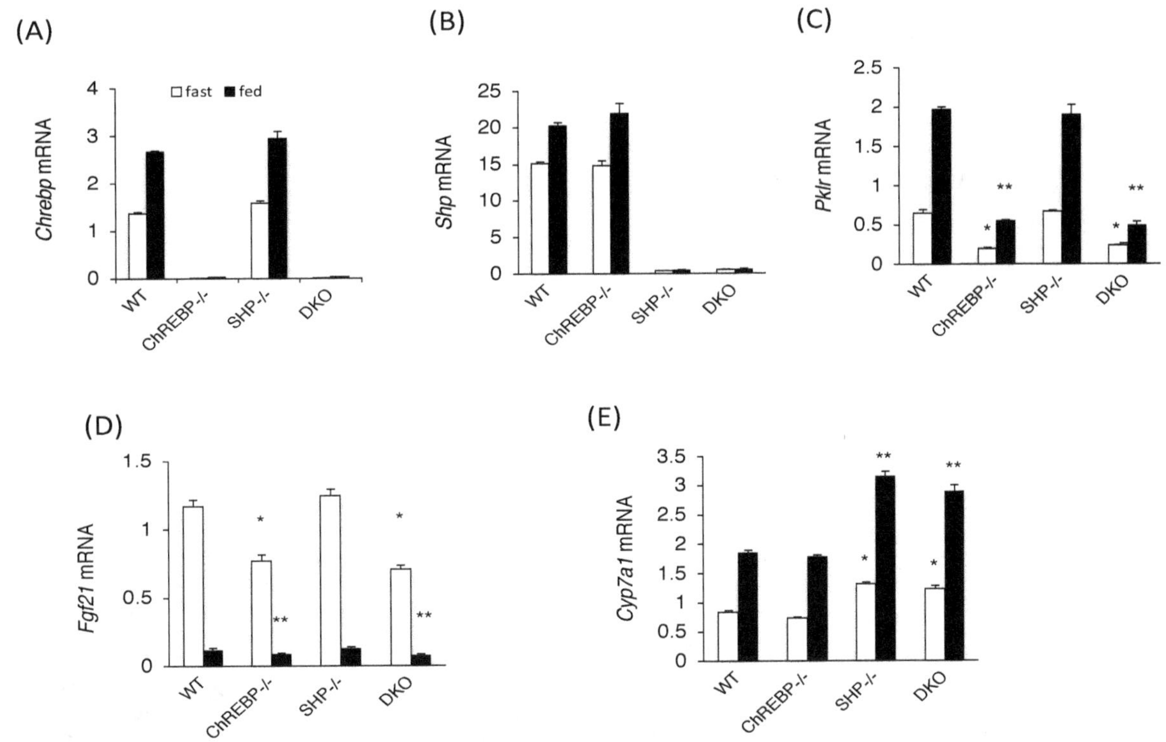

Figure 2. ChREBP and SHP target mRNA levels in wild-type, Chrebp$^{-/-}$, Shp$^{-/-}$, and Chrebp$^{-/-}$ Shp$^{-/-}$ mice. Carbohydrate response element binding protein (Chrebp) (**A**); small heterodimer partner (Shp) (**B**); liver type pyruvate kinase (Pklr) (**C**); fibroblast growth factor 21 (Fgf21) (**D**); and Cholesterol 7 alpha-hydroxylase (Cyp7a1); (**E**) mRNA expression analysis in the livers of wild-type, Chrebp$^{-/-}$, Shp$^{-/-}$, and Chrebp$^{-/-}$ Shp$^{-/-}$ (DKO) mice. Open squares indicate fasted conditions; closed squares indicate fed conditions. Pol2 expression was used as an internal control. Each mRNA levels were corrected with mouse RNA polymerase 2 mRNA. * $p < 0.05$ vs. WT (fast), $n = 4$. ** $p < 0.05$ vs. WT (fed), $n = 4$.

3.3. ChREBP and SHP Respectively Positively and Negatively Controlled VLDL Secretion through Mttp Regulation

We evaluated the effects of *Chrebp* and *Shp* deletion on *Mttp* expression. Hepatic *Mttp* mRNA levels were much lower in Chrebp$^{-/-}$ and DKO mice than in WT mice; however, those in Shp$^{-/-}$ mice were only slightly (only 1.15 times) higher than in WT mice (Figure 3A). Consistent with mRNA levels, MTTP protein levels were significantly much lower in Chrebp$^{-/-}$ and DKO mice than in WT mice (Figure 3B). Moreover, VLDL TG contents of Chrebp$^{-/-}$ and DKO mice were lower than those in WT and Shp$^{-/-}$ mice, while VLDL secretion rates in Chrebp$^{-/-}$ and DKO mice were approximately 0.6 times lower than in WT mice (Figure 3C). In contrast, liver VLDL secretion rates in Shp$^{-/-}$ mice were similar to those in WT mice (Figure 3C). In support of this, the VLDL TG contents and VLDL particle numbers in Chrebp$^{-/-}$ mice and DKO mice were much lower those in WT mice, while those in Shp$^{-/-}$ mice were similar to those in WT mice (Figure 3D,E). Therefore, under normal conditions, the effect of ChREBP on *Mttp* expression was potent but the effect of SHP was physiologically much weaker or lacking.

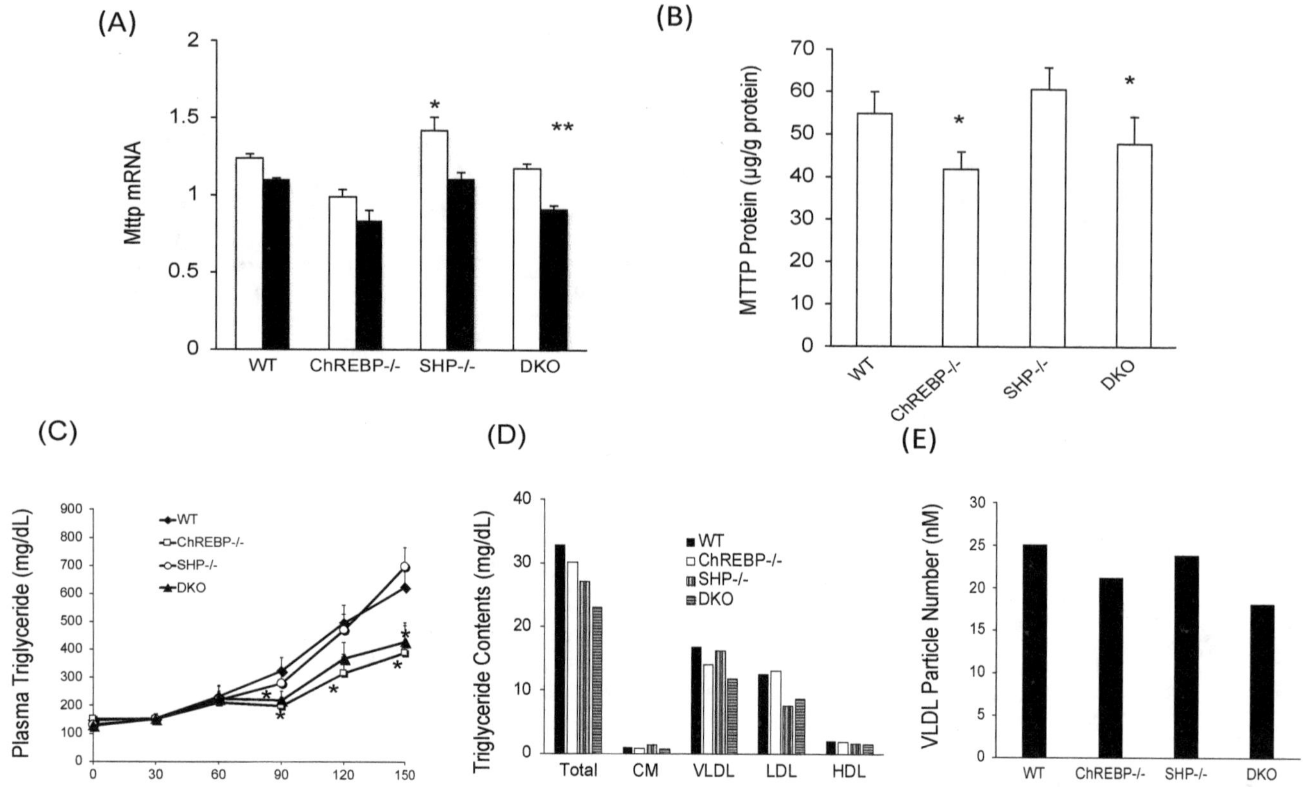

Figure 3. Shp deletion failed to recover decreased Mttp expression, and thereby, VLDL secretion rates mediated by Chrebp deletion. (**A**) Hepatic *Mttp* mRNA levels in the livers of wild-type (WT), Chrebp$^{-/-}$, Shp$^{-/-}$, and DKO mice. Mttp mRNA levels were detected by real-time PCR. Pol2 expression was used as an internal control. * $p < 0.05$ vs. WT (fast), $n = 4$. ** $p < 0.05$ vs. WT (fed), $n = 4$. Data are represented as means ± SD; (**B**) Hepatic MTTP protein expression in the livers of WT, Chrebp$^{-/-}$, Shp$^{-/-}$, and DKO mice. MTTP protein levels were measured by ELISA and corrected for total protein levels. * $p < 0.05$ vs. WT, $n = 5$–7. Data are represented as means ± SD; (**C**) VLDL secretion rates were measured as previously reported [17]. * $p < 0.05$ vs. WT, $n = 5$–7. Data are represented as means ± SD; TG contents in lipoprotein fraction (**D**) and VLDL particle numbers (**E**) were analyzed using gel-permeation high-performance liquid chromatography. Data are representative of six samples pooled.

4. Discussion

In this study, we evaluated whether ChREBP and SHP could coordinately affect VLDL secretion via *Mttp* expression. ChREBP and SHP reciprocally affected *Mttp* mRNA levels; however, the potency of *Mttp* suppression by SHP was much lower than that of *Mttp* induction by ChREBP. Therefore, ChREBP and SHP did not affect the transcriptional activity of each other. Mttp mRNA and protein levels in Chrebp$^{-/-}$ and DKO mice were much lower than those in WT mice; however, those in Shp$^{-/-}$ mice were similar to WT. In agreement with this, VLDL secretion rates of DKO and Chrebp$^{-/-}$ mice were much lower than those of Shp$^{-/-}$ mice, which were the same as those of WT mice. Together, these findings suggest that ChREBP, rather than SHP, regulates *Mttp* expression under normal conditions.

SHP predominantly functions as a transcriptional repressor of gene expression that binds directly to nuclear receptors, such as LRH-1, HNF4α, estrogen receptors, estrogen receptor-related receptors, liver X receptors, peroxisome proliferator-activated receptors, glucocorticoid receptor, thyroid hormone receptor β, retinoic acid receptor α, FXR, pregnane X receptor, constitutive androstane receptor, androgen receptor, nerve growth factor IB, and common heterodimerization partner retinoid X receptors [10]. SHP was previously shown to suppress MTTP expression by binding to HNF4α/LRH-1 sites in the *Mttp* promoter [10,13,35].

Recent reports have proposed a new ChREBP regulatory mechanism (ChREBP-nuclear receptor interaction), in which nuclear factors interact with ChREBP to modify ChREBP transcriptional activity [25–28]. Computer analysis previously revealed that ChREBP contains an LxQLLT sequence that matches the NR binding motif [29]. The rat LxQLLT sequence is localized to a proline-rich region (540–545 a.a.) of ChREBP [29]. SHP binds and represses the transcriptional activities of target genes by utilizing two functional LXXLL-related motifs located in the ligand-binding domain [10]. Some studies have also suggested that the interactions between ChREBP and nuclear receptors, such as FXR and HNF4, play physiological roles in regulating *Pklr* expression [25–28]. HNF4 and FXR positively and negatively regulate ChREBP transcriptional activity, respectively. However, our data revealed that SHP overexpression did not affect *Pklr* mRNA or luciferase activity of the PGL3 3xPKLR ChoRE vector. Moreover, *SHP* deletion did not affect the mRNA levels of ChREBP target genes (*Pklr* and *Fgf21*) in mice. Consistent with this, we found that ChREBP interacted with SHP in the mammalian two-hybrid system, and interactions with SHP did not interfere with the binding between FXR and ChREBP in the mammalian two-hybrid system (data not shown). This indicated that SHP might not affect the interplay between ChREBP and nuclear factors such as FXR and HNF4, and therefore, that it does not modulate ChREBP transcriptional activity.

Reporter assays for the *Mttp* promoter (−211/+81 bp) in the present study revealed that SHP suppressed hepatic *Mttp* expression, but that ChREBP overexpression did not affect luciferase activity controlled by the *Mttp* promoter (−211/+81 bp). This supports the notion that ChREBP does not affect the role of SHP as a corepressor. Taken together with the fact that a *Chrebp* deletion did not affect SHP target gene (*Cyp7a1*) mRNA levels, this suggested that ChREBP does not modulate SHP transcriptional activity. Thus, ChREBP and SHP do not affect the transcriptional activities of each other.

To evaluate ChREBP binding to *Mttp* promoter regions, we searched for putative ChoRE motifs [36–38] in the promoter, exons, and introns. However, we did not detect ChoREs in *Mttp*. Considering that ChREBP regulates the expression of many genes [21,30,32,33,36–39], we propose that it might indirectly induce *Mttp* expression through the activation of other transcription factors. However, further investigation is needed to identify the mechanism underlying the ChREBP induction of *Mttp* expression.

The VLDL secretory pathway is regulated by MTTP, a rate-limiting enzyme. We previously reported that ChREBP positively regulates VLDL secretion [19]. Although SHP controls *Mttp* expression by modulating HNF4 and LRH-1 transcriptional activity, its effect on VLDL secretion was controversial [15,16]. Some studies reported that VLDL secretion in Shp$^{-/-}$ mice on ob/ob or C57BL/6 backgrounds increased relative to WT mice [16], while others showed that VLDL secretion in Shp$^{-/-}$ mice fed a Western diet was similar to that in Shp$^{-/-}$ mice fed a normal diet [15]. Our data were consistent with the latter. They also confirmed that ChREBP regulates VLDL secretion, but that *SHP* deletion did not affect VLDL secretion in either WT or Chrebp$^{-/-}$ mice. Our analyses of MTTP protein levels and VLDL particle numbers also supported these data. Taken together with the fact that SHP overexpression by more than 70 times was needed to suppress ChREBP-mediated *Mttp* induction, these findings suggest that ChREBP plays important roles in VLDL secretion, while those of SHP are much smaller or negligible.

Nutritional conditions affect the development of NAFLD and dyslipidemia. High carbohydrate diets and high fat diets increase Mttp expression [9]. High carbohydrate diets increase de novo lipogenesis and *Mttp* expression [9,18]. As we previously reported, Chrebp deletions prevent hepatic lipid accumulation following consumption of a high carbohydrate diet [30,40]. The prevention from high carbohydrate diet induced fatty liver was due to a decrease in de novo lipogenesis, decreased free fatty acid supply from adipose tissue, and appetite loss from the high sucrose and high fructose diet [30,40–43]. Decreased *Mttp* expression might deteriorate NAFLD in ChREBP$^{-/-}$ mice. As ChREBP$^{-/-}$ mice could not be fed a high carbohydrate diet such as the high sucrose diet [30,41,42], we could not perform an experiment using the high carbohydrate diet. In contrast, a high fat diet increased the FFA supply from dietary fat and induced Mttp expression [17]. The High fat diet suppressed ChREBP transcriptional activity [44]. Moreover, Chrebp deletion did not prevent from high fat diet induced fatty liver owing to decreased fatty acid oxidation [19,43]. As Shp suppress PPAR alpha [45], Shp deletion prevented hepatic lipid accumulation through increased fatty acid oxidation [15]. Consistent with our data, *Mttp* expression was not affected by Shp deletion. Therefore, we analyzed the effects of ChREBP and SHP deletion on *Mttp* expression and VLDL secretion under a normal diet condition. In this study, ChREBP and SHP independently regulated glucose and lipid metabolism. The difference in target genes between ChREBP and SHP might contribute to the different effects of ChREBP and SHP on preventing the development of fatty liver induced by high fat diets in Chrebp$^{-/-}$ and Shp$^{-/-}$ mice (Figure 4).

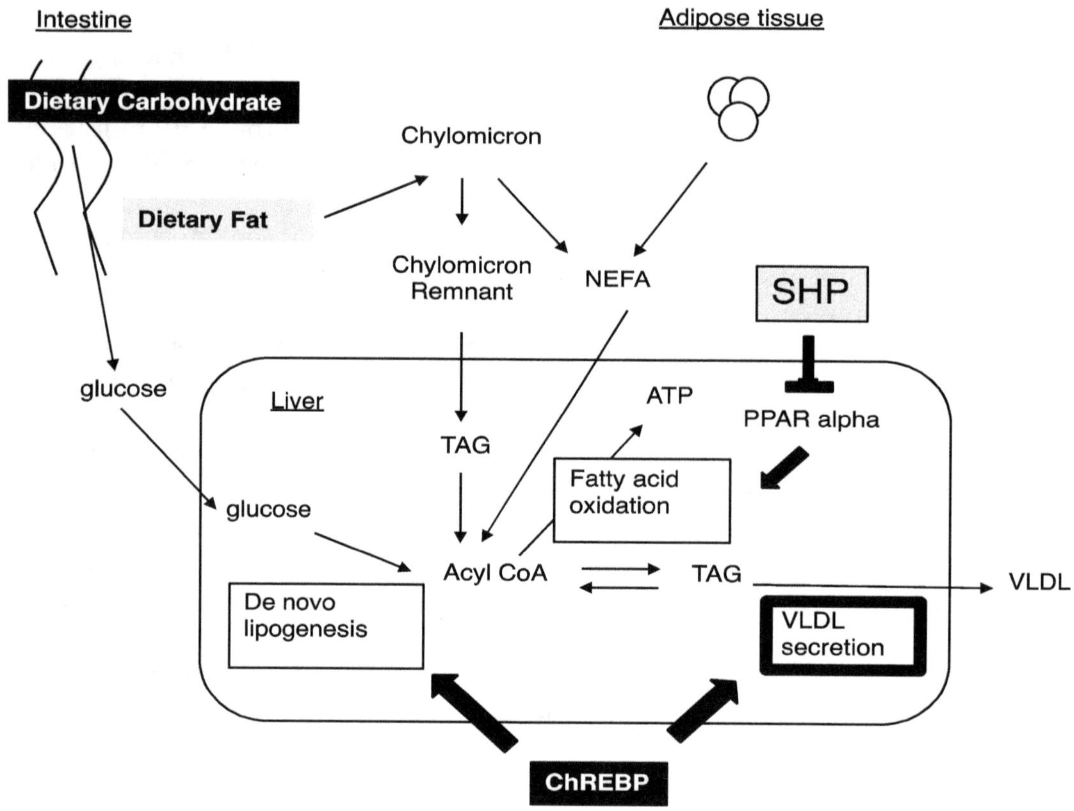

Figure 4. ChREBP and SHP independently regulate hepatic lipid metabolism. High carbohydrate diets increase de novo lipogenesis and VLDL secretion through ChREBP activation. Therefore, Chrebp deletion prevents high carbohydrate diet induced fatty liver [30,40,42,43]. In contrast, SHP suppresses PPAR alpha and an Shp deletion prevents high fat diet induced fatty liver [15,45]. In this study, we clarified that ChREBP, rather than SHP, regulates VLDL secretion through *Mttp* expression (bold line). Thus, ChREBP and SHP independently regulate hepatic lipid metabolism.

5. Conclusions

ChREBP and SHP were shown to modulate hepatic *Mttp* expression, but the capacity of *Mttp* suppression by SHP was much lower than that of *Mttp* induction by ChREBP. Moreover, ChREBP and SHP did not affect the transcriptional activities of each other. Unlike many transcription factors, ChREBP was not regulated by SHP. Finally, ChREBP, rather than SHP, was shown to regulate hepatic VLDL secretion.

Acknowledgments: We thank Sarah Williams, from Edanz Group (www.edanzediting.com) for editing a draft of this manuscript. This work was supported in part by a Grant-in-Aid for Scientific Research from the Japan Society for the Promotion of Science (Iizuka, K.: No. 17K00850, 26500005, Takeda, J.: No. 17K19902), research grants from MSD and Novartis Pharma. (Iizuka, K. and Takeda, J.).

Author Contributions: K.I. conceived and designed the experiments; H.N., T.K., W.W., H.T. and K.T. performed the experiments; H.N. analyzed the data; Y.H. gave a support in the literature review; K.I. and J.T. wrote and revised the paper. All the authors approved the final version of the manuscript.

References

1. Fabbrini, E.; Magkos, F. Hepatic Steatosis as a Marker of Metabolic Dysfunction. *Nutrients* **2015**, *7*, 4995–5019. [CrossRef] [PubMed]
2. Fabbrini, E.; Sullivan, S.; Klein, S. Obesity and nonalcoholic fatty liver disease: Biochemical, metabolic, and clinical implications. *Hepatology* **2010**, *51*, 679–689. [CrossRef] [PubMed]
3. Agius, L. High-carbohydrate diets induce hepatic insulin resistance to protect the liver from substrate overload. *Biochem. Pharmacol.* **2013**, *85*, 306–312. [CrossRef] [PubMed]
4. Westerbacka, J.; Lammi, K.; Häkkinen, A.M.; Rissanen, A.; Salminen, I.; Aro, A.; Yki-Järvinen, H. Dietary fat content modifies liver fat in overweight nondiabetic subjects. *J. Clin. Endocrinol. Metab.* **2005**, *90*, 2804–2809. [CrossRef] [PubMed]
5. Yu, J.; Marsh, S.; Hu, J.; Feng, W.; Wu, C. The Pathogenesis of Nonalcoholic Fatty Liver Disease: Interplay between Diet, Gut Microbiota, and Genetic Background. *Gastroenterol. Res. Pract.* **2016**, *2016*, 2862173. [CrossRef] [PubMed]
6. Donnelly, K.L.; Smith, C.I.; Schwarzenberg, S.J.; Jessurun, J.; Boldt, M.D.; Parks, E.J. Sources of fatty acids stored in liver and secreted via lipoproteins in patients with nonalcoholic fatty liver disease. *J. Clin. Investig.* **2005**, *115*, 1343–1351. [CrossRef] [PubMed]
7. Browning, J.D.; Horton, J.D. Molecular mediators of hepatic steatosis and liver injury. *J. Clin. Investig.* **2004**, *114*, 147–152. [CrossRef] [PubMed]
8. Cuchel, M.; Rader, D.J. Microsomal transfer protein inhibition in humans. *Curr. Opin. Lipidol.* **2013**, *24*, 246–250. [CrossRef] [PubMed]
9. Hussain, M.M.; Nijstad, N.; Franceschini, L. Regulation of microsomal triglyceride transfer protein. *Clin. Lipidol.* **2011**, *6*, 293–303. [CrossRef] [PubMed]
10. Zhang, Y.; Hagedorn, C.H.; Wang, L. Role of nuclear receptor SHP in metabolism and cancer. *Biochim. Biophys. Acta* **2011**, *1812*, 893–908. [CrossRef] [PubMed]
11. Nishigori, H.; Tomura, H.; Tonooka, N.; Kanamori, M.; Yamada, S.; Sho, K.; Inoue, I.; Kikuchi, N.; Onigata, K.; Kojima, I.; et al. Mutations in the small heterodimer partner gene are associated with mild obesity in Japanese subjects. *Proc. Natl. Acad. Sci. USA* **2001**, *98*, 575–580. [CrossRef] [PubMed]
12. Enya, M.; Horikawa, Y.; Kuroda, E.; Yonemaru, K.; Tonooka, N.; Tomura, H.; Oda, N.; Yokoi, N.; Yamagata, K.; Shihara, N.; et al. Mutations in the small heterodimer partner gene increase morbidity risk in Japanese type 2 diabetes patients. *Hum. Mutat.* **2008**, *29*, E271–E277. [CrossRef] [PubMed]
13. Lee, Y.K.; Dell, H.; Dowhan, D.H.; Hadzopoulou-Cladaras, M.; Moore, D.D. The orphan nuclear receptor SHP inhibits hepatocyte nuclear factor 4 and retinoid X receptor transactivation: Two mechanisms for repression. *Mol. Cell. Biol.* **2000**, *20*, 187–195. [CrossRef] [PubMed]
14. Goodwin, B.; Jones, S.A.; Price, R.R.; Watson, M.A.; McKee, D.D.; Moore, L.B.; Galardi, C.; Wilson, J.G.; Lewis, M.C.; Roth, M.E.; et al. A regulatory cascade of the nuclear receptors FXR, SHP-1, and LRH-1 represses bile acid biosynthesis. *Mol. Cell* **2000**, *6*, 517–526. [CrossRef]
15. Park, Y.J.; Kim, S.C.; Kim, J.; Anakk, S.; Lee, J.M.; Tseng, H.T.; Yechoor, V.; Park, J.; Choi, J.S.; Jang, H.C.; et al. Dissociation of diabetes and obesity in mice lacking orphan nuclear receptor small heterodimer partner. *J. Lipid Res.* **2011**, *52*, 2234–2244. [CrossRef] [PubMed]
16. Huang, J.; Iqbal, J.; Saha, P.K.; Liu, J.; Chan, L.; Hussain, M.M.; Moore, D.D.; Wang, L. Molecular characterization of the role of orphan receptor small heterodimerpartner in development of fatty liver. *Hepatology* **2007**, *46*, 147–157. [CrossRef] [PubMed]
17. Lin, M.C.; Arbeeny, C.; Bergquist, K.; Kienzle, B.; Gordon, D.A.; Wetterau, J.R. Cloning and regulation of hamster microsomal triglyceride transfer protein. The regulation is independent from that of other hepatic and intestinal proteins which participate in the transport of fatty acids and triglycerides. *J. Biol. Chem.* **1994**, *269*, 29138–29145. [PubMed]
18. Mock, K.; Lateef, S.; Benedito, V.A.; Tou, J.C. High-fructose corn syrup-55 consumption alters hepatic lipid metabolism and promotes triglyceride accumulation. *J. Nutr. Biochem.* **2017**, *39*, 32–39. [CrossRef] [PubMed]

19. Wu, W.; Tsuchida, H.; Kato, T.; Niwa, H.; Horikawa, Y.; Takeda, J.; Iizuka, K. Fat and carbohydrate in western diet contribute differently to hepatic lipid accumulation. *Biochem. Biophys. Res. Commun.* **2015**, *461*, 681–686. [CrossRef] [PubMed]
20. Uyeda, K.; Repa, J.J. Carbohydrate response element binding protein, ChREBP, a transcription factor coupling hepatic glucose utilization and lipid synthesis. *Cell Metab.* **2006**, *4*, 107–110. [CrossRef] [PubMed]
21. Iizuka, K. The transcription factor carbohydrate-response element-binding protein (ChREBP): A possible link between metabolic disease and cancer. *Biochim. Biophys. Acta* **2017**, *1863*, 474–485. [CrossRef] [PubMed]
22. Abdul-Wahed, A.; Guilmeau, S.; Postic, C. Sweet Sixteenth for ChREBP: Established Roles and Future Goals. *Cell Metab.* **2017**, *26*, 324–341. [CrossRef] [PubMed]
23. Herman, M.A.; Samuel, V.T. The Sweet Path to Metabolic Demise: Fructose and Lipid Synthesis. *Trends Endocrinol. Metab.* **2016**, *27*, 719–730. [CrossRef] [PubMed]
24. Poupeau, A.; Postic, C. Cross-regulation of hepatic glucose metabolism via ChREBP and nuclear receptors. *Biochim. Biophys. Acta* **2011**, *1812*, 995–1006. [CrossRef] [PubMed]
25. Caron, S.; Huaman Samanez, C.; Dehondt, H.; Ploton, M.; Briand, O.; Lien, F.; Dorchies, E.; Dumont, J.; Postic, C.; Cariou, B.; et al. Farnesoid X receptor inhibits the transcriptional activity of carbohydrate response element binding protein in human hepatocytes. *Mol. Cell. Biol.* **2013**, *33*, 2202–2211. [CrossRef] [PubMed]
26. Meng, J.; Feng, M.; Dong, W.; Zhu, Y.; Li, Y.; Zhang, P.; Wu, L.; Li, M.; Lu, Y.; Chen, H.; et al. Identification of HNF-4α as a key transcription factor to promote ChREBP expression in response to glucose. *Sci. Rep.* **2016**, *6*, 23944. [CrossRef] [PubMed]
27. Trabelsi, M.S.; Daoudi, M.; Prawitt, J.; Ducastel, S.; Touche, V.; Sayin, S.I.; Perino, A.; Brighton, C.A.; Sebti, Y.; Kluza, J.; et al. Farnesoid X receptor inhibits glucagon-like peptide-1 production by enteroendocrine L cells. *Nat. Commun.* **2015**, *6*, 7629. [CrossRef] [PubMed]
28. Burke, S.J.; Collier, J.J.; Scott, D.K. cAMP opposes the glucose-mediated induction of the L-PK gene by preventing the recruitment of a complex containing ChREBP, HNF4alpha, and CBP. *FASEB J.* **2009**, *23*, 2855–2865. [CrossRef] [PubMed]
29. McFerrin, L.G.; Atchley, W.R. A novel N-terminal domain may dictate the glucose response of Mondo proteins. *PLoS ONE* **2012**, *7*, e34803. [CrossRef] [PubMed]
30. Iizuka, K.; Bruick, R.K.; Liang, G.; Horton, J.D.; Uyeda, K. Deficiency of carbohydrate response element-binding protein (ChREBP) reduces lipogenesis as well as glycolysis. *Proc. Natl. Acad. Sci. USA* **2004**, *101*, 7281–7286. [CrossRef] [PubMed]
31. Bligh, E.G.; Dyer, W.J. A rapid method of total lipid extraction and purification. *Can. J. Biochem. Physiol.* **1959**, *37*, 911–917. [CrossRef] [PubMed]
32. Iizuka, K.; Horikawa, Y. Regulation of lipogenesis via BHLHB2/DEC1 and ChREBP feedback looping. *Biochem. Biophys. Res. Commun.* **2008**, *374*, 95–100. [CrossRef] [PubMed]
33. Iizuka, K.; Takeda, J.; Horikawa, Y. Glucose induces FGF21 mRNA expression through ChREBP activation in rat hepatocytes. *FEBS Lett.* **2009**, *583*, 2882–2886. [CrossRef] [PubMed]
34. Okazaki, M.; Yamashita, S. Recent Advances in Analytical Methods on Lipoprotein Subclasses: Caluculation of Particle Numbers from Lipid Levels by Gel Permeation HPLC Using "Spherical Particle Model". *J. Oleo Sci.* **2016**, *65*, 265–282. [CrossRef] [PubMed]
35. Hirokane, H.; Nakahara, M.; Tachibana, S.; Shimizu, M.; Sato, R. Bile acid reduces the secretion of very low density lipoprotein by repressing microsomal triglyceridetransfer protein gene expression mediated by hepatocyte nuclear factor-4. *J. Biol. Chem.* **2004**, *279*, 45685–45692. [CrossRef] [PubMed]
36. Jeong, Y.S.; Kim, D.; Lee, Y.S.; Kim, H.J.; Han, J.Y.; Im, S.S.; Chong, H.K.; Kwon, J.K.; Cho, Y.H.; Kim, W.K.; et al. Integrated expression profiling and genome-wide analysis of ChREBP targets reveals the dual role for ChREBP in glucose-regulated gene expression. *PLoS ONE* **2011**, *6*, e22544. [CrossRef] [PubMed]
37. Poungvarin, N.; Chang, B.; Imamura, M.; Chen, J.; Moolsuwan, K.; Sae-Lee, C.; Li, W.; Chan, L. Genome-Wide Analysis of ChREBP Binding Sites on Male Mouse Liver and White Adipose Chromatin. *Endocrinology* **2015**, *156*, 1982–1994. [CrossRef] [PubMed]
38. Ma, L.; Robinson, L.N.; Towle, H.C. ChREBP*Mlx is the principal mediator of glucose-induced gene expression in the liver. *J. Biol. Chem.* **2006**, *281*, 28721–28730. [CrossRef] [PubMed]
39. Iizuka, K. The Role of Carbohydrate Response Element Binding Protein in Intestinal and Hepatic Fructose Metabolism. *Nutrients* **2017**, *9*, 181. [CrossRef] [PubMed]

40. Iizuka, K.; Miller, B.; Uyeda, K. Deficiency of carbohydrate-activated transcription factor ChREBP prevents obesity and improves plasma glucose control in leptin-deficient (ob/ob) mice. *Am. J. Physiol. Endocrinol. Metab.* **2006**, *291*, E358–E364. [CrossRef] [PubMed]
41. Kim, M.; Astapova, I.I.; Flier, S.N.; Hannou, S.A.; Doridot, L.; Sargsyan, A.; Kou, H.H.; Fowler, A.J.; Liang, G.; Herman, M.A. Intestinal, but not hepatic, ChREBP is required for fructose tolerance. *JCI Insight* **2017**, *2*, e96703. [CrossRef] [PubMed]
42. Linden, A.G.; Li, S.; Choi, H.Y.; Fang, F.; Fukasawa, M.; Uyeda, K.; Hammer, R.E.; Horton, J.D.; Engelking, L.J.; Liang, G. Interplay between ChREBP and SREBP-1c Coordinates Postprandial Glycolysis and Lipogenesis in Livers of Mice. *J. Lipid Res.* **2018**, *59*, 475–487. [CrossRef] [PubMed]
43. Burgess, S.C.; Iizuka, K.; Jeoung, N.H.; Harris, R.A.; Kashiwaya, Y.; Veech, R.L.; Kitazume, T.; Uyeda, K. Carbohydrate-response element-binding protein deletion alters substrate utilization producing an energy-deficient liver. *J. Biol. Chem.* **2008**, *283*, 1670–1678. [CrossRef] [PubMed]
44. Kim, J.K.; Lee, K.S.; Chang, H.Y.; Lee, W.K.; Lee, J.I. Progression of diet induced nonalcoholic steatohepatitis is accompanied by increased expression of kruppel-like-factor 10 in mice. *J. Transl. Med.* **2014**, *12*, 186. [CrossRef] [PubMed]
45. Kassam, A.; Capone, J.P.; Rachubinski, R.A. The short heterodimer partner receptor differentially modulates peroxisome proliferator-activated receptor alpha-mediated transcription from the peroxisome proliferator-response elements of the genes encoding the peroxisomal beta-oxidation enzymes acyl-CoA oxidase and hydratase-dehydrogenase. *Mol. Cell. Endocrinol.* **2001**, *176*, 49–56. [PubMed]

Comparison of Prognostic Impact between the Child-Pugh Score and Skeletal Muscle Mass for Patients with Liver Cirrhosis

Hiroki Nishikawa, Hirayuki Enomoto *, Akio Ishii, Yoshinori Iwata, Yuho Miyamoto, Noriko Ishii, Yukihisa Yuri, Kunihiro Hasegawa, Chikage Nakano, Takashi Nishimura, Kazunori Yoh, Nobuhiro Aizawa, Yoshiyuki Sakai, Naoto Ikeda, Tomoyuki Takashima, Ryo Takata, Hiroko Iijima and Shuhei Nishiguchi

Department of Hepatobiliary and Pancreatic disease, Department of Internal Medicine, Hyogo College of Medicine, 1-1, Mukogawacho, Nishinomiyashi, Hyogo 663-8501, Japan; nishikawa_6392@yahoo.co.jp (H.N.); akio0010@yahoo.co.jp (A.I.); yo-iwata@hyo-med.ac.jp (Y.I.); yuho.0818.1989@gmail.com (Y.M.); ishinori1985@yahoo.co.jp (N.I.); gyma27ijo04td@gmail.com (Y.Y.); hiro.red1230@gmail.com (K.H.); chikage@hyo-med.ac.jp (C.N.); tk-nishimura@hyo-med.ac.jp (T.N.); mm2wintwin@ybb.ne.jp (K.Y.); nobu23hiro@yahoo.co.jp (N.A.); sakai429@hyo-med.ac.jp (Y.S.); nikeneko@hyo-med.ac.jp (N.I.); tomo0204@yahoo.co.jp (T.T.); chano_chano_rt@yahoo.co.jp (R.T.); hiroko-i@hyo-med.ac.jp (H.I.); nishiguc@hyo-med.ac.jp (S.N.)

* Correspondence: enomoto@hyo-med.ac.jp

Abstract: Aims: To investigate the influence of skeletal muscle mass index (SMI) as determined by bioimpedance analysis (BIA) (appendicular skeletal muscle mass/(height)^2) on survival by comparing the Child-Pugh score in patients with liver cirrhosis (LC, n = 383, average age = 65.2 years). Patients and methods: In terms of comparison of the effects of SMI and other markers on survival, we used time-dependent receiver operating characteristics (ROC) analysis. Results: The average SMI for male was 7.4 cm^2/m^2 whereas that for female was 6.0 cm^2/m^2 ($p < 0.0001$). As for the Child-Pugh score, five points were in the majority, both in males (51.7%, (106/205)) and females (44.9%, (80/178)). For both genders, the survival curve was well stratified according to SMI ($p < 0.0001$ for males and $p = 0.0056$ for females). In the multivariate analysis for survival, SMI and Child-Pugh scores were found to be significant both in males and females. In time-dependent ROC analyses, all area under the ROCs (AUROCs) for SMI in each time point were higher than those for Child-Pugh scores in males, while in females AUROCs for Child-Pugh scores at each time point were higher than those for SMI. Conclusion: SMI using BIA can be helpful for predicting outcomes, at least in male LC patients.

Keywords: liver cirrhosis; bioimpedance analysis; skeletal muscle mass index; Child-Pugh score; prognosis

---

1. Introduction

The liver is the pivotal organ for metabolism and it metabolizes carbohydrates, lipids, and proteins, which are the so-called "three major nutrients" [1–4]. Liver cirrhosis (LC) is an end-stage form in liver diseases and LC is characterized by several metabolic or nutritional disorders and portal hypertension-related complications such as ascites or varices, all of which can lead to dismal clinical outcome [1–4]. Over the past two or three decades, numerous clinical and biochemical predictors have been proposed in an effort to more accurately predict the prognosis in LC patients and evaluate their short and long-term survival correctly [5–9]. The Child-Pugh scoring system and the Model for End-stage Liver Disease (MELD) scoring system are two major prognostic scoring systems in LC patients [5–9]. In particular, the MELD score is calculated by three easily available and reproducible laboratory tests and is useful for predicting outcomes for patients undergoing liver transplantation (LT) [5]. In our country, LT is not common due to the shortage of transplanted liver and the Child-Pugh scoring system has been preferably used for assessing prognosis in LC patients.

Sarcopenia is a clinical entity as determined by skeletal muscle mass loss and decline of muscle strength and this clinical entity has recently drawn much attention among clinicians owing to its significant deleterious impact on outcomes [10–16]. LC can be associated with secondary sarcopenia because of protein metabolic disorder and/or energy metabolic disorder [11,14,15]. Skeletal muscle mass loss can be linked to poorer clinical outcomes in LC patients, hepatocellular carcinoma (HCC) patients, or patients with other malignancies [17–26]. Skeletal muscle mass can be assessed by computed tomography (CT), magnetic resonance imaging (MRI), dual energy X-ray absorptiometry and bioimpedance analysis (BIA), which are consistent and accurate assessment modalities [14,15,17,19,27,28]. Among these modalities, BIA is particularly attractive since it can noninvasively determine body composition analysis in LC patients [14,15,17,19,27,28].

However, which of two prognostic markers (i.e., the Child-Pugh scoring system and skeletal muscle mass) has stronger influence on clinical outcomes in patients with LC remains unclear. Addressing these questions may be clinically of significance. The aim of this study was to investigate the influence of skeletal muscle mass as determined by data in BIA on survival compared with the Child-Pugh score in patients with LC.

2. Patients and Methods

2.1. Patients

The current study was a single center retrospective study. Between October 2005 and October 2015, a total of 529 LC individuals with BIA data available were admitted at the Division of Hepatobiliary and Pancreatic disease, Department of Internal Medicine, Hyogo College of Medicine, Hyogo, Japan. In our department, BIA (Inbody 720, Tokyo, Japan) was routinely performed in the resting and standing position principally on an outpatient basis for patients who consented to nutritional evaluation. In this analysis, skeletal muscle mass was evaluated using BIA data. Of these patients, patients with severe ascites ($n = 24$) were excluded from this study as body weight, body mass index (BMI), and skeletal muscle mass index (SMI) using BIA may be overestimated in these patients [29,30]. Twenty-three subjects had been lost to follow-up within one year after performing BIA and they were excluded from this analysis for avoiding bias. In the remaining 482 subjects, 99 had HCC on radiological findings at baseline and they were also excluded because presence of HCC can affect the interpretation of BIA data. A total of 383 subjects were therefore analyzed in the current study. Follow-up observation after BIA included periodical blood tests, radiological assessments by ultrasonography (US), CT, or MRI in order to detect HCC incidence every 3–6 months. There was no patient who underwent LT during observation period. LC was diagnosed using pathological findings, radiological findings such as US, CT, or MRI and/or laboratory data including liver fibrosis markers [31–33]. In patients with lower serum albumin level (less than 3.5 g/dL), liver supporting therapies including branched-chain amino acid (BCAA) treatment or late evening snack with BCAA enriched snacks were in consideration [4,34,35]. In patients with hepatitis virus-related LC, antiviral treatments including direct acting antivirals, interferon-based regimens or nucleoside analogues therapy were also in consideration [4,34]. SMI was calculated as reported elsewhere [28]. Briefly, SMI was defined as "appendicular skeletal muscle mass/(height (m))^2" [28]. We retrospectively investigated the influence of SMI on survival in males and females, as compared with Child-Pugh scores, which was well established prognostic marker [7–9]. In terms of the comparison of the effects of SMI and other markers on survival, we used time-dependent receiver operating characteristics (ROC) analysis [36]. We also investigated parameters associated with overall survival (OS) in the univariate and multivariate analyses. HCC diagnosis and treatment choices for HCC were as reported elsewhere [37,38].

The ethical committee meeting in Hyogo College of Medicine acknowledged the current study protocol and this study strictly followed all regulations of the Declaration of Helsinki.

2.2. Statistical Analyses

Categorical parameters were compared by Fisher's exact test. Continuous parameters were compared by unpaired *t*-test, Mann-Whitney *U* test, or Kruskal-Wallis test, as applicable. In continuous parameters, ROC curve analysis for survival was conducted for the purpose of setting the optimal cutoff point that is linked to maximal sum of specificity and sensitivity and we classified continuous parameters into two groups using these cutoff points, which was then treated as dichotomous covariates in the univariate analysis. Survival curve was created by using the Kaplan-Meier method and compared in the log-rank test. Parameters with p value < 0.05 in the univariate analysis were finally subjected to the multivariate analysis in the Cox proportional hazards model. OS was defined as the time interval from the date of performing BIA until death from any cause or the last follow-up visit. Additionally, we analyzed time-dependent ROC curves of SMI, Child-Pugh scores, and variables which revealed to be significant in the multivariate analysis for survival, and compared between area under the ROCs (AUROCs) for above parameters in each time point (two-, three-, four-, five-, six-, and seven-years) [36].

Data are shown as the average $\pm$ standard deviation (SD) unless otherwise mentioned. Statistical significance was set at $p < 0.05$. Statistical analysis was performed with the JMP 11 (SAS Institute Inc., Cary, NC, USA).

3. Results

3.1. Baseline Characteristics

The baseline characteristics of the analyzed subjects (n = 383) are presented in Table 1. They included 205 males and 178 females with an average $\pm$ SD age of 65.2 $\pm$ 10.3 years. The median follow-up periods were 3.2 years (range: 0.2–10.7 years). The average $\pm$ SD value in SMI for male was 7.4 $\pm$ 0.9 cm^2/m^2 whereas that for female was 6.0 $\pm$ 0.7 cm^2/m^2 ($p < 0.0001$). According to the Asian Working Group for Sarcopenia criteria (AWGS), the cut-off values for SMI are 7.0 kg/m^2 for male and 5.7 kg/m^2 for female. [28] The proportion of decreased SMI (D-SMI: less than each cutoff value as defined by AWGS criteria) in male was 36.1% (74/205) and that in female was 34.8% (62/178). A total of 136 patients (35.5%) had D-SMI. As for Child-Pugh scores, five points was in the majority, both in males (51.7%, (106/205)) and females (44.9%, (80/178)). In males, SMI significantly correlated with age (overall significance, $p < 0.0001$), while in females it did not (overall significance, $p = 0.1921$) (Figure 1A,B). In both males and females, SMI significantly correlated with BMI (p values, both <0.0001) (Figure 1C,D). In both males ($p = 0.3716$) and females ($p = 0.1330$), SMI did not significantly correlate with the Child-Pugh classification (Figure 1E,F).

3.2. Cumulative OS Rates for the Entire Cohort, Male and Female According to SMI

For the entire cohort (n = 383), the one-, three-, and five-year cumulative OS rates were 92.7%, 82.4%, and 59.2%, respectively, in patients with D-SMI, and 97.2%, 92.2%, and 84.4%, respectively, in patients without D-SMI ($p < 0.0001$) (Figure 2). For males (n = 205), the one-, three-, and five-year cumulative OS rates were 91.9%, 78.0%, and 53.6%, respectively, in patients with D-SMI, and 96.2%, 92.0%, and 84.7%, respectively, in patients without D-SMI ($p < 0.0001$) (Figure 3A). For females (n = 178), the one-, three-, and five-year cumulative OS rates were 93.6%, 87.7%, and 66.1%, respectively, in patients with D-SMI, and 98.3%, 92.4%, and 83.8%, respectively, in patients without D-SMI ($p = 0.0056$) (Figure 3B).

Table 1. Baseline characteristics (n = 383).

Variables	Number or Average ± SD	Male (n = 205)	Female (n = 178)	p Value (Male vs. Female)
Age (years)	65.2 ± 10.3	64.1 ± 10.8	66.4 ± 9.5	0.0403
Body mass index (kg/m^2)	23.3 ± 3.9	23.4 ± 3.8	23.2 ± 4.0	0.6028
Skeletal muscle mass index (cm^2/m^2)	6.7 ± 1.1	7.4 ± 0.9	6.0 ± 0.7	<0.0001
Causes of liver disease Hepatitis B/Hepatitis C/others	32/235/116	22/122/61	10/113/55	0.2043
Child-Pugh scores, 5/6/7/8/9/10/11	186/93/58/28/13/3/2	106/42/31/15/6/3/2	80/51/27/13/7/0/0	0.2587
Total bilirubin (mg/dL)	1.3 ± 1.1	1.3 ± 1.3	1.2 ± 0.7	0.2319
Serum albumin (g/dL)	3.7 ± 0.53	3.7 ± 0.54	3.6 ± 0.51	0.3897
Prothrombin time (%)	77.0 ± 13.8	77.5 ± 13.4	76.4 ± 14.2	0.4532
Platelets (×10^4/mm^3)	10.6 ± 5.5	10.5 ± 5.3	10.7 ± 5.7	0.8093
Serum sodium (mmol/L)	139.7 ± 2.5	139.3 ± 2.5	140.2 ± 2.6	0.0004
Serum creatinine (mg/dL)	0.74 ± 0.51	0.84 ± 0.65	0.62 ± 0.22	<0.0001
Total cholesterol (mg/dL)	154.0 ± 36.8	152.8 ± 35.4	155.2 ± 38.4	0.5250
Triglyceride (mg/dL)	90.5 ± 45.1	95.5 ± 53.0	84.8 ± 33.0	0.2144
AST (IU/L)	49.3 ± 34.8	49.4 ± 32.3	49.2 ± 37.5	0.9417
ALT (IU/L)	42.6 ± 38.9	43.9 ± 34.2	41.0 ± 43.7	0.0951
Fasting blood glucose (mg/dL)	110.9 ± 34.7	114.8 ± 39.9	106.4 ± 27.0	0.0101
Ascites, yes/no	44/339	25/180	19/159	0.7484

Data are expressed as number or average ± standard deviation (SD). AST: aspartate aminotransferase; ALT: alanine aminotransferase.

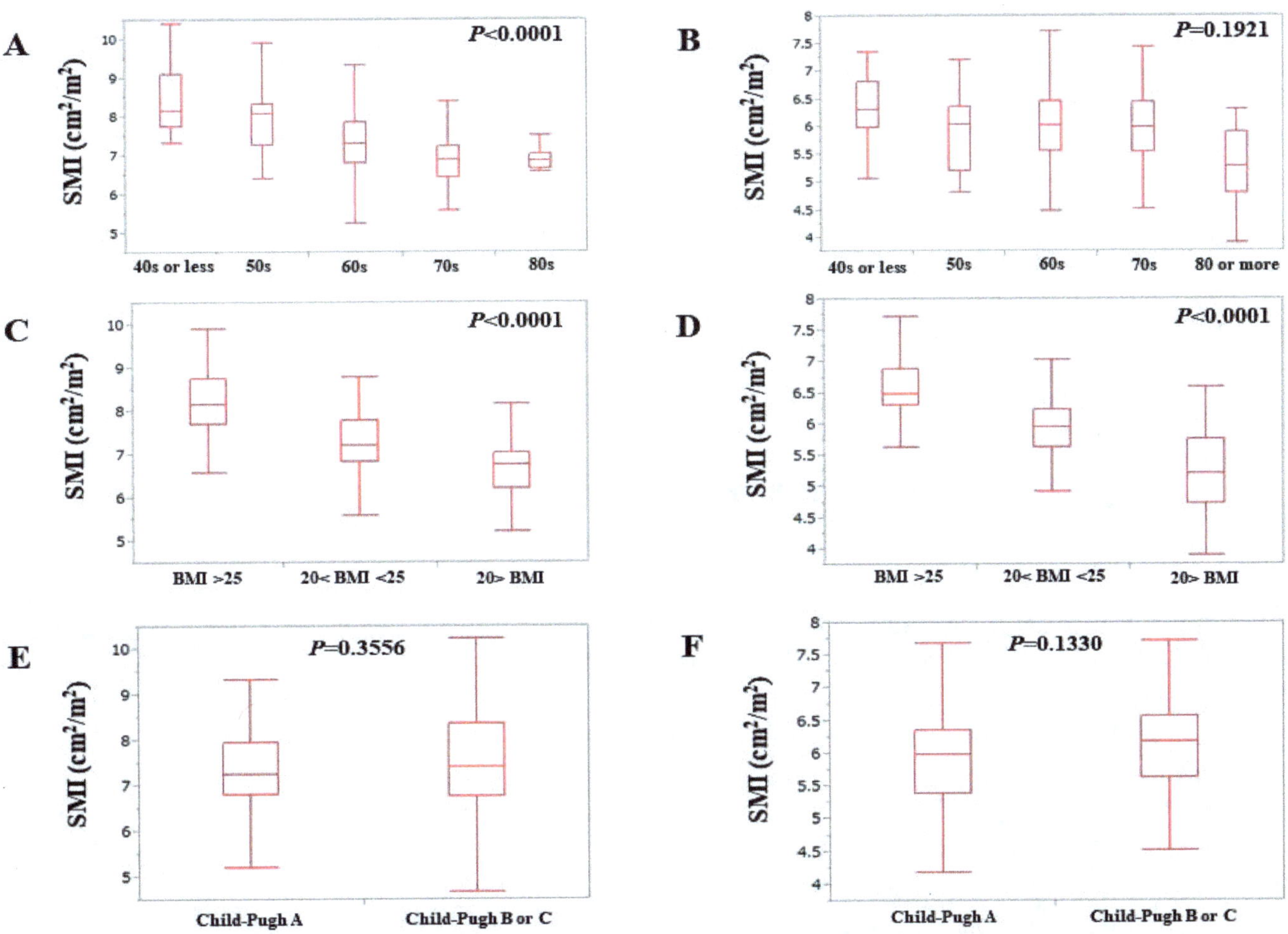

Figure 1. (**A**,**B**) Relationship between SMI and age in males (**A**) and females (**B**). (**C**,**D**) Relationship between SMI and BMI in males (**C**) and females (**D**). (**E**,**F**) Relationship between SMI and Child-Pugh classification in males (**E**) and females (**F**). SMI: skeletal muscle mass index; BMI: body mass index.

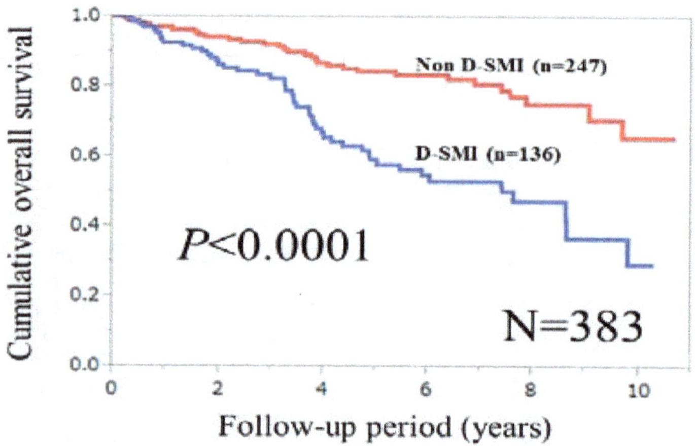

	1-year	3-year	5-year
Non D-SMI	97.2%	92.2%	84.4%
D-SMI	92.7%	82.4%	59.2%

Figure 2. Cumulative overall survival for the entire cohort (n = 383). The one-, three-, and five-year cumulative OS rates were 92.7%, 82.4% and 59.2%, respectively, in patients with decreased SMI (D-SMI), and 97.2%, 92.2% and 84.4%, respectively, in patients without D-SMI ($p < 0.0001$). D-SMI was defined according to the Asian Working Group for Sarcopenia criteria. The cut-off values for SMI are 7.0 kg/m^2 for males and 5.7 kg/m^2 for females. SMI: skeletal muscle mass index; D-SMI: decreased SMI.

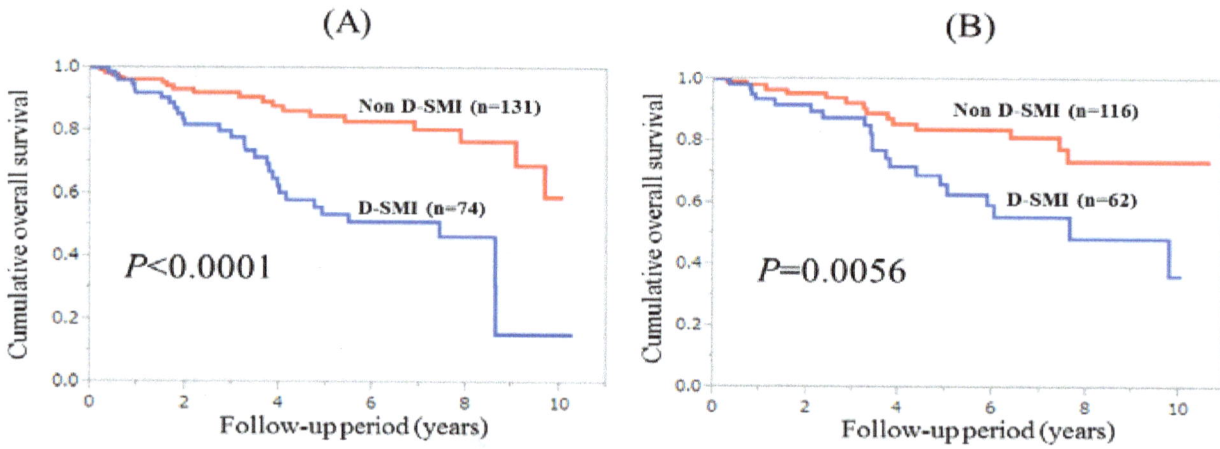

	1-year	3-year	5-year
Non D-SMI	96.2%	92.0%	84.7%
D-SMI	91.9%	78.0%	53.6%

	1-year	3-year	5-year
Non D-SMI	98.3%	92.4%	83.8%
SMI	93.6%	87.7%	66.1%

Figure 3. Cumulative overall survival for males (**A**) n = 205 and for females (**B**) n = 178 in patients with and without D-SMI. SMI: skeletal muscle mass index; D-SMI: decreased SMI.

Using ROC analysis for survival, the optimal cut-off point for SMI was 7.0 cm^2/m^2 in males (AUROC = 0.672, sensitivity = 64.6%, specificity = 69.4%) and 5.4 cm^2/m^2 in females (AUROC = 0.658, sensitivity = 45.7%, specificity = 83.9%). When the cut-off value of 5.4 cm^2/m^2 was adapted to our female patients (cut-off value for female in WAGS; 5.7 cm^2/m^2), similar results were obtained. That is, patients with D-SMI had significantly poorer survival rates than those without D-SMI (p = 0.0076).

3.3. Causes for Death for Males and Females

In male, during the observation period, 48 patients (23.4%) died. The causes for death were liver failure in 28 patients, HCC progression in 10 patients and miscellaneous causes in 10 patients. In female, during the observation period, 35 patients (19.7%) died. The causes for death were liver failure in 28 patients, HCC progression in four patients and miscellaneous causes in three patients.

3.4. *Univariate and Multivariate Analyses of Parameters Contributing to OS for Males*

Univariate analysis identified the following factors as significantly associated with OS for males: age ($p = 0.0041$); SMI ($p < 0.0001$); Child-Pugh score ($p = 0.0252$); aspartate aminotransferase ($p = 0.0150$); alanine aminotransferase (ALT) ($p = 0.0407$); serum albumin ($p = 0.0011$); serum sodium ($p = 0.0133$); serum creatinine ($p = 0.0088$); and BMI ($p = 0.0041$) (Table 2a). Since the Child-Pugh score includes serum albumin, it was not entered into the multivariate analysis, and since age and BMI significantly correlated with SMI, they were also excluded in the multivariate analysis to avoid the effect of collinearity. The hazard ratios (HRs) and 95% confidence intervals (CIs) calculated by using multivariate analysis for the six significant variables ($p < 0.05$) in the univariate analysis are presented in Table 2b. SMI ($p = 0.0005$) and Child-Pugh score ($p = 0.0424$) were found to be significant predictors related to OS in the multivariate analysis (Table 2b).

Table 2. (**a**) Univariate analyses of factors linked to overall survival for males ($n = 205$). (**b**) Multivariate analyses of factors linked to overall survival for male.

(a)

Variables	Number of Each Category	Univariate p Value
Age (years) ≥ 70, yes/no	91/114	0.0041
Cause of liver diseases, B/C/others	22/122/61	0.2746
SMI ≥ 7.0 cm^2/m^2, yes/no	127/78	<0.0001
Child-Pugh score ≥ 6, yes/no	99/106	0.0252
AST ≥ 29 IU/L, yes/no	146/59	0.0150
ALT ≥ 47 IU/L, yes/no	63/142	0.0407
Serum albumin ≥ 3.7 g/dL, yes/no	113/92	0.0011
Total bilirubin ≥ 2.0 mg/dL, yes/no	29/176	0.1539
Prothrombin time $\geq 77.1\%$, yes/no	111/94	0.4521
Platelet count $\geq 9.4 \times 10^4$/mm^3, yes/no	101/104	0.2360
Total cholesterol ≥ 124 mg/dL, yes/no	165/40	0.2398
Triglyceride ≥ 56 mg/dL, yes/no	170/35	0.0649
Serum sodium ≥ 138 mmol/L, yes/no	166/39	0.0133
Fasting blood glucose ≥ 97 mg/dL, yes/no	145/60	0.4942
Serum creatinine ≥ 0.78 mg/dL, yes/no	84/121	0.0088
Body mass index ≥ 23.4 kg/m^2, yes/no	91/114	0.0041
Ascites, yes/no	25/180	0.0712

(b)

Variables	Multivariate Analysis		
	Hazard Ratio	95% CI	p Value
SMI (per one cm^2/m^2)	0.571	0.416–0.777	0.0005
AST (per one IU/L)	1.005	0.987–1.022	0.5683
ALT (per one IU/L)	0.990	0.972–1.008	0.3002
Child-Pugh score (per one point)	1.270	1.020–1.520	0.0424
Serum sodium (per one mmol/L)	0.912	0.807–1.033	0.1481
Serum creatinine (per one mg/dL)	1.104	0.769–1.397	0.4914

CI: confidence interval; SMI: skeletal muscle mass index; AST: aspartate aminotransferase; ALT: alanine aminotransferase.

3.5. *Univariate and Multivariate Analyses of Parameters Contributing to OS for Females*

Univariate analysis identified the following parameters as significantly associated with OS for females: age ($p = 0.0214$); SMI ($p = 0.0076$); Child-Pugh score ($p = 0.0009$); ALT ($p = 0.0104$); serum albumin ($p = 0.0003$); prothrombin time (PT) ($p = 0.0355$); platelet count ($p = 0.0333$); triglyceride ($p = 0.0011$); serum creatinine ($p = 0.0137$); BMI ($p = 0.0270$) and presence of ascites ($p < 0.0001$) (Table 3a). As the Child-Pugh score includes serum albumin, PT, and ascites, they were not entered into the multivariate analysis, and because BMI significantly correlated with SMI, it was also excluded in the multivariate analysis to avoid the effect of collinearity. The HRs and 95% CIs calculated by using multivariate analysis for the seven significant variables ($p < 0.05$) in the univariate analysis are presented in Table 3b. SMI ($p = 0.0016$) and Child-Pugh scores ($p < 0.0001$) were found to be significant predictors related to OS in the multivariate analysis (Table 3b).

Table 3. (**a**) Univariate analyses of factors linked to overall survival for female ($n = 178$). (**b**) Multivariate analyses of factors linked to overall survival for female.

(a)

Variables	Number of Each Category	Univariate p value
Age (years) $\geq$ 77, yes/no	22/156	0.0214
Cause of liver diseases, B/C/others	10/113/55	0.5037
SMI $\geq$ 5.4 cm^2/m^2, yes/no	139/39	0.0076
Child-Pugh score $\geq$ 6, yes/no	98/80	0.0009
AST $\geq$ 80 IU/L, yes/no	20/158	0.0544
ALT $\geq$ 58 IU/L, yes/no	32/146	0.0104
Serum albumin $\geq$ 3.4 g/dL, yes/no	117/61	0.0003
Total bilirubin $\geq$ 2.3 mg/dL, yes/no	10/168	0.7607
Prothrombin time $\geq$ 73.7%, yes/no	103/75	0.0355
Platelet count $\geq$ 9.7 $\times 10^4$/mm^3, yes/no	92/86	0.0333
Total cholesterol $\geq$ 176 mg/dL, yes/no	49/129	0.0558
Triglyceride $\geq$ 72 mg/dL, yes/no	108/70	0.0011
Serum sodium $\geq$ 139 mmol/L, yes/no	143/35	0.4064
Fasting blood glucose $\geq$ 89 mg/dL, yes/no	142/36	0.2428
Serum creatinine $\geq$ 0.63 mg/dL, yes/no	66/112	0.0137
Body mass index $\geq$ 23.4 kg/m^2, yes/no	78/100	0.0270
Ascites, yes/no	19/159	<0.0001

(b)

Variables	Multivariate Analysis		
	Hazard ratio	95% CI	p Value
Age (per one year)	1.018	0.977–1.063	0.3998
SMI (per one cm^2/m^2)	0.450	0.270–0.731	0.0016
ALT (per one IU/L)	0.987	0.967–1.107	0.0506
Platelet count (per one $\times$ 10^4/mm^3)	0.919	0.828–1.008	0.0943
Child-Pugh score (per one point)	1.938	1.400–2.690	<0.0001
Triglyceride (per one mg/dL)	0.998	0.983–1.011	0.7760
Serum creatinine (per one mg/dL)	2.546	0.413–10.860	0.2545

CI: confidence interval; SMI: skeletal muscle mass index; AST: aspartate aminotransferase; ALT: alanine aminotransferase.

3.6. Time-Dependent ROC Analyses for OS in Males

Results for time-dependent ROC analyses at two-, three-, four-, five-, six-, and seven-years of SMI and the Child-Pugh scores for males are shown in Figure 4A. All AUROCs for SMI at each time point were higher than those for Child-Pugh scores, denoting that SMI had consistently superior predictive ability for OS over Child-Pugh scores.

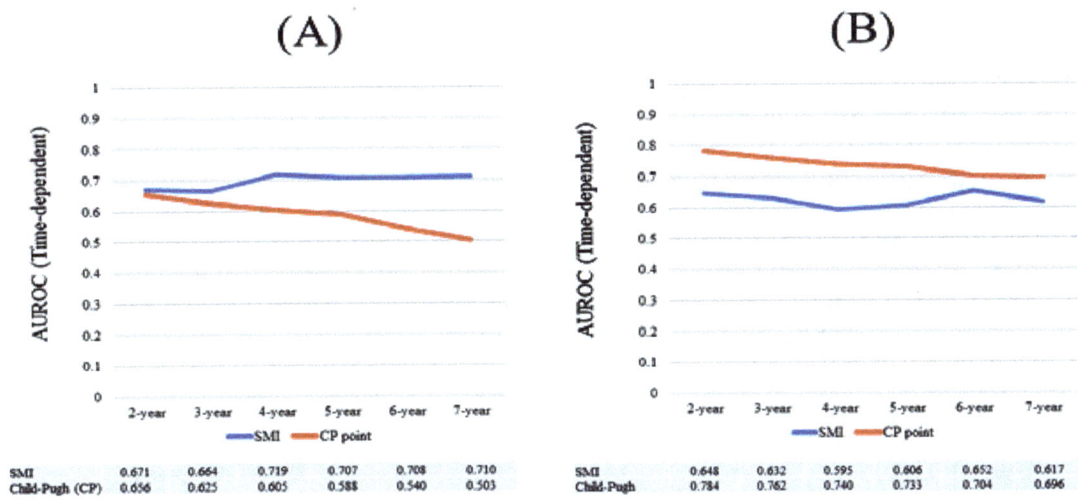

Figure 4. (**A**) Results for time-dependent ROC analyses at two-, three, four-, five-, six-, and seven-years of SMI and Child-Pugh scores for males; (**B**) Results for time-dependent ROC analyses at two-, three-, four-, five-, six-, and seven-years of SMI and Child-Pugh scores for females. ROC; receiver operating characteristics, AUROC; area under the ROC, SMI; skeletal muscle mass index, CP; Child-Pugh.

3.7. Time-Dependent ROC Analyses for OS in Females

Results for time-dependent ROC analyses at two-, three-, four-, five-, six-, and seven-years of SMI and Child-Pugh score for female were shown in Figure 4B. All AUROCs for Child-Pugh scores at each time point were higher than those for SMI, denoting that Child-Pugh scores had consistently superior predictive ability for OS over SMI.

3.8. Time-Dependent ROC Analyses for OS in Male Patients with Child-Pugh A

Results for time-dependent ROC analyses at two-, three-, four-, and five-years of SMI and Child-Pugh scores for male Child-Pugh A patients (n = 148) are shown in Figure 5A. All AUROCs for SMI in each time point were higher than those for Child-Pugh scores, denoting that SMI had consistently superior predictive ability for OS over Child-Pugh scores.

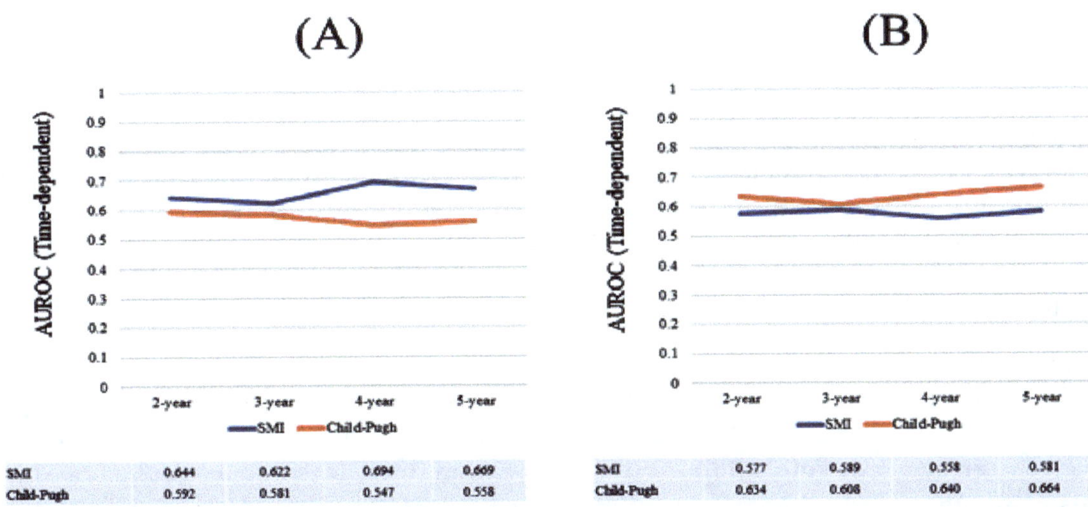

Figure 5. (**A**) Results for time-dependent ROC analyses at two-, three-, four-, and five-years of SMI and Child-Pugh scores for male Child-Pugh A patients; (**B**) Results for time-dependent ROC analyses at two-, three-, four-, and five-years of SMI and Child-Pugh scores for female Child-Pugh A patients. ROC; receiver operating characteristics, AUROC; area under the ROC, SMI; skeletal muscle mass index.

3.9. Time-Dependent ROC Analyses for OS in Female Patients with Child-Pugh A

Results for time-dependent ROC analyses at two-, three-, four-, and five-years of SMI and Child-Pugh scores for female Child-Pugh A patients (n = 131) are shown in Figure 5B. All AUROCs for Child-Pugh score in each time point were higher than those for SMI, denoting that Child-Pugh scores had consistently superior predictive ability for OS over SMI.

3.10. Time-Dependent ROC Analyses for OS in Male Patients with Child-Pugh B or C

Results for time-dependent ROC analyses at two-, three-, four-, and five-years of SMI and Child-Pugh scores for male Child-Pugh B or C patients (n = 57) are shown in Figure 6A. All AUROCs for SMI at each time point were higher than those for Child-Pugh scores, denoting that SMI had consistently superior predictive ability for OS over Child-Pugh scores.

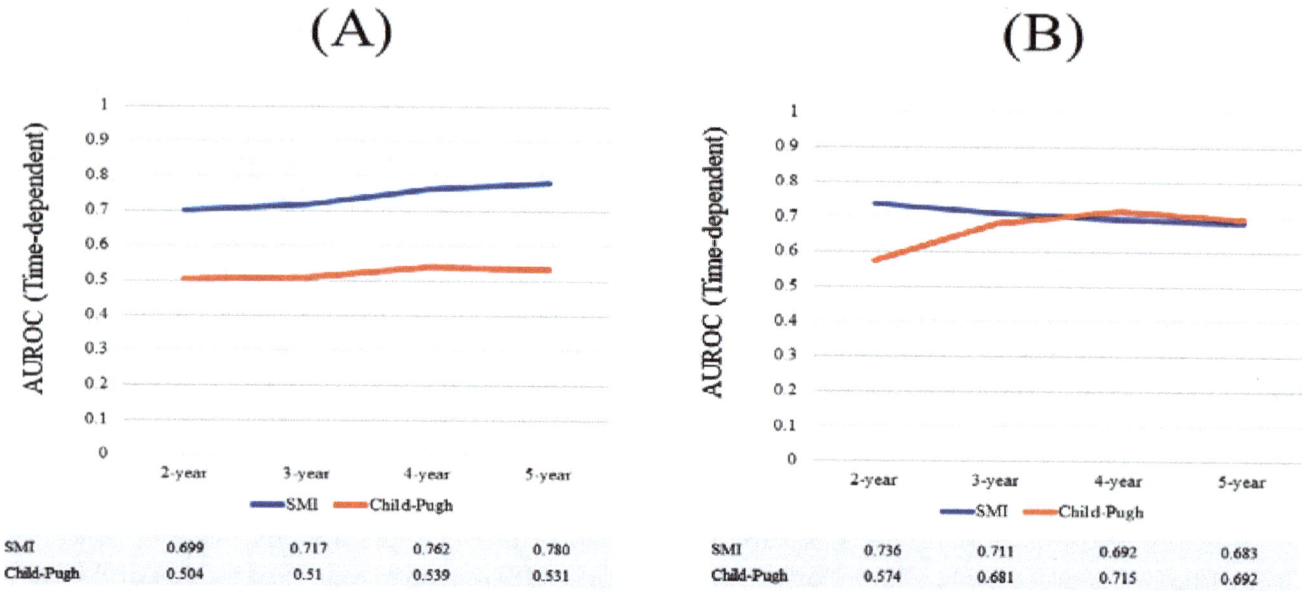

Figure 6. (**A**) Results for time-dependent ROC analyses at two-, three-, four-, and five-years of SMI and Child-Pugh score for male Child-Pugh B or C patients; (**B**) Results for time-dependent ROC analyses at two-, three-, four-, and five-years of SMI and Child-Pugh scores for female Child-Pugh B or C patients. ROC; receiver operating characteristics, AUROC; area under the ROC, SMI; skeletal muscle mass index.

3.11. Time-Dependent ROC Analyses for OS in Female Patients with Child-Pugh B or C

Results for time-dependent ROC analyses at two-, three-, four-, and five-years of SMI and Child-Pugh scores for female Child-Pugh B or C patients (n = 47) are shown in Figure 6B. At four- and five-years, Child-Pugh scores had higher AUROC than SMI.

4. Discussion

To the best of our knowledge, this is the first comparative study in SMI and Child-Pugh scores on clinical outcomes in LC patients. The Child-Pugh scoring system is a well-established prognostic system in LC patients [5–9]. While, SMI in LC has been currently attracting much attention owing to its well predictive performance [14–17,19,27,28]. Investigation into the influence of SMI on outcomes in LC patients is pivotal and, particularly, clarifying which of these two markers has stronger predictive impact for LC is clinically essential in light of creating a novel prognostic system in LC patients. We, therefore, conducted this comparative analysis to address this question. Since skeletal muscle mass significantly can differ between male and female, we analyzed and discussed separately in males and females.

In our results, for males, SMI and Child-Pugh scores were revealed to be significant for OS in the multivariate analysis, and all AUROCs for SMI at each time point were higher than those for Child-Pugh scores. Additionally, in subgroup analyses for male patients with Child-Pugh A or Child-Pugh B or C, SMI had consistently higher AUROCs than the Child-Pugh score. For females, similar results were obtained in the multivariate analysis, however, all AUROCs for Child-Pugh scores at each time point were higher than those for SMI. These results denote that SMI as a predictor can perform well as compared with Child-Pugh score at least in male LC patients. Our current results may provide new information and shed some lights for the better comprehension of prognosis in LC patients. The significant difference in baseline characteristics in such as SMI, age, serum sodium, and serum creatinine between males and females can explain the different results according to gender. In particular, aging can be a significant predictor in LC patients [14,39,40]. Our country is an aging country [39,40]. The reasons for results in time-dependent ROC analysis in females may be attributed to our results that SMI did not significantly correlate with age in females.

In view of our current results, some interventional therapies, including BCAA therapy, testosterone therapy, or exercise, can be considered especially in male LC patients with lower skeletal muscle mass for ameliorating prognosis [13,35,41–43]. However, firm recommendations for LC patients are not currently available. As for cut-off value for BIA, AWGS recommends 2SDs below the average muscle mass of young adults (7.0 cm^2/m^2 for male and 5.7 cm^2/m^2 for female) [28]. In our outcome based ROC analysis, the optimal cut-off points for survival were 7.0 cm^2/m^2 for males and 5.4 cm^2/m^2 for females, which were quite similar to recommendations in AWGS and their recommendations were well validated in our analysis. From the viewpoint of outcome-based analysis, our results may be worthy of reporting.

As described above, it is of note that SMI significantly correlated with age in males, but not in females. In general, changes in muscle mass occur with aging and muscle mass loss is a common condition which is recognized as a part of aging [44]. However, our results showed that the rates of muscle mass decline can vary according to gender, suggesting that factors other than aging, such as diet intake and lifestyle, may influence the maintenance of healthy muscle mass [45]. On the other hand, although the liver transplantation allocation system utilizes MELD score to prioritize organs to the most ill subjects, MELD scores do not perform better than Child-Pugh scores in non-transplant settings. In other words, MELD scores can perform well in decompensated LC rather than compensated LC [8]. Due to the high proportion of patients with Child-Pugh A in our cohort, we did not include MELD scores in the analysis.

Several limitations must be acknowledged in our current analysis. First, this study is a single-center retrospective observational study utilizing data for BIA and parameters reflecting muscle function such as hang grip strength or walking speed were not assessed in this analysis. In future studies, both skeletal muscle mass and muscle function should be evaluated in outcome based analyses. Second, patients with severe ascites were excluded from our analysis because SMI can be overestimated in these patients. Thus, the number of Child-Pugh C patients was rather small and our results cannot be adapted to such patients. Body composition analyses using BIA can be challenging in LC patients with severe ascites. Finally, various treatments for underlying liver diseases were performed during follow-up period in each patient, potentially creating bias. However, our study results denoted that SMI had higher predictive ability, at least in male LC patients. Results in time-dependent ROC analysis support our assertion for the predictive superiority of SMI over Child-Pugh scores in males.

In conclusion, SMI can be accessible for predicting outcomes, at least in male LC patients. Some interventions for male patients with lower SMI may be recommended.

Acknowledgments: The authors would like to thank all medical staff in our hospital for data collection. Financial support is none.

Author Contributions: Hiroki Nishikawa and Hirayuki Enomoto analyzed the data and wrote the paper. Shuhei Nishiguchi supervised this work. The other remaining authors collected data.

Abbreviations

LC: liver cirrhosis; MELD: Model for End-stage Liver Disease; LT: liver transplantation; HCC: hepatocellular carcinoma; CT: computed tomography; MRI: magnetic resonance imaging; BIA: bioimpedance analysis; SMI: skeletal muscle mass index; BMI: body mass index; US: ultrasonography; BCAA: branched-chain amino acid; ROC: receiver operating characteristic curve; OS: overall survival; AUROC: area under the receiver operating characteristic curve; SD: standard deviation; AWGS: Asian Working Group for Sarcopenia criteria; D-SMI: decreased SMI; ALT: alanine aminotransferase; HR: hazard ratios; CI: confidence interval.

References

1. Cheung, K.; Lee, S.S.; Raman, M. Prevalence and mechanisms of malnutrition in patients with advanced liver disease, and nutrition management strategies. *Clin. Gastroenterol. Hepatol.* **2012**, *10*, 117–125. [CrossRef] [PubMed]
2. Charlton, M.R. Branched-chain amino acid enriched supplements as therapy for liver disease. *J. Nutr.* **2006**, *136* (Suppl. 1), 295S–298S. [CrossRef]
3. Kawaguchi, T.; Izumi, N.; Charlton, M.R.; Sata, M. Branched-chain amino acids as pharmacological nutrients in chronic liver disease. *Hepatology* **2011**, *54*, 1063–1070. [CrossRef] [PubMed]
4. Fukui, H.; Saito, H.; Ueno, Y.; Uto, H.; Obara, K.; Sakaida, I.; Shibuya, A.; Seike, M.; Nagoshi, S.; Segawa, M.; et al. Evidence-based clinical practice guidelines for liver cirrhosis 2015. *J. Gastroenterol.* **2016**, *51*, 629–650. [CrossRef] [PubMed]
5. Kamath, P.S.; Wiesner, R.H.; Malinchoc, M.; Kremers, W.; Therneau, T.M.; Kosberg, C.L.; D'Amico, G.; Dickson, E.R.; Kim, W.R. A model to predict survival in patients with end-stage liver disease. *Hepatology* **2001**, *33*, 464–470. [CrossRef] [PubMed]
6. Kim, W.R.; Biggins, S.W.; Kremers, W.K.; Wiesner, R.H.; Kamath, P.S.; Benson, J.T.; Edwards, E.; Therneau, T.M. Hyponatremia and mortality among patients on the liver-transplant waiting list. *N. Engl. J. Med.* **2008**, *359*, 1018–1026. [CrossRef] [PubMed]
7. D'Amico, G.; Garcia-Tsao, G.; Pagliaro, L. Natural history and prognostic indicators of survival in cirrhosis: A systematic review of 118 studies. *J. Hepatol.* **2006**, *44*, 217–231. [CrossRef] [PubMed]
8. Cholongitas, E.; Papatheodoridis, G.V.; Vangeli, M.; Terreni, N.; Patch, D.; Burroughs, A.K. Systematic review: The model for end-stage liver disease—Should it replace Child-Pugh's classification for assessing prognosis in cirrhosis? *Aliment. Pharmacol. Ther.* **2005**, *22*, 1079–1089. [CrossRef] [PubMed]
9. Botta, F.; Giannini, E.; Romagnoli, P.; Fasoli, A.; Malfatti, F.; Chiarbonello, B.; Testa, E.; Risso, D.; Colla, G.; Testa, R. MELD scoring system is useful for predicting prognosis in patients with liver cirrhosis and is correlated with residual liver function: A European study. *Gut* **2003**, *52*, 134–139. [CrossRef] [PubMed]
10. Periyalwar, P.; Dasarathy, S. Malnutrition in cirrhosis: Contribution and consequences of sarcopenia on metabolic and clinical responses. *Clin. Liver Dis.* **2012**, *16*, 95–131. [CrossRef] [PubMed]
11. Cruz-Jentoft, A.J.; Landi, F.; Schneider, S.M.; Zúñiga, C.; Arai, H.; Boirie, Y.; Chen, L.K.; Fielding, R.A.; Martin, F.C.; Michel, J.P.; et al. Prevalence of and interventions for sarcopenia in ageing adults: A systematic review. Report of the International Sarcopenia Initiative (EWGSOP and IWGS). *Age Ageing* **2014**, *43*, 748–759. [CrossRef] [PubMed]
12. Sinclair, M.; Gow, P.J.; Grossmann, M.; Angus, P.W. Review article: Sarcopenia in cirrhosis—Aetiology, implications and potential therapeutic interventions. *Aliment. Pharmacol. Ther.* **2016**, *43*, 765–777. [CrossRef] [PubMed]
13. Hanai, T.; Shiraki, M.; Nishimura, K.; Ohnishi, S.; Imai, K.; Suetsugu, A.; Takai, K.; Shimizu, M.; Moriwaki, H. Sarcopenia impairs prognosis of patients with liver cirrhosis. *Nutrition* **2015**, *31*, 193–199. [CrossRef] [PubMed]
14. Nishikawa, H.; Shiraki, M.; Hiramatsu, A.; Moriya, K.; Hino, K.; Nishiguchi, S. JSH guidelines for sarcopenia in liver disease (first edition): Recommendation from the working group for creation of sarcopenia assessment criteria in the JSH. *Hepatol. Res.* **2016**, *46*, 951–963. [CrossRef] [PubMed]
15. Santilli, V.; Bernetti, A.; Mangone, M.; Paoloni, M. Clinical definition of sarcopenia. *Clin. Cases Miner. Bone Metab.* **2014**, *11*, 177–180. [CrossRef] [PubMed]
16. Nardelli, S.; Lattanzi, B.; Torrisi, S.; Greco, F.; Farcomeni, A.; Gioia, S.; Merli, M.; Riggio, O. Sarcopenia is Risk Factor for Development of Hepatic Encephalopathy After Transjugular Intrahepatic Portosysthemic Shunt Placement. *Clin. Gastroenterol. Hepatol.* **2017**, *15*, 934–936. [CrossRef] [PubMed]

17. Itoh, S.; Shirabe, K.; Matsumoto, Y.; Yoshiya, S.; Muto, J.; Harimoto, N.; Yamashita, Y.; Ikegami, T.; Yoshizumi, T.; Nishie, A.; et al. Effect of body composition on outcomes after hepatic resection for hepatocellular carcinoma. *Ann. Surg. Oncol.* **2014**, *21*, 3063–3068. [CrossRef] [PubMed]
18. Carrara, G.; Pecorelli, N.; De Cobelli, F.; Cristel, G.; Damascelli, A.; Beretta, L.; Braga, M. Preoperative sarcopenia determinants in pancreatic cancer patients. *Clin. Nutr.* **2016**. [CrossRef] [PubMed]
19. Fujiwara, N.; Nakagawa, H.; Kudo, Y.; Tateishi, R.; Taguri, M.; Watadani, T.; Nakagomi, R.; Kondo, M.; Nakatsuka, T.; Minami, T.; et al. Sarcopenia, intramuscular fat deposition, and visceral adiposity independently predict the outcomes of hepatocellular carcinoma. *J. Hepatol.* **2015**, *63*, 131–140. [CrossRef] [PubMed]
20. Zhuang, C.L.; Huang, D.D.; Pang, W.Y.; Zhou, C.J.; Wang, S.L.; Lou, N.; Ma, L.L.; Yu, Z.; Shen, X. Sarcopenia is an Independent Predictor of Severe Postoperative Complications and Long-Term Survival after Radical Gastrectomy for Gastric Cancer: Analysis from a Large-Scale Cohort. *Medicine* **2016**, *95*, e3164. [CrossRef] [PubMed]
21. Harimoto, N.; Shirabe, K.; Yamashita, Y.I.; Ikegami, T.; Yoshizumi, T.; Soejima, Y.; Ikeda, T.; Maehara, Y.; Nishie, A.; Yamanaka, T. Sarcopenia as a predictor of prognosis in patients following hepatectomy for hepatocellular carcinoma. *Br. J. Surg.* **2013**, *100*, 1523–1530. [CrossRef] [PubMed]
22. Antoun, S.; Borget, I.; Lanoy, E. Impact of sarcopenia on the prognosis and treatment toxicities in patients diagnosed with cancer. *Curr. Opin. Support Palliat. Care* **2013**, *7*, 383–389. [CrossRef] [PubMed]
23. Iritani, S.; Imai, K.; Takai, K.; Hanai, T.; Ideta, T.; Miyazaki, T.; Suetsugu, A.; Shiraki, M.; Shimizu, M.; Moriwaki, H. Skeletal muscle depletion is an independent prognostic factor for hepatocellular carcinoma. *J. Gastroenterol.* **2015**, *50*, 323–332. [CrossRef] [PubMed]
24. Kamachi, S.; Mizuta, T.; Otsuka, T.; Nakashita, S.; Ide, Y.; Miyoshi, A.; Kitahara, K.; Eguchi, Y.; Ozaki, I.; Anzai, K. Sarcopenia is a risk factor for the recurrence of hepatocellular carcinoma after curative treatment. *Hepatol. Res.* **2016**, *46*, 201–208. [CrossRef] [PubMed]
25. Suzuki, Y.; Okamoto, T.; Fujishita, T.; Katsura, M.; Akamine, T.; Takamori, S.; Morodomi, Y.; Tagawa, T.; Shoji, F.; Maehara, Y. Clinical implications of sarcopenia in patients undergoing complete resection for early non-small cell lung cancer. *Lung Cancer* **2016**, *101*, 92–97. [CrossRef] [PubMed]
26. Harimoto, N.; Yoshizumi, T.; Shimokawa, M.; Sakata, K.; Kimura, K.; Itoh, S.; Ikegami, T.; Ikeda, T.; Shirabe, K.; Maehara, Y. Sarcopenia is a poor prognostic factor following hepatic resection in patients 70 years of age and older with hepatocellular carcinoma. *Hepatol. Res.* **2016**, *46*, 1247–1255. [CrossRef] [PubMed]
27. Hamaguchi, Y.; Kaido, T.; Okumura, S.; Kobayashi, A.; Hammad, A.; Tamai, Y.; Inagaki, N.; Uemoto, S. Proposal for new diagnostic criteria for low skeletal muscle mass based on computed tomography imaging in Asian adults. *Nutrition* **2016**, *32*, 1200–1205. [CrossRef] [PubMed]
28. Chen, L.K.; Liu, L.K.; Woo, J.; Assantachai, P.; Auyeung, T.W.; Bahyah, K.S.; Chou, M.Y.; Chen, L.Y.; Hsu, P.S.; Krairit, O.; et al. Sarcopenia in Asia: Consensus Report of the Asian Working Group for Sarcopenia. *J. Am. Med. Dir. Assoc.* **2014**, *15*, 95–101. [CrossRef] [PubMed]
29. Dasarathy, S. Consilience in sarcopenia of cirrhosis. *J. Cachexia Sarcopenia Muscle* **2012**, *3*, 225–237. [CrossRef] [PubMed]
30. Montano-Loza, A.J. Clinical relevance of sarcopenia in patients with cirrhosis. *World J. Gastroenterol.* **2014**, *20*, 8061–8071. [CrossRef] [PubMed]
31. Kudo, M.; Zheng, R.Q.; Kim, S.R.; Okabe, Y.; Osaki, Y.; Iijima, H.; Itani, T.; Kasugai, H.; Kanematsu, M.; Ito, K.; et al. Diagnostic accuracy of imaging for liver cirrhosis compared to histologically proven liver cirrhosis. A multicenter collaborative study. *Intervirology* **2008**, *51*, 17–26. [CrossRef] [PubMed]
32. Zarski, J.P.; Sturm, N.; Guechot, J.; Paris, A.; Zafrani, E.S.; Asselah, T.; Boisson, R.C.; Bosson, J.L.; Guyader, D.; Renversez, J.C.; et al. Comparison of nine blood tests and transient elastography for liver fibrosis in chronic hepatitis C: The ANRS HCEP-23 study. *J. Hepatol.* **2012**, *56*, 55–62. [CrossRef] [PubMed]
33. Tsochatzis, E.A.; Gurusamy, K.S.; Ntaoula, S.; Cholongitas, E.; Davidson, B.R.; Burroughs, A.K. Elastography for the diagnosis of severity of fibrosis in chronic liver disease: A meta-analysis of diagnostic accuracy. *J. Hepatol.* **2011**, *54*, 650–659. [CrossRef] [PubMed]
34. Kumada, H.; Okanoue, T.; Onji, M.; Moriwaki, H.; Izumi, N.; Tanaka, E.; Chayama, K.; Sakisaka, S.; Takehara, T.; Oketani, M.; et al. Guidelines for the treatment of chronic hepatitis and cirrhosis due to hepatitis C virus infection for the fiscal year 2008 in Japan. *Hepatol. Res.* **2010**, *40*, 8–13. [CrossRef] [PubMed]

35. Kappus, M.R.; Mendoza, M.S.; Nguyen, D.; Medici, V.; McClave, S.A. Sarcopenia in Patients with Chronic Liver Disease: Can It Be Altered by Diet and Exercise? *Curr. Gastroenterol. Rep.* **2016**, *18*, 43. [CrossRef] [PubMed]
36. Heagerty, P.J.; Zheng, Y. Survival model predictive accuracy and ROC curves. *Biometrics* **2005**, *61*, 92–105. [CrossRef] [PubMed]
37. European Association for the Study of the Liver; European Organisation for Research and Treatment of Cancer. EASL-EORTC Clinical Practice guidelines: Management of hepatocellular carcinoma. *J. Hepatol.* **2012**, *56*, 908–943.
38. Kudo, M.; Izumi, N.; Kokudo, N.; Matsui, O.; Sakamoto, M.; Nakashima, O.; Kojiro, M.; Makuuchi, M.; HCC Expert Panel of Japan Society of Hepatology. Management of hepatocellular carcinoma in Japan: Consensus-Based Clinical Practice Guidelines proposed by the Japan Society of Hepatology (JSH) 2010 updated version. *Dig Dis.* **2011**, *29*, 339–364. [CrossRef] [PubMed]
39. Asahina, Y.; Tsuchiya, K.; Tamaki, N.; Hirayama, I.; Tanaka, T.; Sato, M.; Yasui, Y.; Hosokawa, T.; Ueda, K.; Kuzuya, T.; et al. Effect of aging on risk for hepatocellular carcinoma in chronic hepatitis C virus infection. *Hepatology* **2010**, *52*, 518–527. [CrossRef] [PubMed]
40. Osaki, Y.; Nishikawa, H. Treatment for hepatocellular carcinoma in Japan over the last three decades: Our experience and published work review. *Hepatol Res.* **2015**, *45*, 59–74. [CrossRef] [PubMed]
41. Davuluri, G.; Krokowski, D.; Guan, B.J.; Kumar, A.; Thapaliya, S.; Singh, D.; Hatzoglou, M.; Dasarathy, S. Metabolic adaptation of skeletal muscle to hyperammonemia drives the beneficial effects of l-leucine in cirrhosis. *J. Hepatol.* **2016**, *65*, 929–937. [CrossRef] [PubMed]
42. Sinclair, M.; Grossmann, M.; Hoermann, R.; Angus, P.W.; Gow, P.J. Testosterone therapy increases muscle mass in men with cirrhosis and low testosterone: A randomised controlled trial. *J. Hepatol.* **2016**, *65*, 906–913. [CrossRef] [PubMed]
43. Dasarathy, S. Cause and management of muscle wasting in chronic liver disease. *Curr. Opin. Gastroenterol.* **2016**, *32*, 159–165. [CrossRef] [PubMed]
44. St-Onge, M.P. Relationship between body composition changes and changes in physical function and metabolic risk factors in aging. *Curr. Opin. Clin. Nutr. Metab. Care* **2005**, *8*, 523–528. [PubMed]
45. Syddall, H.; Evandrou, M.; Cooper, C.; Sayer, A.A. Social inequalities in grip strength, physical function, and falls among community dwelling older men and women: Findings from the Hertfordshire Cohort Study. *J. Aging Health* **2009**, *21*, 913–939. [CrossRef] [PubMed]

Permissions

All chapters in this book were first published by MDPI; hereby published with permission under the Creative Commons Attribution License or equivalent. Every chapter published in this book has been scrutinized by our experts. Their significance has been extensively debated. The topics covered herein carry significant findings which will fuel the growth of the discipline. They may even be implemented as practical applications or may be referred to as a beginning point for another development.

The contributors of this book come from diverse backgrounds, making this book a truly international effort. This book will bring forth new frontiers with its revolutionizing research information and detailed analysis of the nascent developments around the world.

We would like to thank all the contributing authors for lending their expertise to make the book truly unique. They have played a crucial role in the development of this book. Without their invaluable contributions this book wouldn't have been possible. They have made vital efforts to compile up to date information on the varied aspects of this subject to make this book a valuable addition to the collection of many professionals and students.

This book was conceptualized with the vision of imparting up-to-date information and advanced data in this field. To ensure the same, a matchless editorial board was set up. Every individual on the board went through rigorous rounds of assessment to prove their worth. After which they invested a large part of their time researching and compiling the most relevant data for our readers.

The editorial board has been involved in producing this book since its inception. They have spent rigorous hours researching and exploring the diverse topics which have resulted in the successful publishing of this book. They have passed on their knowledge of decades through this book. To expedite this challenging task, the publisher supported the team at every step. A small team of assistant editors was also appointed to further simplify the editing procedure and attain best results for the readers.

Apart from the editorial board, the designing team has also invested a significant amount of their time in understanding the subject and creating the most relevant covers. They scrutinized every image to scout for the most suitable representation of the subject and create an appropriate cover for the book.

The publishing team has been an ardent support to the editorial, designing and production team. Their endless efforts to recruit the best for this project, has resulted in the accomplishment of this book. They are a veteran in the field of academics and their pool of knowledge is as vast as their experience in printing. Their expertise and guidance has proved useful at every step. Their uncompromising quality standards have made this book an exceptional effort. Their encouragement from time to time has been an inspiration for everyone.

The publisher and the editorial board hope that this book will prove to be a valuable piece of knowledge for researchers, students, practitioners and scholars across the globe.

List of Contributors

Jean-Pascal De Bandt, Prasanthi Jegatheesan and Naouel Tennoune-El-Hafaia
EA4466 PRETRAM, Faculté de Pharmacie de Paris, USPC, 75006 Paris, France

Peter Witters
Metabolic Center, University Hospitals Leuven, B-3000 Leuven, Belgium
Department of Development and Regeneration, Faculty of Medicine, KU Leuven, B-3000 Leuven, Belgium

David Cassiman
Department of Gastroenterology-Hepatology and Metabolic Center, University Hospitals Leuven, B-3000 Leuven, Belgium

Eva Morava
Metabolic Center, University Hospitals Leuven, B-3000 Leuven, Belgium
Department of Development and Regeneration, Faculty of Medicine, KU Leuven, B-3000 Leuven, Belgium
Hayward Genetics Center, Tulane University School of Medicine, New Orleans, LA 70112, USA

Merethe Brevik-Andersen, Derek Tobin and Yan Qin
BASF AS, NO-1327 Lysaker, Norway

Jacqueline K. Innes
Human Development and Health Academic Unit, Faculty of Medicine, University of Southampton, Southampton SO16 6YD, UK

Philip C. Calder
Human Development and Health Academic Unit, Faculty of Medicine, University of Southampton, Southampton SO16 6YD, UK
National Institute for Health Research Southampton Biomedical Research Centre, University Hospital Southampton NHS Foundation Trust and University of Southampton, Southampton SO16 6YD, UK

Mahmud Mahamid
Endoscopy Unit, Nazareth Hospital EMMS, 16100 Nazareth, Israel
Azrieli Faculty of Medicine, Bar-Ilan University, 13195 Safed, Israel

Nicola Luigi Bragazzi
School of Public Health, Department of Health Sciences, University of Genoa, 16132 Genoa, Italy

Naim Mahroum, Howard Amital, Abdulla Watad and Yarden Yavne
Department of Medicine 'B', Sheba Medical Center, Tel-Hashomer, Israel, Sackler Faculty of Medicine, Tel-Aviv University, 52621 Tel-Aviv, Israel

Kasem Shalaata
Azrieli Faculty of Medicine, Bar-Ilan University, 13195 Safed, Israel
Internal Medicine Department, Nazareth Hospital EMMS, 16100 Nazareth, Israel

Mohammad Adawi
Ziv and Padeh Medical centers, 13195 Safed, Israel

Brandon J. Perumpail
Department of Medicine, Drexel University College of Medicine, Philadelphia, PA 19129, USA

Andrew A. Li, George Cholankeril, Radhika Kumari and Aijaz Ahmed
Division of Gastroenterology and Hepatology, Stanford University School of Medicine, Stanford, CA 94305, USA

Daisuke Uchida, Akinobu Takaki, Takuya Adachi and Hiroyuki Okada
Department of Gastroenterology and Hepatology, Okayama University Graduate School of Medicine, Dentistry and Pharmaceutical Sciences, 2-5-1 Shikata-cho, Kita-ku, Okayama 700-8558, Japan

Claudia Mandato
Pediatrics, Santobono - Pausilipon Pediatric Hospital, 80100 Naples, Italy

Antonella Di Nuzzi and Pietro Vajro
Department of Medicine, Surgery and Dentistry "Scuola Medica Salernitana", Pediatrics Section, University of Salerno, 84081 Baronissi (Salerno), Italy

Shilpa Tiwari-Heckler, Hongying Gan-Schreier, Wolfgang Stremmel, Walee Chamulitrat and Anita Pathil
Department of Internal Medicine IV, Gastroenterology and Hepatology, University of Heidelberg, Im Neuenheimer Feld 410, 69120 Heidelberg, Germany

Eric R. Yoo
Department of Medicine, Santa Clara Valley Medical Center, San Jose, CA 95128, USA

Hiroki Nishikawa, Takashi Nishimura, Hirayuki Enomoto, Yoshinori Iwata, Akio Ishii, Yuho Miyamoto, Noriko Ishii, Yukihisa Yuri, Ryo Takata, Kunihiro Hasegawa, Chikage Nakano, Kazunori Yoh, Nobuhiro Aizawa, Yoshiyuki Sakai, Naoto Ikeda, Tomoyuki Takashima, Shuhei Nishiguchi and Hiroko Iijima
Division of Hepatobiliary and Pancreatic disease, Department of Internal Medicine, Hyogo College of Medicine, Hyogo 6638501, Japan

Christine H. Yang and John A. Kerner Jr.
Division of Pediatric Gastroenterology, Hepatology and Nutrition, Lucile Packard Children's Hospital, Palo Alto, Stanford, CA 94304, USA

Aijaz Ahmed
Division of Gastroenterology and Hepatology, Stanford University School of Medicine, Stanford, CA 94305, USA

Monika Cahova and Miriam Bratova
Centre for Experimental Medicine, Institute for Clinical and Experimental Medicine, Department of Metabolism and Diabetes, Videnska 1958/9, 14021 Prague 4, Czech Republic

Petr Wohl
Centre of Diabetology, Institute for Clinical and Experimental Medicine, Department of Metabolism and Diabetes, Videnska 1958/9, 14021 Prague 4, Czech Republic

Kenji Imai, Koji Takai, Satoshi Watanabe, Tatsunori Hanai, Atsushi Suetsugu, Makoto Shiraki and Masahito Shimizu
Department of Gastroenterology/Internal Medicine, Gifu University Graduate School of Medicine, Gifu 501-1194, Japan

Marcin Krawczyk
Department of Medicine II, Saarland University Medical Center, Saarland University, 66421 Homburg, Germany
Laboratory of Metabolic Liver Diseases, Centre for Preclinical Research, Department of General, Transplant and Liver Surgery, Medical University ofWarsaw, 02-097 Warsaw, Poland

Dominika Maciejewska, Karina Ryterska, Maja Czerwińka-Rogowska, Dominika Jamioł-Milc, Karolina Skonieczna-Żydecka and Ewa Stachowska
Department of Biochemistry and Human Nutrition, Pomeranian Medical University, 71-210 Szczecin, Poland

Joanna Raszeja-Wyszomirska
Liver and Internal Medicine Unit, Department of General, Transplant and Liver Surgery of the Medical University ofWarsaw, 02-097 Warsaw, Poland

Piotr Milkiewicz
Liver and Internal Medicine Unit, Department of General, Transplant and Liver Surgery of the Medical University of Warsaw, 02-097 Warsaw, Poland
Translational Medicine Group, Pomeranian Medical University, 71-210 Szczecin, Poland

Miriam Hoene
Department of Internal Medicine IV, Division of Endocrinology, Diabetology, Angiology, Nephrology and Clinical Chemistry, University Hospital Tübingen, 72076 Tübingen, Germany

Andras Franko, Marketa Kovarova, Hans-Ulrich Häring, Andreas Peter, Benjamin A. Jaghutriz and Martin Heni
Department of Internal Medicine IV, Division of Endocrinology, Diabetology, Angiology, Nephrology and Clinical Chemistry, University Hospital Tübingen, 72076 Tübingen, Germany
Institute for Diabetes Research and Metabolic Diseases of the Helmholtz Center Munich, University of Tübingen, 72076 Tübingen, Germany
German Center for Diabetes Research (DZD e.V.), 85764 Neuherberg, Germany

Dietrich Merkel and Cyrus Papan
Sciex Germany GmbH, 64293 Darmstadt, Germany

Alfred Königsrainer
Department of General, Visceral and Transplant Surgery, University Hospital Tübingen, 72076 Tübingen, Germany

Stefan Lehr
German Center for Diabetes Research (DZD e.V.), 85764 Neuherberg, Germany
Institute for Clinical Biochemistry and Pathobiochemistry of DDZ, University of Düsseldorf, 40225 Düsseldorf, Germany

Anika Nier, Annette Brandt and Ina Bergheim
Department of Nutritional Sciences, Molecular Nutritional Science, University of Vienna, A-1090 Vienna, Austria

Ina Barbara Conzelmann and Yelda Özel
Department of Nutritional Medicine, (180), University of Hohenheim, D-70599 Stuttgart, Germany

Janin Henkel, Christin Stuhlmann, Madita Vahrenbrink and Gerhard P. Püschel
Department of Nutritional Biochemistry, Institute of Nutritional Science, University of Potsdam, D-14558 Nuthetal, Germany

Eugenia Alfine and André Kleinridders
German Institute of Human Nutrition, Junior Research Group Central Regulation of Metabolism; D-14558 Nuthetal, Germany
German Center for Diabetes Research (DZD), D-85764 München-Neuherberg, Germany

Juliana Saín
Department of Nutritional Biochemistry, Institute of Nutritional Science, University of Potsdam, D-14558 Nuthetal, Germany
Department of Biological Sciences, Food Science and Nutrition, Faculty of Biochemistry and Biological Sciences, National University of the Litoral (UNL), Santa Fe S3000, Argentina

Korinna Jöhrens
Institute of Pathology, Carl Gustav Carus University Hospital Dresden; D-01307 Dresden, Germany

Daniela Weber and Jeannette König
Department of Molecular Toxicology, German Institute of Human Nutrition; D-14558 Nuthetal, Germany

José P. Castro
Department of Molecular Toxicology, German Institute of Human Nutrition; D-14558 Nuthetal, Germany
Department of Medicine, Division of Genetics, Brigham and Women's Hospital and Harvard Medical School, Boston, MA 02115, USA

Wenke Jonas
Department of Experimental Diabetology, German Institute of Human Nutrition; D-14558 Nuthetal, Germany
German Center for Diabetes Research (DZD), D-85764 München-Neuherberg, Germany

Hiroyuki Niwa, Takehiro Kato, Wudelehu Wu, Hiromi Tsuchida, Ken Takao, Yukio Horikawa and Jun Takeda
Department of Diabetes and Endocrinology, Graduate School of Medicine, Gifu University, Gifu 501-1194, Japan

Katsumi Iizuka
Department of Diabetes and Endocrinology, Graduate School of Medicine, Gifu University, Gifu 501-1194, Japan
Gifu University Hospital Center for Nutritional Support and Infection Control, Gifu 501-1194, Japan

Hiroki Nishikawa, Hirayuki Enomoto, Akio Ishii, Yoshinori Iwata, Yuho Miyamoto, Noriko Ishii, Yukihisa Yuri, Kunihiro Hasegawa, Chikage Nakano, Takashi Nishimura, Kazunori Yoh, Nobuhiro Aizawa, Yoshiyuki Sakai, Naoto Ikeda, Tomoyuki Takashima, Ryo Takata, Hiroko Iijima and Shuhei Nishiguchi
Department of Hepatobiliary and Pancreatic disease, Department of Internal Medicine, Hyogo College of Medicine, 1-1, Mukogawacho, Nishinomiyashi, Hyogo 663-8501, Japan

Index

www.ingramcontent.com/pod-product-compliance
Lightning Source LLC
LaVergne TN
LVHW081018210926
848485LV00004B/890